HEALTH CARE AND THE COMMON GOOD

A Catholic Theory of Justice

José I. Lavastida, S.T.D.

University Press of America,® Inc.
Lanham • New York • Oxford

Copyright © 2000 by
University Press of America,® Inc.
4720 Boston Way
Lanham, Maryland 20706

12 Hid's Copse Rd.
Cumnor Hill, Oxford OX2 9JJ

All rights reserved
Printed in the United States of America
British Library Cataloging in Publication Information Available

Library of Congress Cataloging-in-Publication Data

Lavastida, José I.
Health care and the common good : a Catholic theory of
Justice / José I. Lavastida.
p. cm.
Includes bibliographical references.
1. Medical ethics—United States. 2. Medical care—Social aspects—United States. 3. Medical care—Religious aspects—United States. I. Title.
R725.5.L384   1999   174'.2—dc21   99-048697 CIP

ISBN 0-7618-1524-4 (cloth: alk. ppr.)
ISBN 0-7618-1525-2 (pbk: alk. ppr.)

♾™ The paper used in this publication meets the minimum requirements of American National Standard for Information Sciences—Permanence of Paper for Printed Library Materials, ANSI Z39.48—1984

Contents

Introduction	1
UNIT ONE: HEALTH CARE IN THE U.S.A.	7
Chapter One: A Description of Health Care in the U.S.	9
An Introduction to Health Care Delivery	9
A Brief History of the System	11

The first century. The period of the large hospitals. The introduction of the scientific method. The social and organizational structure of the system. The period of limited resources, restriction of growth, and regulation of effort.

The Constant Mirage: The Establishing of a National Health Plan	21
Public Health Care in the U.S.	26
Medicare	26
Medicaid	29
Aid to Families With Dependent Children	32
Veterans Health Administration	34
Private Health Care in the U.S.	36
Private Health Insurance	36
Employer-Based Health Insurance	39

Community Hospitals and Clinics	43
Home Health Care	46

Chapter Two: Access to Health Care in the U.S.   **49**

Defining Access to Health Care	49
Who Has Access to Health Care in the U.S.	53
A Study of the Factors That Limit Access to Health Care	63
Social Factors	63
Poverty and the inadequacies of Medicaid.	
The problem with the uninsured.	
Cultural Factors	71
Institutional Factors	76
Market justice and health care. Role of primary care.	
Geographical Factors	81

UNIT TWO: THEORIES AND PRINCIPLES INFLUENCING
HEALTH CARE DELIVERY IN THE U.S.   **83**

Chapter Three: The Fundamental Question of Rights and Obligations   **85**

The Concept of a Right to Health Care	85
Defining the Meaning of "Right"	85
Defining the Meaning of "Health"	87
Balancing the Notion of "Rights"	94

Chapter Four: The Fundamental Answers Based on the Philosophical Foundations of American Health Care   **99**

Origins of American Thought Before Modern Theories	100
The Utilitarian Philosophy	105

Main Tenets of Utilitarianism	105
Issues Raised by Utilitarianism Concerning Health Care	107

Rationing health care. Managed care and the market. Diagnosis-related groups. The presidential commission.

Modern Utilitarian Thinkers and a Critique of Their Main Ideas	118

John Stuart Mill. Joseph Fletcher. Tom Beauchamp.

The Libertarian Philosophy	123
Main Tenets of Libertarianism	123
Issues Raised by Libertarianism Concerning Health Care	125

The role of government. Health care as a market commodity.

Modern Libertarian Thinkers and a Critique of Their Main Ideas	131

Robert Nozick. Robert Sade. H. Tristram Engelhardt.

The Egalitarian Philosophy	137
Main Tenets of Egalitarianism	137
Issues Raised by Egalitarianism Concerning Health Care	139

A basic minimum of health care. A multi-tiered system of health care.

Modern Egalitarian Thinkers and a Critique of Their Main Ideas	143

Gene Outka. Robert Veatch. Bernard Williams. John Rawls.

UNIT THREE: A CATHOLIC THEORY OF JUSTICE	**157**
Chapter Five: The Common Good	**159**
A Historical Survey of the Common Good	159

The Common Good in the Magisterium
    of the Catholic Church 170
The Classic Texts 171
    Rerum novarum. Quadragesimo anno.
The Transition in Catholic Social Thought 173
    Mater et magistra. Pacem in terris.
The Second Vatican Council and Post Conciliar
    Teaching 175
    Gaudium et spes. Populorum progressio.
    Octogesima adveniens. The Synod
    document "Justice in the World."
The Social Teaching of Pope John Paul II 179
    Laborem exercens. Sollicitudo rei socialis.
    Centesimus annus.
The National Conference of Catholic Bishops
    of the United States 182

The Present Day Debate on the Common Good . . . 186

Chapter Six: Distributive Justice 193

A Historical Survey of the Notion of Justice 193
The Common Good and Distributive Justice 197

Magisterial Documents and Distributive Justice . . . 199
The Classic Texts 199
    Rerum novarum. Quadragesimo anno.
The Transition in Catholic Social Thought 204
    Mater et magistra. Pacem in terris.
The Second Vatican Council and Post Conciliar
    Teaching 207
    Gaudium et spes. Populorum progressio.
    Octogesima adveniens. The Synod
    document "Justice in the World."
The Social Teaching of Pope John Paul II 211
    Laborem exercens. Sollicitudo rei socialis.
    Centesimus annus.
The National Conference of Catholic Bishops
    of the United States 216

The Present Day Debate on Distributive Justice 218

Chapter Seven: Towards a Catholic Theory of Justice 227

A Social Understanding of the Person 228

A Humane Understanding of Society: The
    Common Good 231

A Just Distribution According to Human Needs 235

UNIT FOUR: REFORMING ACCESS TO HEALTH CARE 239

**Chapter Eight: The Problems and the
Proposals for Reform** 241

Main Problems Affecting Access to Health Care 241
The Uninsured 242
Poverty 242
Cultural and Racial Factors 243
Market Mentality 243

Proposals for Health Care Reform 245
Tax Reforms 245
    *The Heritage Foundation proposal.
    President Bush's proposal.*
Universal Access Retaining Present Mixed System 249
    *Basic Health Care for All Americans Act.
    Health Access America. Consumer Choice
    Health Plan. National Leadership Commission
    on Health Care.*
Universal Coverage Increasing Public Coverage While
    Keeping Private Employment-Based
    Coverage 255
    *MediPlan. The Pepper Commission. The
    President's Health Security Plan.*
Unified National Financing with Administration
    by Private Insurers 259
    *The Health Security Partnership. Health
    U.S.A. Act. Catholic Health Association*

proposal.
Single Payer National Health Insurance 265
The Physicians for a National Health Program. The Universal Health Care Act.

Chapter Nine: Common Good, Distributive Justice and Health Care **271**

Moral Basis for Health Care Reform 272
The nature of health care. Stewardship of resources. Universal access. Comprehensive similar benefits. Integrity in the physician-patient relationship.
Application of Moral Basis to the American Context 280
Patient as the priority. A comprehensive approach to health care. The role of government. Care over administration. Promote local responsibility. Terminology needs to change.
Distributive Justice in Practice 290
Health care is not simply a market commodity. Rationing is not the solution. The dilemma of equity versus utility.

Chapter Ten: Four Proposals for Promoting Just Access to Care **303**

Universal Access 303
A Single-Payer System 305
Greater Involvement of the States 308
Preventive Over Defensive Care 309

Conclusion 311

Bibliography 315

INTRODUCTION

For the last four decades the United States of America has been undergoing dramatic changes in health care. These changes have come about mostly as a consequence of technological and medical developments which have made medical science a reliable ally of modern society. People today are taught to see health care as an integral part of life, and in many instances they have faced medical situations which have allowed them to understand that without timely and effective health care they probably would not be alive today. We have experienced tremendous developments in neo-natal care, allowing infants, who otherwise would not have survived, to turn into healthy children, while at the same time allowing more and more people to see their great-grandchildren and beyond, due to the life-sustaining techniques at the other end of the age spectrum.

These developments have not come without a cost. There certainly has been a financial cost, as we have seen health care costs soar in recent decades, while at the same time there has been a social cost due to the fact that the prevailing attitude in American society concerning medical care has emphasized the notion of health care as a market commodity at the expense of a more socially minded notion that would promote an ethical obligation to provide universal coverage and equitable care. More and more people in today's American society find themselves with no health care coverage and with little or no access to a coherent, effective, and service oriented health care system.

There is an urgent need today to re-evaluate the status of access to health care in the United States and to suggest ethical alternatives that could facilitate the re-structuring of a health care system that would be true to its very nature, namely the promoting and the securing of the experiential and functional health of all citizens.

This work will study the situation related to access to health care in the United States of America. Access to care is the most significant factor when dealing with the quality of health care that the nation is receiving. Even universal coverage for health care needs is not the ultimate determinant of how well citizens are cared for medically.

2 Health Care and the Common Good

Universal coverage does not always translate into universal access. Historically Americans have been more concerned with the whole issue of personal rights and whether health care should be considered a right or not. The underlying assumption about rights has been influenced primarily by philosophical notions that tend to leave out a social conception of rights while emphasizing individualistic understandings. This has affected the way health care has been structured in the country, and has now created a situation in which an erosion of the values that would promote a societal obligation to provide equitable health care has taken place. At the same time the solutions that have been offered which promote a continuation of individualistic attitudes in regards to health care have not improved the situation regarding access to care. Actually the situation has deteriorated to a point that there is a critical need to investigate ways in which society as a whole can become the catalyst for health care reform. This can only be accomplished if a societal obligation to provide just health care is recognized.

The problems that have been raised in regards to the development of a notion of a societal obligation to provide equitable health care are related to the difficulties in finding the principles upon which such obligation would be based, especially considering today's pluralistic society. In this work the principles of the common good and distributive justice will be presented as two of the ones that, when understood within the framework of their social dimensions, can provide the bases for a notion of social obligation that could be accepted by society as a whole.

The methodology that will be followed will include in the first chapter a history of the health care system in the United States of America while at the same time describing how the system (or lack of system) is presently structured. There will be a study of the different ways that access to health care has been monitored in the country and an analysis of the statistics. Chapter two will search for the philosophical roots of the present system and the ethical values that have brought about the kind of health care provision that exists in the United States. None of the philosophies that have influenced the present structure of health care has given a comprehensive satisfactory answer to the problem when considering their accomplished results. Chapter three will discuss the two principles of the common good and distributive justice, especially as considered in the social teaching of the Catholic Church. There will be a study of both principles according to the contemporary debate and a discussion of the issues raised by both topics. Finally a theory of justice will be introduced based on the way the Catholic Church has understood these two principles. In the fourth and final chapter, this theory will be applied to the current problems in relation to the lack of access to health care in American society with four specific proposals that, if implemented, would help promote just access to health care.

The methodology described in the above paragraph will approach the problem through first analyzing the history, then synthesizing or bringing together the different solutions, both philosophical and practical, that have been attempted in order to reform health care in the nation, and finally presenting and analyzing the ways the problems with access to health care could be solved when using an ethical approach which would be nourished according to the guidance offered by the teaching of the Catholic Church.

The main sources for the work have been organized in the bibliography by highlighting the general sources first and then the ones used in each chapter. The first chapter relies heavily upon the historical works of J. Duffy (1976), F.R. Packard (1931), G. Marks and W.K. Beatty (1973), P. Starr (1982), and J. Bordley and H.J. McGehee (1976). The historical description of the development of medicine in the United States has been divided into five significant periods after carefully studying these diverse studies mentioned above, since there is no clear consensus as to how to divide the history of health care in the United States.

The description of the public elements in the American system of health care are based mainly on the documents of the Social Security Amendments of 1965: the U.S. Congress Public Law 89-97, the 89th Congress House of Representatives Bill 6675 of July 30, 1965, and the Green Books from the House of Representatives Ways and Means Committee for 1992, 1993, and 1994. Another main source for this information was the Encyclopedia of Social Work, 19th edition (1995).

Most of the material on the private elements of health care in the U.S. has been taken from different journal articles of which we would like to highlight the ones by E. Friedman (1991) and N.S. Jecker (1993).

In the section on access to health care in the United States the statistical data is taken mainly from those offered by the National Center for Health Statistics, Hyattsville, Maryland of the Public Health Service Department. The textbook *Changing the U.S. Health Care System,* by R.M. Andersen, T.H. Rice, and G.F. Kominski (1996) also provided invaluable help, especially in the categories that study access to health care.

Much of the material in chapter two concerning the problem with the definition of health comes from the article by S. Kelman (1975). The book by M.A. Glendon (1991) is also very important in the development of the section on balancing the whole notion of rights. The material having to do with the different philosophical theories has as its main sources the most important works of the philosophical writers considered. Most of the works mentioned and studied have become key books or articles in describing and defining the most important and controversial positions of their authors.

In chapter three the main sources for the discussion on the papal encyclicals are the ones by D.J. O'Brien, T.A. Shannon (1992) and C. Carlen (1981). The first book is the one that suggests the classification of the papal encyclicals and other documents from the National Conference of Catholic Bishops in the U.S. into a five-fold structure.

In the section on the present day debate on the common good, several works provided important material. Among them are the ones by R. Bellah, et al (1985), M.J. Sandel (1996), A. MacIntyre (1984^2), and the article by D. Hollenbach (1989).

In the section on the present day debate on distributive justice some significant sources are the works of D. Hollenback (1988), M. Walzer (1983), and the article by D. Hollenback found in C.H. Reynolds and R.V. Norman (1988).

When developing a Catholic theory of justice, the works by J Maritain (1947, 1941), M. Novak (1989), and M.J. Sandel (1996) are significant.

In describing the different proposals for reform in chapter four, one of the main sources was the documentation of the different House and Senate bills that were introduced in Congress. Much of this material comes from the depository in the Law Library of the Supreme Court of the state of Louisiana. The bills are always referred to by the Congress number and the session, as well as the microfiche number assigned to them. Other proposals come directly from articles written by the proponents, or from the documents of the commission that sponsored such proposal of reform. It is important also to mention the contribution of R. Veatch particularly through his article on *Resolving Conflicts Among Principles: Ranking, Balancing, and Specifying* (1995). He offers a model to follow in order to solve problematic situations when utility and equity go against each other. Also throughout the different chapters, whenever possible, recent newspapers and periodical articles have been utilized in order to share the most recent information available.

Even with the vast amount of information and sources available which cover the topic discussed in this work, one is left with the sensation that there is always more to be aware of. With this in mind we want to discuss this important topic with the hope that what we say may help in continuing the social conversation about this critical issue of just access to health care and contribute to the establishment of a national system that will be more efficient, equitable, and effective for the well being of all.

UNIT ONE

HEALTH CARE IN THE UNITED STATES OF AMERICA

The United States of America is relatively a young country. Yet, in its 221 years of history, there have been great developments and success stories that have had an influence in the whole world. One of these stories has been the development of health care. The advances in this field have been nothing less that spectacular in a very short period of time. Nevertheless, it is worthwhile to reflect on the development of health care in the country with special concern for how this growth and importance attributed to health care, have made it reach a level of recognition in which it is impossible to consider our lives without access to it.

The first section of this work aims at examining our health care system especially in what relates to how people access medical services, and the differences that have developed in this access according to a variety of factors. It will briefly describe the history of the system, how it is structured today, and the problems that are related to access to health care. Chapter one will describe the system, and chapter two will deal specifically with access and how it is measured.

ONE

A DESCRIPTION OF HEALTH CARE
IN THE UNITED STATES

In order to understand the different problems related to access to health care in the United States of America, it is important to understand how the system itself works. One of the significant factors of the current system, is that it combines public and private features which interrelate with and affect one another, and foster the development of very concrete problems for the citizen who has any kind of health need.

This chapter will deal specifically with a brief history of health care in the United States and an explanation of both the public and private aspects of health care in the country.

A. AN INTRODUCTION TO HEALTH CARE DELIVERY

In the Shakespearean play *The Tempest*, one of the characters is portrayed as saying, "What's past is prologue." This line is meant as a reminder that the events of the past usually end up setting the stage for the future. The history of health care delivery in the United States of America offers a perfect example of this. Without an understanding of the different stages that the system has gone through and how these are interconnected, it is impossible to comprehend the actual state of health care in the country.

Obviously there are many ways to write an account of the history of health care in America. A detailed account that would consider the numerous and important people who have shaped the system would be one way to proceed. On the other hand, another possible way would be to consider the scientific breakthroughs throughout the years and how they have affected the total system. A third way would be to study the voluminous legislation related to health care in the country throughout the different decades. Each one of these accounts would cover very important elements concerning the evolution of health care that would provide a partial picture of the whole.[1]

It seems that historians of the system themselves, have had a very difficult time assigning consistent divisions that would provide a historical account. For the purposes of this work, which does not have as its main focus the people who have influenced the system, nor the breakthroughs or the legislation pertinent to health care development, the best approach will be dividing its history into five great significant periods. By doing this, there will be greater freedom in mentioning people, technological innovations, and enacted laws that have brought the system to where it is today.

There are five significant periods in the history of health care delivery in the United States: 1) The first century, which begins in the middle of the eighteenth century and goes roughly to the middle of the nineteenth; 2) The period of the large hospitals, which begins around 1850; 3) The introduction of the scientific method, which begins around the turn of the century (1900); 4) The period of the interest in the social and organizational structure of the system, which began with the Second World War; and 5) The period of limited resources, restriction of growth, and regulation of effort, which has only begun in the last couple of decades.[2] In examining these five distinct periods in the history of health care in America, it will be possible to have a better understanding of the present. In essence, each one of these periods has become the prologue for the next one, thus calling us to be aware of the kind of prologue we are preparing today for the future. We shall examine each period individually.

---

[1]Different authors that have tried to write a history of American medicine have emphasized different approaches. There seems to be little agreement as to what would be a good way to divide the history of health care delivery in the U.S. (Cf. DUFFY J., *The Healers: A History of American Medicine.* Univ. of Ill. Press, Urbana, 1976; PACKARD F.R., *History of Medicine in the United States.* Paul B. Hoeber Inc., New York, 1931 [2 volumes]; MARKS G. and BEATTY W.K., *The Story of Medicine in America.* Charles Scribner's Sons, New York, 1973; STARR P., *The Social Transformation of American Medicine.* Basic Books, Inc., New York, 1982; BORDLEY J., III and MCGEHEE Harvey A., *Two Centuries of American Medicine.* W.B. Saunders Co., Philadelphia, 1976.

[2]For the division into five distinct periods the author has used some of the material found in BORDLEY and MCGEHEE, *op. cit.,* and in WILLIAMS S.J. and TORRENS P.R., (ed.) *Introduction to Health Services.* John Wiley & Sons, New York, 1980, p. 4.

1. A Brief History of the System

a. The first century

The whole first century of American medicine, which we will consider roughly from 1750 until the 1850's when the first large hospitals appeared, was greatly influenced by the model of eighteenth-century England. Medicine's social structure reflected the hierarchical structure of society. Physicians considered themselves members of a learned profession preferring to observe, speculate and prescribe, rather than getting involved with their own hands. This was the work of surgeons, who since 1745 were members of the same guild as barbers. However, since the physicians in America did not serve within a society which was so highly stratified as the one in England, and since the guilds, so powerful in England, had no force in the colonies, Americans came to regard anybody who practiced medicine as a doctor. The distinction between profession and trade became blurred in America.[3] It was common for the clergy to blend medical and religious services for their congregations. Yet, as Americans who had served in the colonies as apprentices with a colonial practitioner, sought a medical education in cities such as Leyden, London, and Edinburgh, the ones who returned home brought with them the desire to establish medicine as a profession that would enjoy the same standards and dignity that the profession had in Europe. This kind of development promoted the separation of medicine from religion, and helped in developing the formation of the medical profession. It would be mistaken, though, to attribute to religion in the colonies the magical practices in medicine connected with the Medieval Church. As the English historian Keith Thomas has shown, it was religion which repudiated the magical practices allowed by the medieval church at a time when science had not yet given an explanation of disease that was adequate. Contrary to what many times is common opinion, it was the development of religious thought, and not medical progress, that initially brought the decline in magical healing practices in the United States.[4]

Apprenticeship served in the early years as the principal form of medical training, since very few people would travel to Europe for medical education. Even with the establishment of the first schools in American

---

[3]STARR P., *The Social Transformation of American Medicine*, p. 39.

[4]Ibid., p. 35.

soil, apprenticeship retained its importance. Practitioners who were successful in the medical practice would take young men as assistants. They would allow them to read from their books, and take care of their household chores. By the end of three years they would be given a certificate of proficiency and good character. In 1765 it was the College of Philadelphia, later to become the University of Pennsylvania, that became the first medical school in the colonies. Institutions like this acquired their personalities according to the people who became influential as professors. For example, the College of Philadelphia came to existence due to the initiative of a young, European-trained American physician by the name of John Morgan. He proposed the hierarchical system of Europe as a model for medicine in the colonies, specifically calling for the separation of physic from surgery and pharmacy. No more was a physician required to handle a knife than a general of the army should be required to dig trenches.[5]

Other personalities included the revolutionary leader and physician Benjamin Rush, who devised a system that reflected the adhesion to tradition present in the English medical thought when he claimed that there was only one kind of fever in the world, induced by capillary tension, and that the only cure needed was to bleed the patients. Physicians were encouraged to practically bleed their patients to death, and to do it without any fear, since this was the only way to recovery. Heavy doses of mercurous chloride, which was called cathartic calomel, was given to the patients in order to help them "cleanse" their bodies from toxic elements. Practices such as these continued until the early part of the nineteenth century.

Another medical school that came into existence during this time was the medical department of King's College in New York City, which began in 1768. Between the College of Philadelphia and King's College in New York City, only 51 medical degrees were awarded between 1765 and 1776 when they had to suspend their programs due to the war.[6] By the year 1810, five medical schools were functioning in the United States. The medical students in the country numbered about 650, of whom about 100 of them received degrees on that year. The population of the country was about seven million people, and there were only three public general

---

[5]STARR P., *The Social Transformation of American Medicine*, p. 41.

[6]BORDLEY J., MCGEHEE H. A., *Two Centuries of American Medicine*, p. 10.

A Description of Health Care in the U.S. 13

hospitals to serve them: the Pennsylvania Hospital in Philadelphia, the New York Hospital in New York City, and Charity Hospital in New Orleans.[7]

After the War of 1812, medical schools began to grow all around the country. These were established in cities like Baltimore, Lexington, Cincinnati, and even rural communities in places like Vermont and New York state. Their faculties were made up of practitioners who lived in the area and offered their services. Due to the loss of physicians during the Revolutionary War, and the lack of new graduates during the war years, these schools began to lower their standards in order to attract students. The degree of *Bachelor of Medicine* was done away with, and the doctoral degree was given after only two years.[8] The growth of these schools continued over the next three decades, and by 1850 there were forty-two such schools in the country. In order to offer a comparison, France at the same time only had three such schools.[9] Even in such large numbers, these schools were still considered undergraduate schools of lower standing than the school of arts. The medical education was two years shorter than an education in the arts.

There were some major organized alternatives to the medical practice in the first century of medicine in the country. The strongest and most radical such movement was organized by the New Englander Samuel Thomson. His radical movement of botanic medicine became known as the Thomsonian movement. It was a system based on very few simple principles. Every disease was brought about by one general cause and could be treated with one general remedy. The cause was "cold", the remedy was "heat." The main medications were Indian tobacco, red pepper, and steam and hot baths. His movement was directed as a critique, not of science itself, but of the particular way that medical knowledge was being controlled. Thomson accused doctors of deliberately deceiving people by keeping them in ignorance. For him, the "natural" remedies were sufficient. This was not superstition or magical belief. Actually this movement was a creative misreading of the

---

[7]BORDLEY J., MCGEHEE H. A., *Two Centuries of American Medicine*, p. 11.

[8]Ibid., pp. 16-17.

[9]STARR P., *The Social Transformation of American Medicine*, p. 42.

14   Health Care and the Common Good

Enlightenment and a defender of rationalism.[10]

There were other cults and movements that came to existence at this time as well. The Grahamites, for example, founded in the 1830's by Sylvester Graham of Pennsylvania, blamed calomel as the cause of many illnesses, and advocated hygienic measures as the best guarantor of good health. The cult of *hydropathy* was brought to the United States from Germany in the 1840's, and promoted different kinds of waters as therapeutic. Also of great importance at the time was the cult of *homeopathy,* founded by Samuel C. Hahnemann at the end of the eighteenth century. This cult believed in curing disease by administering a medicine that would produce in the patient the very symptoms of the illness being treated, but with controlled doses of the agent causing the disease. Its followers subsisted and gained strength well into the next century. Many homeopaths were graduates of orthodox medical schools and respected members of their communities, which made them a greater threat to the established profession.[11] Because of these semi-occult movements, popular belief in America during the early nineteenth century began to reflect a type of rationalism that demanded for a democratization of science. Behind this notion was the democratic ideal which rejected and was highly suspicious of any kind of occult knowledge.[12]

The kinds of problems that physicians faced in the first century of medical history in America were very different from those of today. Infectious diseases were very common. The mortality rate among children was very high. Epidemics like yellow fever and cholera were paramount. In the yellow fever epidemic of 1793 in Philadelphia, it is estimated that 8,000 of about 45,000 inhabitants contracted the illness.[13]

There was little progress made in the United States regarding the fields of hygiene and preventive medicine in this first century. There was very little knowledge of the agents that caused disease, and also there was

---

[10]STARR P., *The Social Transformation of American Medicine,* pp. 52-53.

[11]BORDLEY J., MCGEHEE H. A., *Two Centuries of American Medicine,* pp. 42-44.

[12]STARR P., *The Social Transformation of American Medicine,* p. 56.

[13]BORDLEY J., MCGEHEE H. A., *Two Centuries of American Medicine,* p. 31.

A Description of Health Care in the U.S. 15

very little participation of the government in health matters. The individual states were in charge of health care for the people, and even by the end of the nineteenth century, of the thirty-eight states which comprised the union, only twelve had state boards of health.[14] It was not until 1872 that the American Public Health Association was founded in order for the government of the Union to play an active role in public hygiene and the prevention of illnesses.

b. The period of the large hospitals

The first institution in the British colonies of North America that could be called a "hospital" seems to have been St. Philip's Hospital in Charlestown in Carolina, built in 1736 to serve the poor of St. Philip's parish church. It functioned more as a house of correction, even though it did take care of the sick who lacked financial resources and had a physician hired at an annual salary. Yet, the typical institution of the time which bore the name "hospital" included among its many functions the provision of suitable lodging for the poor, provision of housing to the sick who were badly accommodated in their homes thus making caring for them more difficult, providing a haven for people with mental illnesses who became the terror of their neighbors, providing medical, surgical, and nursing care for the poor, and offering the opportunity for medical apprentices to practice by applying dressings and rendering other assistance.[15] These institutions for the most part were dismal places, where poor people lived in crowded, unsanitary, and poorly ventilated areas.[16]

It was not until the second half of the nineteenth century, when the first large hospitals, like Bellevue Hospital in New York City and Massachusetts General Hospital in Boston, began to function in a different way. This development marked the institutionalization of health care in the United States. It was during this time that the economic expansion of the period promoted the rapid institutional development of organizations of all kinds, including hospitals. As the market mentality penetrated the institution of the hospital, its function of caretaking began to change into

---

[14]BORDLEY J., MCGEHEE H. A., *Two Centuries of American Medicine*, p. 47.

[15]Ibid., pp. 55-56.

[16]WILLIAMS S.J., TORRENS P.R., *Introduction to Health Services*, p. 173.

providing active treatment. This caused it to change its ideals from benevolence to a professionalism that gave physicians much greater control and power. There was a shift in values that occurred at this time from more gentlemanly ones to utilitarian considerations.[17]

In a broader historical frame, the growth of hospitals can be seen as part of the general movement of change in the social structures of the time from "communal" to "associative" relations. Communal relations refer to bonds which stress group solidarity; associative relations refer to economic exchanges that come about when associations have shared interests or ends. This shift happened not only in the development of new organizations that from their beginnings fostered associative relations to the demise of institutions or organizations that fostered communal relations, but it also happened that organizations that used to emphasize the communal relation became increasingly associative.[18]

There were four major developments during this time that were particularly significant in bringing about the transformation of hospitals.[19] The first one was advances in medical science, like for example the discovery of anesthetics such as ether, used by Long in 1842 and then by Morton in 1846, and the increase of surgical procedures that followed; and the elaboration of the germ theory with the discoveries of antiseptic and sterilizing techniques, pioneered by Pasteur in 1861 and followed up by Lister when in 1867 he introduced carbonic acid spray in surgery rooms as an antiseptic to keep wounds and incisions clean.

A second development was specialized technology. The first hospital laboratory began to function in 1889, and in 1896 *x-rays* films were used for diagnostic purposes for the first time. Blood types were discovered in 1901, making blood transfusions safe, and the electrocardiogram was developed during this time and first used in 1903. It is obvious that such technology could only benefit the growth of institutions where such delicate and complicated instrumentation could be kept. At the same time, this development promoted the growth of specialization in the medical profession, since it was difficult to be competent in all areas of medical practice.

---

[17]STARR P., *The Social Transformation of American Medicine*, p. 148.

[18]Ibid.

[19]WILLIAMS S.J., TORRENS P.R., *Introduction to Health Services*, pp. 175-177.

A Description of Health Care in the U.S. 17

A third development which helped the transformation of hospitals during the end of the nineteenth century was professional nursing. The transformation of nursing into a profession is credited to Florence Nightingale, who was sent by England to Crimea to take care of the wounded soldiers in 1854. In the United States Dorothea Dix was appointed Superintendent of Nursing for the Union Army. She recruited nurses who then had to undergo a one-month training program. The benefits of good nursing soon became obvious by offering better care for less money than the one given by the previously untrained women hired to do that kind of work. Nursing schools in the country went from 22 with 600 graduates in 1883, to 400 with 10,000 graduates in 1898. Efficient and skilled care provided by trained nurses, made hospitals acceptable to all people and not just the poor.

A fourth important development during this time of the growth of hospitals was the advances in medical education. Up to this time, there were no standards of academic training for physicians. There was little laboratory instruction or research. In 1910 a report entitled *Medical Education in the United States and Canada,* better known as the Flexner report due to its main author Abraham Flexner,[20] appeared. This report had a major impact and played a decisive role leading to changes in the content and methods of instruction emphasizing the scientific basis of medicine. Schools that did not meet the standards established by the Flexner report were forced to close. Four years of study plus clinical training in the hospital ward became standard.

c. The introduction of the scientific method

We have seen how the Flexner report was so influential in the growth of the hospitals. This report was also an example of the introduction of the scientific method into the mainstream of medical education. With epidemics and infectious diseases under control by the beginning of the twentieth century, the predominant attention concerning health problems turned to the individual acute conditions that affected people one by one. It was recognized that something like heart disease could not be dealt with a *one-shot-affair* attitude. It was acknowledged

---

[20]He was not a physician but his report acknowledges the *"generous assistance from Dr. William H. Welch of Johns Hopkins and Dr. Simon Flexner of the Rockefeller Institute."* Simon was Abraham's brother, who had seen medical education from both ends of the spectrum having been a medical student at the University of Louisville, the largest of the American schools.

that this kind of illness was connected with personal habits acquired sometimes since childhood, and directly related to life style. The solution for such health problems could not be a single lecture to the individual on the evils of a bad diet or the dangers of cigarette smoking. The whole aim of medicine shifted at this time into trying to bring major changes in the individual's knowledge of the disease, and his patterns of behavior. Most of the discoveries and the research achieved during this time came from an effort to make medicine more understandable and integral in the individual's life. The scientific advances of the time contributed to the easier and safer diagnosis and treatment of acutely ill patients.

In 1901 the American scene changed dramatically with the founding of the Rockefeller Institute by John D. Rockefeller. This organization was conceived, not by physicians or scientist, but by laymen who thought that the time was right for an institute devoted exclusively to medical research.[21] The purpose of the Rockefeller Institute was to help and encourage investigations in the areas of hygiene, medicine and surgery, and disease prevention. Areas immediately under study included "pathology and bacteriology, physiology and pharmacology, biological chemistry, and experimental surgery."[22] Great advancements were made in the areas of bacterial and pathologic research; culturing living cells, tissues, and organs; syphilis, yellow fever, Oroya fever, and trachoma; rheumatic fever and heart disease among others.[23]

d. The social and organizational structure of the system

Even though the period between the 1900 and 1940 was one of rapid growth and development in scientific technology, it was nothing compared to what happened with the coming of World War II. There were two very important concerns shaping health care at the time of the beginning of the war: the first one was how to organize the best talent and resources available at the time for the care of the wounded; the second one was how to deal with the systemic health care problems generated by the war.

---

[21]MARKS G., BEATTY W.K., *The Story of Medicine in America*, pp. 276-277.

[22]Ibid., p. 279.

[23]Ibid., p. 280.

A Description of Health Care in the U.S. 19

As part of the mobilization effort for the war, millions of men and women entered the military and in return received all kinds of health services. These services were provided without a charge by physicians hired by the government, and, more importantly, these services continued to be provided as a right and not a charity to those in the service who could no longer take care of themselves. World War II also accustomed the country to a large-scale health care program, and encouraged the growth of the health insurance industry. Considerable activity occurred concerning the development of pensions, disability programs, and health insurance plans as the health insurance industry began to flourish. This type of industry provided the American people with a new form of social organization: the *third party* or fiscal intermediary. Attention was directed to the financing of health care, resulting in the foundation of insurance plans like Blue Cross and Blue Shield. During this time there was an increase of the concentration of power in the federal government with the advent of acts like the Hill-Burton Act, which was designed to help in the construction and the modernization of American hospitals after the war. A Hill-Burton facility would agree to provide, in return for an aggregate of nearly $6.5 billion in government grants and loans, "a reasonable volume of free or reduced-cost care."[24] It was also during this time that huge amounts of money were budgeted for the National Institutes of Health—a government agency that had been established in 1930 with the purposes of research.[25] More recently, the development of the role of the federal government has been seen with the passing of Medicare legislation in 1965. One of the things that transpired during this period after World War II was that the principle of health care as a right and not a privilege began to be discussed more openly and had wide acceptance among the American people.

e. The period of limited resources, restriction of growth, and regulation of effort

All throughout the four previous periods discussed above, there was a general notion that the health care system would always be encouraged to expand and grow in complexity and size. Underneath this notion there was the strong believe that there would always be sufficient

---

[24]DOWELL M.A., *"Hill-Burton: The Unfulfilled Promise,"* Journal of Health Politics, Policy and Law. 12(1): 155, 1987 Spring.

[25]WILLIAMS S.J., TORRENS P.R., *Introduction to Health Services,* p. 4.

resources to support the expansion. Since the early 1980's, and in part due to the amazing and costly technological advances, this unlimited sense of growth in the future has been critically challenged. It is clear that the country has to budget its resources according to the well-being of the people, and even though health care is certainly one of those elements that has a direct impact on such well-being, it is impossible to provide with limited resources for what seems to be an unlimited demand for health care services. There is a growing realization today that supplying more health care to the population does not mean that the demand will decrease due to better health care, but on the contrary, health care related treatments tend to increase the demand for services. It would be absurd to allocate all of the national budget into certain categories of public assistance while totally overlooking others. There is a disproportion of the amount of the gross domestic product (GDP) dedicated to health care as compared to many other public needs. This has evolved into several concerns which have to do with the rationing of health care and the ethical questions connected to such rationing. In fact, there has been much discussion in the last two decades about a restructuring of the whole health care system in the country, with health care reform and cost reduction being the predominant concerns of the 1980's. With the advent of the 1990's, the ethics of health care reform have come to the fore in the debate about health care delivery in the nation, and proposals that address not only practical matters, but the very essence of health care itself, will become very important in the next century if any real solutions to the system are to be offered. Some authors have written about the beginning of a new era in the history of medicine in the United States—an era, which began in the 1990's, concerned with values and priorities.[26]

With the absence of a national health plan, the problems created by the limited resources of health care, the need to control costs and growth, and the efficient regulation of effort have become increasingly more difficult to correct. Which brings us to the question: "Why has it been so difficult to establish a national health plan?" We now turn to this question.

---

[26]KISSICK W.L., *Medicine's Dilemmas. Infinite Needs Versus Finite Resources*, p. 75.

A Description of Health Care in the U.S.   21

2. The Constant Mirage: The Establishing of a National Health Plan

The theme related to a right to health care will be addressed later. For now, it is sufficient to realize that one of the conditions which makes a country favorable to a national health plan is the recognition of a right to health care on the part of its people. There is no national health plan in the United States, even though this has been a topic of much debate throughout the history of the country.

Serious modern concern regarding the issue of whether there is a right to health care, can be traced roughly to the *Universal Declaration of Human Rights* of the United Nations General Assembly which was proclaimed on December 10, 1948. The United States signed this declaration which, among other things, contains a recognition of a *right to health care*. Even with this, such a right is not recognized in the United States, which makes America, together with South Africa, the only two countries of all the industrialized democracies of the world that do not recognize such a right.[27]

Yet, laws in this country implicitly granting positive rights to health care have been passed, and serious discussion on positive rights have been going on since 1813.[28]

In order to understand why there is no national health plan in the U.S., it is necessary to understand the social structure and development of the nation, and also the factors that came into play at the different times when a national policy for health care was being discussed.

There are several factors which affect the evolution of any kind of public system in a particular society. It is a well known fact, that the way in which power is distributed in a particular society tends to set limits on the different professions, and shapes the types of relationships that will develop. In the medical delivery system of the United States the distribution of power set the limits on the autonomy of the medical profession and the relations that would ensue among the state, the doctors, the working class, and the upper income groups. This class structure, helps to explain historically, which illnesses would be most subject to treatment, and which groups would have the most access to medical care.

---

[27]DOUGHERTY C., *American Health Care. Realities, Rights, and Reforms*, p. 26.

[28]BEAUCHAMP T.L., FADEN R.R., *"The Right to Health and the Right to Health Care,"* Journal of Medicine and Philosophy 4(2): 125, June 1979.

Another factor which helped influence the development of the health care delivery system in the United States was the commercial and business spirit of the American people. J. Rogers Hollingsworth, in comparing the medical systems of Great Britain and the United States has this to say:

> Throughout the history of the U.S., foreign observers have been struck by the extent to which a large proportion of physicians have viewed their practice as a business enterprise and by the way the desire to accumulate wealth has influenced the medical profession. And therefore it should be no surprise that the profit motive is more important in shaping the contemporary structure of the medical delivery system in the U.S. than in any other advanced capitalist society.[29]

Even when many of the leaders of the medical profession in the country have spoken favorably for national insurance, the grass roots of the medical profession have remained opposed to it. The reason for this seems to be that for the majority of physicians the source of payment for health care is as important an issue as the method of payment to be used. The fear seems to be that if the source of payment were to change, the fee-for-service method would have to be altered.

A third factor influencing the way the health care delivery system developed in the United States has to do with a lack of a sense of community. Since there has been throughout its history great differences concerning ethnic, racial, and religious factors, Americans in general have been less concerned with the well-being of their fellow citizens than their European counterparts. When there is a society with such a great ethnic and religious diversity as in the U.S., there is a tendency to emphasize individual responsibility for medical needs at the expense of the communal responsibility.[30] In such a society, medical care tends to be consumed more in the private rather than in the public sector. This racial and ethnic heterogeneity found in America helped the development of a medical delivery system in the private sector.

It has already been mentioned that the distribution of power among particular interest groups in society is the key to understanding how

---

[29]HOLLINGSWORTH J.R., *A Political Economy of Medicine: Great Britain and the United States*, p. 66.

[30]Ibid.

A Description of Health Care in the U.S.   23

health care is financed in different countries. This is so since the power of the various groups active in society constraints the kind of structure that emerges. When the financing of health care services becomes a salient issue in the country, the structure that emerges depends greatly on whether the consumers or the providers are better organized. If the consumers are better organized than the providers of health care, there is a better chance of the emergence of a national health insurance plan with the state playing a prominent role in its organization and regulation. When the opposite is true, that is, where the providers are better organized than the consumers of health care, the structure that emerges tends to rely on the private sector and a national health insurance program is usually slow to develop or totally nonexistent.[31]

A case could be made that, had the working class been better organized at the different times when the debate of a national health insurance came to the forefront, the U.S. might have adopted the legislation. The poor organization of workers, the low level of class consciousness, and the philosophical divisions over the issue, prevented national health insurance from becoming a reality. At several times when national health insurance was being implemented in many industrialized societies, the U.S. continued to reject emphatically such a development. Even at times when it seemed certain that the time was right for a national policy regarding health care insurance, something else interfered preventing the passage of such legislation. Analyzing the history of the discussions of national health insurance is helpful in showing those moments.

It was during the years 1912-1920 that the American Association for Labor Legislation (AALL) organized the first major campaign for a national health insurance plan. Originally this group was composed of academics and intellectuals which were later joined by professional organizations of nurses, public health officials and others. Theodore Roosevelt included national health insurance as an important part of his platform for the 1912 presidential campaign running on the Bull Moose ticket. By the year 1920 there had been public health insurance proposals introduced in 16 states. The American Medical Association ignored the movement in the beginning. The President of the American Federation of Labor (AFL) also opposed it since he contended that such widely available benefits for laborers could undermine the ability of the union to attract

---

[31]HOLLINGSWORTH J.R., *A Political Economy of Medicine: Great Britain and the United States,* p. 110.

workers since the unions had been established precisely upon their ability to negotiate such benefits. People who led industries were also against obligatory health insurance since they simply did not want to pay for it. Last but not least, the commercial insurance industry provided the strongest opposition since national health insurance would include funeral benefits. This was one of the most lucrative parts of commercial insurance, since the top companies sold approximately $200 million worth of funeral insurance every year.[32] By the time the United States entered World War I in 1917, physicians had come out strongly against the idea, and the propagandists labeled it a Prussian plot, since it was similar to the German system of social insurance.[33]

Right after the First World War, national health insurance was labeled a Bolshevik plot until the Great Depression of the 1930's brought the issue to the table once again. This time a notable absence in the proposal for national health insurance was the whole part of funeral benefits.[34] There were massive demonstrations across the country in 1937, and in response to these the original draft of the Social Security Act included health coverage. There was a conference in Washington D.C. organized by the more progressive government elements in order to discuss the proposed national health program. Nothing came out of this effort, and with the emergence after the 1938 elections of a new group of Republicans and Dixiecrats, the advances in the push for national health insurance were halted and sabotaged until the beginning of World War II. With the pressing concerns about the war, the debate on national health insurance vanished from the scene to give way to greater preoccupations.

In the year 1942 a national poll was taken which indicated that three out of every four Americans were in favor of national health insurance.[35] By this time, though, the coordinated movement which had begun during the Depression, had been sapped.

President Truman revived the debate on national health insurance in 1945. He announced his support for a similar proposal to the one that

---

[32]WEISS L.D., *No Benefit: Crisis in America's Health Insurance Industry*, p. 10.

[33]Ibid.

[34]Ibid.

[35]Ibid., p. 12.

had been made back in the late 1930's. This time the public reaction was mixed, and it varied according to the socioeconomic status of the people. Those with higher incomes reacted strongly against it, while those with lower incomes were supportive of it. Once again, the American Medical Association was openly against it, and labeled it "socialized medicine." With such attacks the proposal died, and with the beginning of the conflict in Korea, Americans turned their attention to other problems.

During the late 1950's and early 1960's the health care needs of the elderly received much attention. Once again there was strong support for a national health insurance. In 1965 Medicare was enacted into law as a compromise legislation, and perhaps, in the opinion of some authors, "met the needs of the health care providers better than the needs of the elderly."[36] The American Medical Association and the American Hospital Association, working together, achieved the elimination of legislated control over the reimbursement for services, thus gaining maximum control over the operations of the Medicare program.[37]

By the end of the 1960's Walter Reuther, the president of the United Automobile Workers (UAW), led the call for a comprehensive national health insurance plan. Public support was so strong at this time, that the American Medical Association and the American Hospital Association decided not to fight it, but to propose their own alternative plans. In 1967 Senator Edward Kennedy (D-MA) introduced the first of a long series of health bills in Congress. His bill would have nationalized health insurance but would have left all health services in the private sector. The response by the Republican administration of President Nixon was to fund a national program of health maintenance organizations. With this prepaid group practices, a plan that could be accepted by health care providers and the commercial health insurance industry was presented as an alternative.

With the combined impact of the recession and inflation in the 1970's, the whole movement for national health insurance was halted.

In the 1990's new efforts were introduced by the Democratic administration of President Clinton, only to be completely defeated by a combination of public ignorance of the issues involved, a highly complicated and bureaucratic plan that called for managed competition

---

[36]WEISS L.D., *No Benefit: Crisis in America's Health Insurance Industry*, p. 14.

[37]STARR P., *The Social Transformation of American Medicine*, p. 375.

and universal access to health care, and an enormous campaign by the commercial insurance industry against the plan.

After this brief historical account on the debate about national health insurance, it should not be a surprise that the whole issue has become a well known mirage for many Americans who favor a national health insurance plan. This historical account can only speculate as to what "could have happened" if national health insurance would have passed at any of the historical moments previously discussed. The reality of the American health care delivery is that, in the midst of all those debates, there has come about the emergence of a health care that combines public and private elements in a way that requires an individual account and explanation of both: public and private health care. In the next two sections we will try to explain the different ways that people in the United States gain access to health care delivery.

B. PUBLIC HEALTH CARE IN THE UNITED STATES

Within Public Health in the United States, we will consider Medicare, Medicaid, Aid to Families With Dependent Children, and the Veterans Health Administration.

1. Medicare

Social Security is the term used in the United States to refer to a group of programs which have been developed by the federal government in order to provide economic security for people in their old age, disabled workers, and workers' survivors in cases of worker's death. One of the programs embraced by Social Security is the Medicare Program. This program helps pay for the health care of eligible elderly and disabled people.

The securing of medical benefits within Social Security has a history of its own. During the year 1950, after the quest for a comprehensive and universal health insurance plan had been defeated in the national scene, there was a proposal made to Oscar Ewing, then the federal security administrator, that Social Security beneficiaries be insured for health and medical care. The most important political figures of the time in the House Ways and Means Committee did not dare to deal with this proposal in 1951 or 1952. It was until 1957 that the bill was introduced in Congress by a member of the powerful House committee. This member was Alfred Forand, (D-RI), and the bill was popularly called "the Forand Bill." It failed to pass in 1957, 1958, and 1959. There was an effort made at the same time to expand the public assistance for medical services for people in need, but the American Medical Association strongly opposed such proposal in 1956. It was in 1960 that Senator John F. Kennedy, then the presidential candidate for the Democratic Party, embraced the idea of providing health insurance for the elderly through the Social Security program. Even with Kennedy's support as President, the idea failed to pass for four more years. In its place a federal-state plan for the needy called the Kerr-Mills Bill passed in 1960. It was Arthur Flemming, then the Secretary of Health, Education and Welfare—a Republican—who offered a plan called "Medicare." This term was later transferred to the Social Security proposal and it stuck. The fight between the proponents and the opponents of Medicare was a long and intense one. After President Kennedy's assassination in November 1963, President Johnson tried to get the legislation enacted in early 1964, but once again the House Ways and Means Committee and its chairman Wilbur D. Mills, (D-AR), opposed the push. The proposal went into a deep freeze all throughout that year. After President Johnson was re-elected at the end of 1964, and was supported by the new Congress, Medicare and Medicaid legislation was assured in 1965.[38]

Medicare, as it exists today, is comprised of two parts: Hospital Insurance, which represents Part A of Title XVIII of the Social Security Act, and Supplementary Medical Insurance which represents Part B. The Health Care Finance Administration (HCFA) is the government entity responsible for the administration of both parts.

There are three main categories of people eligible for Hospital Insurance benefits under Medicare.[39] These are: 1) all persons 65 years and older who are eligible for cash benefits either through Old-Age and Survivors Insurance or the Railroad Retirement System; 2) all disabled workers, disabled widows and widowers 50 years and older, and insured worker's adult children whose disability originated before the age of 22; 3) insured workers and their families who need dialysis or a kidney

---

[38]COHEN W.J., *"The Long, Difficult Road to Enactment,"* Health Progress 66:22, Jul-Aug 1985.

[39]The information in this section is taken from *The Social Security Amendments of 1965*, U.S. Congress, Public Law 89-97, 89th Congress, H.R. 6675, July 30, 1965; and from the *Encyclopedia of Social Work*, 19th ed. NASW Press, Washington D.C., 1995.

transplant.

There are four kinds of benefits provided under Hospital Insurance which are: hospital services, skilled nursing facility services, home health care, and hospice care. The services in the hospital include supplies and assistance normally required for inpatient care. These usually include room and board, operating facilities, laboratory tests and x-rays, drugs, dressings, nursing services, and the assistance of interns and residents who are in training. Personal conveniences and private services such as duty nurses, televisions and telephones are excluded. In the same way, the insurance only covers the cost of semi-private accommodations, unless private ones are medically required. The Hospital Insurance covers the cost of hospital care up to 90 days in a single illness spell. In addition, there is a "lifetime reserve" of 60 additional days for every insured person. To receive home health services, the insured person has to be confined to a home, require intermittent skilled nursing care for physical or speech therapy, and be under the care of a physician.

Supplementary Medical Insurance helps in paying certain medical services especially physicians' fees. All beneficiaries of Medicare have to choose whether they wish this supplementary coverage or not. There are certain periods provided under the law to enroll, and there is a monthly premium that has to be paid ($36.60 in 1993).

In order to finance Old-Age and Survivors Insurance and Disability Insurance as well as the Hospital Insurance component of Medicare, the government levies a payroll tax on employers, employees, and the self-employed, up to a maximum taxable earnings amount of $57,600 in 1993 for Old-Age and Survivors Insurance and Disability Insurance, and $135,000 for Hospital Insurance. The tax rate has been 7.65% since 1990 for employees and employers, and 15.3% for the self-employed.

Even when recently there has been a growing concern about the current spending levels and the possibility of the fund going bankrupt,[40] Medicare has helped tremendously in providing health care for the elderly and the disabled. It has for the most part become the most efficient part

---

[40]EDDY D.M., *"Health System Reform. Will Controlling Costs Require Rationing Services?"* Journal of the American Medical Association 272(4): 324-325, July 27, 1994.

of the health care system in the U.S. and the most popular.[41] This has improved the well-being of a growing section of the population. Even though some problems with Medicare will be addressed later, for the most part it has helped in securing a more just distribution of medical resources for the elderly and the disabled.

2. Medicaid

Unlike Medicare, the Medicaid program is run by the federal and state governments.[42] Medicaid is basically an all-encompassing name to describe forty-nine different programs designed to serve the poor.[43] It was authorized by Title XIX of the Social Security Act in order to pay for the health care of the *categorically needy* and the *medically needy*. The first ones are those receiving help from the Aid to Families with Dependent Children (AFDC) program, which will be discussed later, and the ones receiving Supplementary Security Income (SSI) because of their being aged, blind, or disabled. On the other hand, the *medically needy* are those people who have sufficient money to live on, but not enough money to pay for health care.

For the Medicaid program, it is up to each individual state to determine the eligibility requirements—income and otherwise—for classification as *medically needy*. As it should be expected, the requirements vary greatly from state to state. Title XIX, though, requires the state to provide a set of twenty-one services in order to be eligible to receive federal funds. Some of these services covered include: inpatient

---

[41]ANGELL M., *"The Beginning of Health Care Reform: The Clinton Plan,"* New England Journal of Medicine 329(21): 1570, Nov. 18, 1993.

[42]The information in this section has been taken from *The Social Security Amendments of 1965*, U.S. Congress, Public Law 89-97, 89th Congress, H.R. 6675, July 30, 1965; and from the *Encyclopedia of Social Work*, 19th ed. NASW Press, Washington D.C., 1995, as well as from the following works: BORDLEY J., MCGEHEE H. A., *Two Centuries of American Medicine*, pp. 435-437; JONAS S., *An Introduction to the U.S. Health Care System*, 3rd ed., pp. 132-133; KOVNER A.R., *Health Care Delivery in the United States*, pp. 248-249; RAFFEL M.W., RAFFEL N.K., *The U.S. Health System, Origins and Functions*, 3rd. Ed., pp. 257-259.

[43]The state of Arizona, out of the 50 states, does not have a Medicaid program.

and outpatient hospital services, skilled nursing facilities services, physician services, home health care, family planning services, and early periodic screening, diagnosis, and treatment of children under twenty-one who are eligible. The individual state also may elect to pay for dental services, prescription drugs, eyeglasses, intermediate care facility services, among other services.

Medicaid is financed from general revenues with the federal government covering from 50% in the most wealthy states to about 77% in those states with the lowest personal income per capita. The law allows for the federal government to cover a maximum of 83% of the state's cost for Medicaid. The states administer the program following the federal regulations and guidelines. Medicaid is the largest single state-administered program, and its expenditures account for approximately 10% of what is budgeted in the state's general fund.[44]

There are many problems with Medicaid. A combination of low-income eligibility requirements and low fees for providers leads to very limited coverage in most states. Many providers choose not to participate in the program, or limit the number of Medicaid recipients they are willing to take. Some states also have set their income thresholds for eligibility below the federal poverty level. This makes that many poor individuals become ineligible for Medicaid. The fortunes of Medicaid began to change when in the late 1980's Congress established a law requiring Medicaid coverage of pregnant women and young children with incomes of 185% above the poverty line.[45] This caused resistance to the program from the states, who already felt a burden trying to make ends meet with their limited funds.

Even when care is given through Medicaid, it is often far from comprehensive, and much of the Medicaid payments go to nursing-home care. One common practice in some states is to keep the income eligibility requirements unchanged, thus the rise in incomes that takes place to keep pace with inflation, ends up affecting poor people who all of a sudden find themselves outside the income range required to receive Medicaid benefits. States have also begun to impose limits as to the number of days for in-hospital care, and the amounts available to pay physicians, hospitals,

---

[44]CURTIS R., *"The Role of State Governments in Assuring Access to Care,"* Inquiry 23(3):280, Fall 1986.

[45]FRIEDMAN E., *"The Uninsured. From Dilemma to Crisis,"* Journal of the American Medical Association 265(19):2492, May 15, 1991.

and nursing homes. Sometimes hospitals and nursing homes end up having to reclassify patients, for example from a skilled nursing facility to an intermediate care facility, in order to lower costs and services covered.

Eligibility to receive Medicaid benefits has become a labyrinth in the United States. It is estimated that as a result of all these problems from 21 to 28 million people among the poor or low-income population, remain uninsured. Being part of the working force is not always a solution to this problem, since half of those low-income Americans who are employed, do not have health insurance of any kind, and are ineligible for Medicaid benefits.[46] In fact, the working poor and their families have been practically eliminated from Medicaid coverage.[47] In 1989 it was estimated that only 40% of the population living in poverty was covered by Medicaid.[48] A particularly vulnerable population has been the children who represent about 36% of the country's 37 million or so uninsured individuals.[49] The proportion of low-income Americans covered by Medicaid has also decreased drastically throughout the years.[50]

---

[46]MENZEL P.T., *Strong Medicine: The Ethical Rationing of Health Care*, p. 118.

[47]STEVENS P.E., *"Who Gets Care? Access to Health Care as an Arena for Nursing Action,"* Scholarly Inquiry for Nursing Practice 6(3):189, Fall-Winter 1992.

[48]FRIEDMAN E., *"The Uninsured. From Dilemma to Crisis,"* Journal of the American Medical Association 265(19):2492, May 15, 1991. This was still the case in 1992 (See STEVENS P.E., *"Who Gets Care? Access to Health Care as an Arena for Nursing Action,"* Scholarly Inquiry for Nursing Practice 6(3):189, Fall-Winter 1992.)

[49]STEVENS P.E., *"Who Gets Care? Access to Health Care as an Arena for Nursing Action,"* Scholarly Inquiry for Nursing Practice 6(3):189, Fall-Winter 1992.

[50]BUTLER J.A., ROSENBAUM S., PALFREY J.S., *"Ensuring Access to Health Care for Children with Disabilities,"* New England Journal of Medicine 317(3):164, July 16, 1987.

32 Health Care and the Common Good

3. Aid to Families with Dependent Children (AFDC)

At the time of the Great Depression during the 1930's, the Congress of the United States enacted Aid to Dependent Children (ADC). This was done after the rejection of several proposals, that would have covered all poor children regardless of the structure of the families in which they lived. In 1935 Congress made ADC part of the Social Security Act. The idea behind ADC was to offer financial assistance to children who lacked care or support due to the absence or incapacity of a parent. In 1962 this program was renamed Aid to Families with Dependent Children (AFDC).[51] Most of the people applying for this program are mothers. AFDC is jointly administered and funded by the federal government and the states. The program exists today in all fifty states, the District of Columbia, Guam, Puerto Rico, and the Virgin Islands, but participation in it is strictly voluntary. In order to receive federal funds, the states or other territories and commonwealth must comply with the requirements of the Social Security Act.

One of the requirements in order for the state to qualify, requires that a plan be developed by the state outlining the way it complies with the federal AFDC standards. This becomes like a contract between the individual state and the federal government. There are broad federal guidelines, and each state can set its own standards of need, income limits, benefit levels and administrative procedures. Each state can decide whether to include pregnant women, to establish conditions related to the suitability of the home as part of the eligibility requirements, to count food stamps and other subsidies as income, to require under-aged parents to live with a guardian, or to provide help to those over 18 who are going to school.

Even with the many federal requirements, states have managed to keep considerable control over the design of their AFDC programs. This has contributed throughout the years to much administrative

---

[51]The information on this section is taken from the U.S. House of Representatives, Committee on Ways and Means. *Overview of entitlement programs. Background material and data on programs within the jurisdiction of the Committee on Ways and Means.* Washington D.C.: U.S. Government Printing Office. Green Books for 1992 (May 15), 1993 (July 7), and 1994 (July 15). Also from the *Encyclopedia of Social Work*, 19th ed. NASW Press, Washington D.C., 1995.

A Description of Health Care in the U.S. 33

discretion and discrimination.[52]

Federal and State funding for AFDC in 1993 totaled $25.2 billion. This sum has increased consistently throughout the years.[53] The share of this amount paid by the federal government was a total of $14.7 billion, or about 1% of the total federal budget. The program is funded through an open-ended federal appropriation to the states that is drawn from income tax money. Federal reimbursements vary inversely according to the per capita income of the state in question. Of the $25.2 billion spent in 1993, 88 percent went for benefits and 12 percent for administration costs. This ratio has remained constant, and it militates against the popularly held idea that administrative costs absorb a disproportionate amount of the program's expenditures.

In order to qualify for assistance in this program some of the factors considered have to do with family composition, income, age of the children, and the willingness of the applicant to collaborate and participate in the welfare-to-work program and in trying to obtain paternity and child support. Children will qualify for AFDC help if a parent is deceased, absent from the home, or with a mental or physical incapacity that is expected to last more than 30 days. Sometimes couples may qualify as well if a parent works less than 100 hours a month, but generally, AFDC payments are available to families that do not work at all.[54]

The program is meant to serve children from birth, even though in many states help is being given as well to assist pregnant mothers. At the moment when the youngest child reaches age 18 (or 19 if enrolled in school), the benefits from the program cease. Recent proposals by Congress may impose a lifetime limit for all AFDC recipients, thus tightening the rules and promoting job training and employment programs for those in welfare. AFDC mothers who lack work skills or who have any kind of illness may be placed in serious financial difficulties.

There is a requirement established by the Social Security Act which demands that each state develop a standard of need. There is no clear definition from the federal government about what this standard

---

[52]TRATTNER W.I., *From Poor Law to Welfare State: A History of Social Welfare in America*, (4th ed.).

[53]It was $16.5 billion in 1985 and $21.2 billion in 1990.

[54]RHODES R.P., *Health Care: Politics, Policy, and Distributive Justice*, p. 83.

should be. This standard is meant to determine the benefit levels for AFDC recipients in each state, but due to the lack of definition about these standards there are great inequalities according to the state. For example, some states include as part of their need standards all basic goods such as food, clothing, shelter, utilities, personal care items, and household maintenance supplies. About half of the states include transportation, and about one-fourth of them include educational expenses, medicine chest supplies, and household equipment. Most states prefer a low standard since this reduces the welfare rolls, benefit levels, and costs. The need standard for a three-person family ranges from a high of $1,648 a month in the state of New Hampshire to a low of $320 a month in the state of Indiana.

There were about 13.6 million AFDC recipients in 1992, with 9.2 million of those being children. These children accounted for 14 percent of the U.S. population under the age of 18 and 63 percent of the children in poverty. The racial composition in 1992 of the beneficiaries overall was 38.9 percent white, 37.2 percent blacks, and 17.8 percent were Hispanics. The remaining 6.2 percent were Asian, Native Americans, or other races. Yet, this composition varied according to state. For example, in Washington D.C. the percentage of whites was 0.8 percent while in the state of Maine it was 98.2 percent white. Some of these patterns should be studied more closely. For example, between 1983 and 1992 the number of African American female-headed families with children grew faster than the number of such white families, yet, in that same time the percentage of African American families receiving AFDC benefits dropped from 43.8 percent to 37.2 percent. The percentage of the white families covering the same time period decreased less rapidly, from 41.8 percent to 38.9 percent.

4. Veterans Health Administration

The United States has today the most comprehensive and complete system of services for veterans in the world.[55] There is a long history of national and popular support for people who have served, and are currently serving, in the armed forces. Health services for veterans are provided by the Veterans Health Administration (VHA) through a

---

[55]YOSHIKAWA T.T., *United States Department of Veterans Affairs: Health care for the aging veteran*, pp. 431-437.

comprehensive range of health and mental health care services.[56] These include acute medical, surgical, and psychiatric inpatient and outpatient care; intermediate hospital, nursing home, and home care; noninstitutional extended care; and a range of special programs and services in outpatient settings. All of the facilities of the VHA are accredited by the Joint Commission on Accreditation of Healthcare Organizations (JCAHO).

Every year more than 2.5 million veterans receive medical care in one of the 171 medical centers and 340 outpatient clinics run by the VHA. There they are provided with state-of-the-art, high-technology health care, and also with preventive care through a Preventive Medicine Program which has been in place since 1985. This program focuses on eleven risk factors for which veterans tend to have large morbidity and mortality rates. These are such factors as hypertension, high cholesterol, breast cancer, and colorectal cancer.

The VHA is also noted for operating one of the most comprehensive mental health services in the country. Under the Readjustment Counseling Service, which was established in 1979 in order to treat Vietnam War veterans, outreach and counseling services have been established all around the country. These centers most recently have extended their services to Persian Gulf War veterans.

The VHA also provides a broad range of long-term-care services through institutional and residential care services that recognizes the needs of a rapidly aging veteran population. The institutional long-term care consists of VHA nursing home units, community nursing homes, state nursing homes, and domiciliary programs. The noninstitutional long-term care includes hospital-based home care, adult day health care, community residential care, and respite care.

It is projected that by the year 2020 women will constitute 11% of all veterans. Women use fewer services through the VHA than men. During 1992 only 2% of all patients treated at a VHA facility were women. Nevertheless, studies have found that women served by the VHA were as satisfied as their male counterparts regarding medical care.

---

[56]WORTHEN D.M., *"The Partnership Between the VA and U.S. Medical Schools,"* VA Practitioner, June 1984, pp. 53-58. The information in this section is also taken from the following documents: Veterans Administration, *Annual report, 1984.* Washington D.C.: U.S. Government Printing Office; Veterans Health Services and Research Administration. *Integrated psychiatric care planning guidelines, criteria and standards.* Washington, D.C.: Department of Veterans Affairs, 1991.

Medical centers and clinics of the VHA report treating more than 19,000 veterans with human immunodeficiency virus (HIV) or acquired immune deficiency syndrome (AIDS). This is approximately 6% of the cumulative number of adult cases of AIDS in the nation.

C. PRIVATE HEALTH CARE IN THE UNITED STATES

Under this main heading we will consider private commercial health insurance, employer-based health insurance, community hospitals and clinics, home health care and acute care.

1. Private Health Insurance

Private health insurance in the United States is provided basically by three groups: the Blue Cross/Blue Shield plans, commercial insurance companies, and independent plans.

Historically, the year 1929 has generally marked the birth of modern health insurance. It was during that year that Justin Ford Kimball established at Baylor University Hospital of Dallas, Texas, a hospital insurance plan. Through this plan schoolteachers, for 50 cents a month, were provided the assurance of 21 days of paid hospitalization per year in a semiprivate room. This later became known as the Blue Cross around the country. It emphasized not the cost, but service, by providing hospital accommodations and even a very specific frame of 21 days of benefits.[57] At its annual meeting in 1931, the American Hospital Association requested Kimball to describe the Baylor plan for them. Other hospitals as well developed interest, and by 1936 there were 21 other hospital insurance plans in over eleven states.[58] Part of the reason for this surge was that, due to the Depression, patients loads in hospitals were diminishing, unpaid bills were escalating, and hospital income was declining. These new health plans offered hospitals a way to stabilize their incomes. Since insurance was regulated at a state level, many of these plans felt the state pressure to organize as insurance companies. The AHA and the local hospitals thought they had a better idea by pursuing nonprofit status and exemptions from state insurance regulations. The

---

[57]RAFFEL M.W., RAFFEL N.K., *The U.S. Health System, Origins and Functions*, 3rd. Ed., p. 243.

[58]Ibid., p. 244.

A Description of Health Care in the U.S. 37

benefits included exemption from the general insurance laws of the state, status as a charitable organization, exemption from maintaining the reserves required of commercial insurers, and tax exemption. The justification offered to offset all these benefits was the promise to serve the community, and especially the low income population.[59] At the same time there was a move to develop an agency to coordinate this rapidly growing movement. This agency was developed within the framework of the AHA, and eventually became an independent body called the Blue Cross Commission and, later, the Blue Cross Association.

As Blue Cross plans began to show their feasibility of covering hospital expenses through insurance, there were pressures that developed to do the same for physician services. In 1939 the California Medical Association established the California Physicians Service, later to be known as the Blue Shield plans for payment of physician's bills. The California plan provided complete payment for physician's services for $1.70 monthly.[60] The two organizations, namely Blue Cross and Blue Shield, rapidly developed very strong links, which enabled each to serve the needs of the other while actively opposing alternative forms of health care organizations such as cooperatives.[61]

Originally, these plans covered employees and not their dependents, but eventually common sense and equity had it that dependents should be covered too.

The state of New York was the first to adopt this kind of legislation, and by 1938 Blue Cross had enrolled 1.4 million people. By the end of the war in 1945 this Blue Cross enabling legislation had been adopted by 35 states in the Union. In this way the individual Blue Cross plans across the country were born. These plans grew in a phenomenal fashion during the next few years, but by the early 1950's private commercial hospital insurance grew at an even faster rate. By 1951 Blue Cross had 37 million people enrolled nationally, while the commercial health insurance companies had 40 million enrollees. This trend continued with Blue Cross not being able to compete effectively during the 1950's

---

[59]WEISS L.D., *No Benefit: Crisis in America's Health Insurance Industry*, p. 11.

[60]RAFFEL M.W., RAFFEL N.K., *The U.S. Health System, Origins and Functions*, 3rd. Ed., pp. 244-245.

[61]STARR P., *The Social Transformation of American Medicine*, p. 309.

and 1960's. By 1969 there were 67 million people enrolled with Blue Cross under the age of 65, yet that represented only 37% of the market. The rest were practically all insured by the commercial insurance companies.[62]

During the 1950's major medical insurance plans began to develop very rapidly. The coverage offered by these commercial insurance companies included a wide range of hospital services, both inpatient and outpatient, drugs, appliances, ambulance services, and others. They however included a deductible and coinsurance as well as an upper limit on the amount of expenses. A deductible is the amount paid by the insured before coverage can take effect. Coinsurance payment refers to the part of the total cost that is expected to be covered by the insured. Based on these two elements, there are basically an infinite variety of benefit packages within commercial health insurance companies. Some of the variations as well, have to do with the services provided, for example, the number of hospital days allowed, the amount of money paid for surgical and medical care, whether home and office health care is provided, and whether dental, vision, and major medical expenses are covered. During the past twenty years it has become increasingly clear that these differential levels of allowable insurance reimbursements made by hospitals or medical practitioners, have created a pattern of unequal access to health care. For those individuals who are inadequately protected, it may require large out-of-pocket expenses for medical care that is essential. When those individuals are poor, the consequence may be exclusion from needed medical care.[63]

The commercial companies cover today a little more than half of the people who have private health insurance. Some companies, like Prudential and Equitable, restrict their business to group coverage. Other companies offer insurance primarily based on individual policies. Different from Blue Cross / Blue Shield, each individual company is independent from the others, each being a business by itself.

---

[62]WEISS L.D., *No Benefit: Crisis in America's Health Insurance Industry*, p. 12.

[63]BAYER R., CALLAHAN D., CAPLAN A.L., JENNINGS B., *"Toward Justice in Health Care,"* American Journal of Public Health 78(5): 586, May 1988.

A Description of Health Care in the U.S. 39

What these commercial insurance companies would do is to charge employers or individuals an annual premium, and then would pay health care providers on a fee-for-service basis. A set amount established by the insurance plan or negotiated between the insurer and the provider of care was paid by the insurance company to the provider every time the beneficiaries made use of a covered service.

Historically, commercial insurance companies entered the market cautiously. They had lost money during the Depression, and were concerned with the comprehensive benefits offered by Blue Cross / Blue Shield. It was a Supreme Court decision which recognized fringe benefits as a legitimate part of the bargaining process plus the freezing of industrial wages during the war, that finally convinced commercial insurance companies to compete.

During the 1980's, though, tremendous changes occurred affecting the relationship between insurers and providers. Health maintenance organizations have made an impact by delivering services on a capitated basis instead of a fee-for-service basis. Capitation is the system by which a flat fee is paid to a primary care physician to provide a stipulated range of services for the patient for a given time, which is usually a year. The difference under capitation is that the fee is the same regardless of how much or how little care the patient needs or uses. By 1988 HMO's accounted for 18% of all private insurance. Another type of insurance called preferred provider organizations (PPO's), which limit beneficiaries to a list of physicians or give economic incentives to utilize physicians who have offered discounts to the insurer, have grown as well accounting for 11% of the private insurance market in 1988.[64]

2. Employer-Based Health Insurance

A distinctive practice in the United States is to link private health insurance to the work place.[65] This system came into existence after the defeat of the proposals for national health insurance that happened prior to World War II during the 1930's and 1940's. Before this arrangement took effect, private health insurance plans, for the most part, offered contracts that would provide medical services by a single physician to a

---

[64]KOVNER A.R., *Health Care Delivery in the United States,* p. 252.

[65]JECKER N.S., *"Can an Employer-based Health Insurance System Be Just?,"* Journal of Health Politics, Policy and Law 18(3):657, Fall 1993.

group of subscribing individuals. These individuals had to pay for the plan, but the plans themselves were sponsored by the employers for their employees or by labor unions, lodges, fraternal orders, and consumer groups. Hospital care was generally excluded from such plans. Each physician in the plan would be paid in advance a fixed amount per enrolled person per year. These plans were not widely available, and depended on favorable circumstances as for example, a strong union, a forward-looking employer, or a cohesive immigrant group.[66]

Right after World War II began, there was a growth in interest on the part of employers to offer group health plans. One of the reasons for this was that civilian labor was in very short supply during the war years, and the War Labor Board imposed a ceiling on wages in 1942 in order to prevent inflation. This same board also decided that a 5% increase in fringe benefits would not be considered inflationary. With this in mind, employers responded by expanding employee benefits by including in them health insurance. In this way they could lure new workers and retain their existing employees by offering a competitive market. To offer health insurance as part of employment benefits became even more attractive in 1961 when the U.S. Treasury allowed employers to deduct from profits, and count as wages, what was contributed by the company towards employees' health plans.[67] With this new law employers could deduct health care insurance payments from their profits, and at the same time employees would receive a nontaxable benefit. The end result was that part of the health care costs for insurance was underwritten by the government since a dollar contributed to health insurance lowered the employer's federal income tax, but did not raise the employee's tax. The motivations for this federal tax subsidy were several: There were the concerns with assuring financial solvency to hospitals, or those of sustaining physician's income, or providing financial security to individuals and families who banded together in order to undercut the efforts of introducing a government-sponsored health insurance program.[68] To summarize, employer-based health insurance became in a short period of time the cornerstone of health insurance, and appropriate for a nation

---

[66]JECKER N.S., *"Can an Employer-based Health Insurance System Be Just?,"* Journal of Health Politics, Policy and Law 18(3):659, Fall 1993.

[67]Ibid.

[68]Ibid.

"steeped in the Puritan work ethic."[69]

Employer-based health insurance kept growing steadily after the war and well into the 1970's.[70] That is when the percentage of employed Americans without health insurance began to increase. Employment has been shifting from manufacturing jobs to service oriented jobs, and the strength of the labor unions has declined. The jobs that used to offer health services have been stagnant, while jobs without health benefits have grown. As a matter of fact, the National Medical Expenditure Survey found that in the year 1987 the uninsured population was composed of 46.4% of working adults, 6.8% of nonworking spouses of working adults, and 23.6% of children of working adults. This means that 76.8% of the uninsured population were people who had employment or were nuclear-family dependents of the employed.[71] This percentage grew to 85% in 1988.[72]

On the other hand, having employer-based health insurance does not necessarily mean that there is access to health care. Health care benefits and access to them are not uniform. One of the greatest challenges to the employer-based health insurance has come from what has been termed the "domino effect" which comes about from basing health care on an already unjust work distribution. In other words, if it can be shown that the way jobs are distributed in the United States has already some elements of injustice, then to use the work distribution as the basis to provide health care will in itself be flawed as well. This "domino effect" factor seems to affect women especially. In 1980, for example, of the 58.4 million men fifteen years of age or older who had a salary income, 65.4% (or basically 38.2 million men) had an employer or union that provided for all or part of the health insurance. In contrast, of the 50.1 million women workers in the same category, only 49.7% (or 24.9

---

[69]FRIEDMAN E., *"The Uninsured. From Dilemma to Crisis,"* Journal of the American Medical Association 265(19):2492, May 15, 1991.

[70]STARR P., *The Logic of Health Care Reform: Why and How the President's Plan Will Work*, p. 60.

[71]FRIEDMAN E., *"The Uninsured. From Dilemma to Crisis,"* Journal of the American Medical Association 265(19):2493, May 15, 1991.

[72]JECKER N.S., *"Can an Employer-based Health Insurance System Be Just?,"* Journal of Health Politics, Policy and Law 18(3):660, Fall 1993.

million women) had any outside contribution for health care. The entire cost of the insurance was paid for 29.6% of the working men but only for 22.9% of the women.[73] Working women tended to be involved more often in nonunion jobs which are less likely to provide health insurance coverage. Union membership differences between men and women are evident. For example, in the 25-34 age group, 13% of the women belong to unions, while 19% of the men workers do. This gap widens when we consider the 35-54 age group with 19.2% of the women belonging to unions compared to 29.8% of the men.[74]

In recent years there has been a tremendous erosion in the connection between employment and health insurance. Between 1988 and 1994, for example, there was a decrease of 4 million people who were covered by employment-based insurance.[75] Employers are not necessarily the villains, since health insurance products for small businesses tend to be both limited and expensive. This restricts the ability of smaller businesses to spread the risks over a large number of employees, thus resulting in higher premiums in the case that an employer has to incur large costs. The number of employers offering health coverage is dropping dramatically.[76]

Another factor affecting women is the rate in which women change jobs. This has an impact on health insurance since there is a tendency to lose your insurance as you change jobs, and many times other insurances are not willing to take people with a pre-existing condition. Also low-paying jobs, which include clerical, retail, and service work categories, are less likely to offer a health care insurance package, and women predominate in such jobs.[77] The same holds true for part-time jobs. Only 16% of part-time workers, male or female, are enrolled in

---

[73]JECKER N.S., *"Can an Employer-based Health Insurance System Be Just?,"* Journal of Health Politics, Policy and Law 18(3):662, Fall 1993.

[74]Ibid., p. 663.

[75]SCHROEDER S.A., *"The Medically Uninsured - Will They Always Be With Us?,"* New England Journal of Medicine 334(17):1132, 1996.

[76]Business Week. November 26, 1990, p. 187.

[77]JECKER N.S., *"Can an Employer-based Health Insurance System Be Just?,"* Journal of Health Politics, Policy and Law 18(3):663-664, Fall 1993.

group health plans through work, while 72% of full-time workers have such health coverage.[78]

In recent times the whole concept of the employer mandated insurance has been called into question. To provide health insurance through the place of employment, tends to hold the rest of the economy hostage to health care. The competition that comes about from large, profit-making businesses who compete trying to lower health insurance costs, can threaten the quality of the health care provided.[79] Some people have questioned the practicality of changing the system of employer-based insurance at this point in history. As the problem with insurance coverage grows, though, more and more firms are beginning to question why did they ever become involved in choosing doctors and hospitals for their employees when they do not choose other important needs such as schools and housing.[80] It is becoming more evident today that the current system of employer-based health insurance came about through accidental and historical events, and in no way through a careful, deliberate, and morally conscious process. Many patterns of injustice have arisen because of this.[81]

3. Community Hospitals and Clinics

For many people in the United States local hospitals and clinics end up providing for most of the health care needs. This applies to rural and urban populations, but it is especially true within the urban, inner city neighborhoods. These community hospitals include general short-term institutions under not-for-profit auspices, as well as investor-owned facilities. These hospitals constitute about 83% of the total number of

---

[78]STEVENS P.E., *"Who Gets Care? Access to Health Care as an Arena for Nursing Action,"* Scholarly Inquiry for Nursing Practice 6(3):190, Fall-Winter 1992.

[79]ANGELL M., *"The Beginning of Health Care Reform: The Clinton Plan,"* New England Journal of Medicine 329(21):1570, November 18, 1993.

[80]STARR P., *The Logic of Health Care Reform: Why and How the President's Plan Will Work*, p. 56.

[81]JECKER N.S., *"Can an Employer-based Health Insurance System Be Just?,"* Journal of Health Politics, Policy and Law 18(3):670-671, Fall 1993.

hospitals in the United States, and account for 90% of all hospital admissions in one year. About 60% of them are owned by not-for-profit groups, 15% by for-profit or investor-owned groups, and 26% by state and local governments. Not-for-profit simply means that the hospital or institution is not required to pay taxes on its income or property, nor does it distribute any leftover monies to any individual as profit.

The community hospital provides a variety of diagnostic services as well as therapeutic ones. It deals with medical and surgical cases. It is usually thought of as an acute, short-term institution. The responsibility within a community hospital rests with a board of trustees whose members are elected. These trustees, typically do not receive any payment for their services as trustees. Among their jobs are: determining the policies of the institution, hiring senior administrators, and appointing physicians to the medical staff.

These community hospitals can be small or large, teaching or non-teaching, depending on the size of the population served and the range of services provided. Around the country there are many large hospitals in small communities. Their existence can be justified because of the fact that most of the times they are referral hospitals. This means that people from other communities, where there are limitations on the services provided by a local hospital, are referred to larger ones that can justify and maintain the expense of some services not provided at the smaller ones.

When community hospitals are labeled *teaching hospitals,* this simply means that there is the presence in the hospital of an approved residency or internship program for medical students. Historically, most teaching hospitals have been public general hospitals in which large number of indigent patients are cared for. Residents and medical students learned by treating these patients. In a sense it can be said that these indigent patients paid for their care by providing their bodies to be used for training purposes. Until the advent of Medicaid, with which poor people were entitled to private care, many complained about this reality, and resented the experimental dimension of such care. By 1966 this practice changed, and all patients, whether they payed or not, were considered teaching patients.[82]

There are three types of state government general hospitals. First, there are hospitals owned and operated by the state as part of a state university. The university in question and its medical school have control

---

[82]RAFFEL M.W., RAFFEL N.K., *The U.S. Health System, Origins and Functions,* 3rd. Ed., p. 155.

A Description of Health Care in the U.S.   45

of this institution. Second, there is the hospital connected with the state's penal system. The third type of hospital is found in some states in order to serve the poor.

The investor-owned community hospitals, or as they are also known, for-profit or proprietary institutions, are owned by one person, a group in partnership, or a corporation. These hospitals are often called in the United States "private" hospitals. This term can be misleading. This is so because in other countries private means nongovernmental, and with the capability of being for-profit or not-for-profit. Most proprietary hospitals in the U.S. were developed by physicians in order to meet the needs of the local community. Some of those very small institutions today, have given way to larger institutions that have responded to the population shifts, the increased costs, and the necessities of modern medical practice. Hospitals that have been named *"doctors' hospital,"* may be profit or nonprofit. Some of them were established to meet the community needs, as mentioned above, but some came about as a result of professional conflicts within an already existing hospital, or by a group of doctors that had no hospital privileges at a certain institution.[83]

Among the proprietary hospitals, the most important ones are the corporately owned institutions. There are several corporations that build, own, and operate several hospitals in the United States and abroad. Humana Inc. of Louisville for example owns over 85 hospitals in the country.[84]

One interesting element concerning hospitals is the developments taking place among rural hospitals. Rural areas are the ones that fall outside the metropolitan statistical areas. There are different ways that a rural population can be determined such. An area is defined a rural area if it contains a city with a population of at least 50,000 people with a total metropolitan population of at least 100,000. In 1986, for example, 46% of the nation's hospitals were rural. Seventy-one percent of them had fewer than 100 beds. The breakdown of these rural hospitals was as follows: ten percent were investor-owned, forty-nine percent were private not-for-profit institutions, and forty-one percent were public facilities

---

[83]RAFFEL M.W., RAFFEL N.K., *The U.S. Health System, Origins and Functions,* 3rd. Ed., p. 157.

[84]Ibid., p. 158.

operated by state or local governments.[85] There has been a pattern in recent years of a decrease in admissions to rural hospitals, with most hospitals having a 50% occupancy average rate. Many of these hospitals have closed, depriving local residents of access to health care. Issues of financial viability, quality of care, and difficulties attracting qualified and skilled professionals have plagued these hospitals in recent years.

4. Home Health Care

Even as late as the mid 1900's, many people were still receiving most of their health care at home. It was a fairly common practice for physicians to visit the homes of the patients. After several decades of reliance on hospitals and hospital staffs, it is evident that there is a tremendous growth in home health care today. At times the motivation appears to be mainly economic, with an emphasis on cost-containment, but certainly this is not the only motivation. There is a re-discovery of other elements of health care which have to do with social and psychological factors that have catapulted home health care to a new level of utilization.

There is evidence of the reliance upon home health care from very early on in American history. As far back as 1796, the Boston Dispensary addressed the issue about the importance of the ill not being deprived of their families, and how they could be taken care at home.[86] During the late 1800's nursing services at the home were organized by lay persons, who provided skilled nursing care to the ill and their families. In 1877 the Women's Branch of the New York City Mission employed a graduate nurse with the purpose of providing care to the sick in their own homes. This was the first time this kind of hiring happened. When health care shifted to long term care instead of controlling epidemics, hospitals became overcrowded, and sought ways to deal with the bed shortage. The University of Syracuse began a program in 1941 to provide health care to the patients that were discharged from the hospital with a need of follow up. In 1946 a nationwide committee established by the National Organization of Public Health Nursing made several recommendations concerning home care. The recommendations had to do with having the health department support and administer also the care of the sick at home.

---

[85]KOVNER A.R., *Health Care Delivery in the United States*, p. 150.

[86]SPIEGEL A.D., *Home Healthcare: Home Birthing to Hospice Care*, p. 2.

A Description of Health Care in the U.S. 47

Even after these recommendations, home health care continued to develop without much organization.

It was not until 1947, when Dr. E.M. Bluestone began a hospital based homecare program at Montefiore Hospital in New York, that a more organized effort began to provide home health care. Dr. Bluestone's notion of a hospital was one "without walls." This meant that it would not limit its care to the people within the hospital building. He expressed it clearly when he said: "If you have a 500 bed hospital and 50 patients on homecare, you have a 550 bed hospital."[87] There is a description of his program in the February 1949 issue of the American Journal of Public Health.[88]

In 1961 the Community Health Services and Facilities Act gave permission to the Surgeon General of the United States to make project grants to public or nonprofit agencies in order to develop services outside the hospital. This Act had authority from 1962 to 1967, and during that period of time $42 million was used to conduct nearly 300 projects. Of this money, about 15% was used for homecare activities.[89]

The Medicare legislation in 1965 greatly influenced the expansion of home health care. Originally the federal requirement in order to be considered a homecare agency was to provide nursing services plus one additional service such as physical therapy, occupational therapy, speech therapy, medical social service, or home health aide service. This requirement of "nursing-plus-one" seemed to be too much to ask since in 1963, of the 1,100 agencies offering home care, only 250 qualified for Medicare.[90] In order to deal with this, the federal government assisted homecare agencies in raising their level of care. After spending $16 million of government funds, there were 1,275 home health agencies that

---

[87]RYDER C.F., *Changing Patterns in Home Care*, p. 2.

[88]CHERKASKY M., *The Montefiore Hospital Home Care Program*, American Journal of Public Health 39(2): 163-166, February 1949.

[89]SPIEGEL A.D., *Home Healthcare: Home Birthing to Hospice Care*, p. 9.

[90]WARHOLA C.F., RYDER C.F., *Planning for Home Health Services: A Resource Handbook*, p. 6.

were approved for Medicare participation in 1966.[91] In 1970 homecare benefits were declared mandatory for Medicaid as well. Even though the amount of dollars of Medicaid spent on home care increased greatly, still the percentage of Medicaid expenditures for home services is only 1%.[92] Home health services are also included under Title XX of the Social Security Act.

Recently there has been some discussion concerning home health care, and whether to consider it a more narrow service of skilled services, usually for acute, episodic bouts with illness, or to consider it a broader professional and supportive service. Today the latter, more inclusive definition, is the one most favored. This broad-service oriented home health care combines traditional health care and non-traditional social services. It is clear that the level of governmental involvement will affect which factors will be emphasized in the future of home health care. There is some hesitation from the part of the government to expand home health benefits because of the uncertainty over potential costs. Nursing home care or other institutional settings may prove to be more economical.

---

[91]WARHOLA C.F., RYDER C.F., *Planning for Home Health Services: A Resource Handbook*, p. 6.

[92]Ibid.

TWO

ACCESS TO HEALTH CARE
IN THE UNITED STATES

The old axiom which states that "before affirming or denying, first we must define," will be very relevant in this chapter. In order to evaluate the present state of access to health care in the United States, it is important to arrive at a better understanding of what is meant by "access." We will first try to explain the different elements of such a definition, and then give an statistical account and interpretation of who has access to health care in America. Finally, there will be a discussion of the different aspects which limit access to health care.

A. DEFINING ACCESS TO HEALTH CARE

As with everything that relates to human beings, there are many subjective elements that enter into play when we talk about access to health care. One initial distinction that needs to be made is that access to care is not the same as access to coverage. To find out the difference we only need to ask many pregnant Medicaid clients that have not received care, since four out of ten obstetricians no longer take new Medicaid clients or any Medicaid clients at all. Or we could ask many families that receive AFDC who have found out that 44% of pediatricians either limit their Medicaid clientele or refuse them altogether. Or ask a woman who has coverage but lives in a southern county of the state of Illinois, where there is no single obstetrician practicing. In all these cases, coverage does not guarantee access to health care.[93]

It is important to realize that access to health care can be defined according to the philosophical system embraced at a particular moment in the history of the country. We will specifically deal with the philosophical theories of justice in chapter two, but for now we can mention that the definition of "access" will vary according to the different philosophies.

---

[93]FRIEDMAN E., *"Making Room in the Marketplace,"* Health Progress 71(10):16, December 1990.

For example, for a libertarian, access to care may simply mean that no one should be legitimately prevented from obtaining health care. In such a way, having a right to access has nothing to do with having health care provided to all persons, or having a system that equitably distributes care. For an egalitarian, access to care may refer to the ability to obtain specific goods or services to which every person should have an equal claim. The problem is that usually these goods or services are not specified clearly, and may vary from place to place and from country to country.[94] For a utilitarian, access to health care may mean to have the possibility of obtaining services and goods according to the distribution of resources that will maximize the well being of the majority of the needy population. It is clear that our conception of access will be affected by the philosophical theory of justice from which we depart.

Still, it is possible to mention some objective parameters that can be applied to the whole question of access regardless of the philosophical theory that directs the delivery of health care. Access can be defined experientially in terms of the very concrete and specific problems encountered by the people in their attempt to receive medical assistance. There are several categories that can help us in understanding the experience. Access can be divided into potential access, realized access, equitable and inequitable access, effective access, and efficient access. The first one is defined operationally in terms of having a regular source of health care. When considering potential access there is an assumption that a person with such access is likely to encounter less difficulties when seeking health care than a person without such regular source of care. The second category—realized access—is based on the rates of utilization which take into consideration the actual care-seeking behavior of people. Realized access may be positive or negative. It will be positive when there is a successful attainment of the goods or services. It will be negative when difficulties arise in seeking health care. Substantial differences have been revealed when positive measures are analyzed, and physician involvement has been found to be clearly different depending on whether patients were insured or not.[95] There are two main types of measures of realized (also called actual) access: Subjective measures are related to the

---

[94]BEAUCHAMP T.L., CHILDRESS J.F., *Principles of Biomedical Ethics*, p. 355.

[95]BASHSHUR R.L., HOMAN R.K., SMITH D.G., *"Beyond the Uninsured: Problems in Access to Care,"* Medical Care 32(5):410-411, May 1994.

satisfaction with treatment, while the objective measures are related with the various utilization rates.[96]

There have been two main objections to using utilization rates based on need as the sole or primary measure of realized access. The first objection has to do with the fact that focusing on utilization rates based on need tends to ignore at least one other necessary condition for equity of access to health care. Variations in the potential access variables can have equity implications even if they are not considered important variables in reference to utilization rates. Even if health care seeking behavior is not affected by some variables as seen by the end-result of utilization rates, still they can affect other outcomes, as for example, what else someone can do with his or her time and money.

A second objection is that utilization rates do not necessarily reflect differences in attitudes from different sub-groups toward health care. The fact that some specific procedure is not utilized by a certain sub-group, does not necessarily imply that there is some inequity or injustice, but it may simply denote a different approach to health care which may be present in certain groups within our society.[97]

Other authors clearly admit the importance of utilization rates in analyzing access to health care, yet they are concerned about the way in which certain process variables may vary with the geographical area, the income group, or the race in consideration. Some refer to these variations as the "humaneness" of the care provided, and how these are likely to be captured better by subjective measures of realized access even when they do not affect the objective ones based on utility rates. Two authors—Sloan and Bentkover—put it this way: "Many, for example, would view the long waits the poor experience in clinics as an injustice, irrespective of the effect patient waiting might have on utilization rates."[98] The basic idea behind this comment is that health care cannot be considered equitable if it is much more difficult for some people to receive care, even when they are willing to make the necessary adjustments and eventually receive the care they need. Potential access factors are usually

---

[96]DANIELS N., *"Equity of Access to Health Care: Some Conceptual and Ethical Issues,"* Milbank Memorial Fund Quarterly - Health and Society 60(1):56, Winter 1982.

[97]Ibid., p. 60.

[98]Ibid., p. 62.

divided into three categories.[99] The first one has to do with structural features in the health care system. These will include, for example, the availability of physicians or hospitals in different areas of the country, which can be measured by physician-patient ratios. The second category is related to features of individuals who are members of the population. These include predisposing factors such as age, cultural background, and health status, and such enabling factors such as income or insurance coverage. There are studies that have found that some people avoid using health care services due to a perceived or actual inability to afford those goods or health services. The very expectation of being refused health care many times underlie the avoidance of services.[100] A third category related to potential access can be called "process" factors. These have to do with the stages that must be undertaken when seeking health care. Part of the analytic task when considering access to health care is to determine the importance of each of these factors, and how the variations of these factors end up affecting realized access to care.

The analytic test for the causal importance of a variable related to potential access must be reformulated in a way that its effect on the equity of access can be shown. There is equitable access to health care when need rather than structural, individual, or process factors determine entry to the system. In order for access to be equitable, the potential access variables, as operationally defined, must all be related to health status in the proper way. Equitable distribution of health care services is achieved when illness, as defined by the patient and his or her family or by the health professional, is the major determinant of the allocation of resources.[101] Inequitable access occurs when social characteristics and enabling resources, such as ethnic background or income, determine who gets health care.

---

[99]DANIELS N., *"Equity of Access to Health Care: Some Conceptual and Ethical Issues,"* Milbank Memorial Fund Quarterly - Health and Society 60(1):62, Winter 1982.

[100]BASHSHUR R.L., HOMAN R.K., SMITH D.G., *"Beyond the Uninsured: Problems in Access to Care,"* Medical Care 32(5):413, May 1994.

[101]DANIELS N., *"Equity of Access to Health Care: Some Conceptual and Ethical Issues,"* Milbank Memorial Fund Quarterly - Health and Society 60(1):58-59, Winter 1982.

Effective access to health care can be conceived as the link between realized access, which means the utilization of health services, and health outcomes, which relates to health status and consumer satisfaction. Its purpose is to assess the benefit of medical care as manifested by the improvements in health outcomes.

Finally, efficient access category links resources utilized to health services and associated health outcomes. Its purpose is to achieve the minimization of costs of health services while at the same time maximizing health status or consumer satisfaction. It consists of two components: allocative and productive. Allocative efficiency requires the attainment of the most valued mix of outputs possible, while productive efficiency means producing a level of outcome at a minimum cost.

There is a broad social consensus emerging in the United States that all citizens should be able to achieve equal access to health care. This would include appropriate insurance coverage for all, with no temporal gaps of coverage nor unjust exclusionary clauses. Later in the text we will develop how this consensus partially rejects the absolutism of some traditional philosophical strands upon which the United States was founded.

This emerging consensus suggests that there are principles of justice that must govern the distribution of health care, and in that way, guarantee fair equality of opportunity for all. There is a need for a foundation that would promote health care as a social obligation. This obligation could be summarized as the provision of health care to all citizens with no obstacles—whether financial, racial, geographical, or any other—to access health care services and goods. There are numerous instances or examples today in our society of disregard for this obligation, and also plenty of situations in which health care is not available to all citizens regardless of their situation in life and other particulars. In the next part of the chapter we will take a look at the trends in access related to health care in the United States, using the access categories already mentioned in this section.

B. WHO HAS ACCESS TO HEALTH CARE IN THE UNITED STATES?

If we try to analyze the data of recent trends concerning the access categories that we have already defined, it is evident that potential access to health care in the U.S. for persons under 65 years of age has decreased. The most obvious way to measure this is by analyzing the

54 Health Care and the Common Good

uninsured population. There are some experts that feel that the term "uninsured" is misleading. Many times one may hear people say that the uninsured are young, healthy, middle class people who are just out of college or between jobs. Yet, recent surveys show a somewhat different picture. In these surveys age distribution of the uninsured is quite similar to that of the general population which is under 65 years of age. Actually the uninsured tend to be poorer than the general population, with 60% of them having incomes either below the federal poverty level or less than twice that level, as compared with 35% of the general population.[102]

Recent reports that have been based on a review of this problem conclude that the uninsured have less access to care, use less care, cannot obtain specific health care services, are twice as likely to be hospitalized for conditions that can be averted by outpatient care (such as acute asthma attacks), and have a higher risk of death when admitted to the hospital.[103] The proportion of uninsured people in the U.S. increased from 13% in 1980 to 17% in 1995.[104] (Refer to Table 1 in the next page for this and the information that follows). Overall Medicaid coverage increased from 6% to 11% during the same period, but this was offset by a decline in private insurance coverage which went from 79% in 1980 to 71% of the population in 1995. The percentage of the uninsured in the category of people within 15 to 44 years of age, went up from 14% during 1980 to 21% in 1995. The proportion of coverage by private insurance went down in every age group from 1980 to 1995. For adults in the 45-64 age range it went down from 84% to 80%. In the 15-44 age range it went down from 79% to 71% covered. Most dramatic was the decline in the Under 15 category, which went down from 75% to 65%. Nevertheless, since 1980, Medicaid has covered an increasing proportion of the children, which was 10% in 1980 and reached 21% in 1995. This reflects the expanded Medicaid income eligibility which was enacted by Congress in the 1980's in order to extend Medicaid's beneficial effects to more low-income pregnant women and their children. Even though only 51% of poor

---

[102]SCHROEDER S.A., *"The Medically Uninsured-Will They Always Be With Us?"* New England Journal of Medicine 334(17): 1130-1131, (1996).

[103]Ibid.

[104]The statistical data is taken from the National Center for Health Statistics, Health United States, 1996-97, Hyattsville, Md.: Public Health Service, 1996-97, p.269.

TABLE 1: HEALTH CARE COVERAGE BY AGE, RACE/ETHNICITY, AND INCOME

	Percentage of the Population								
	Private Insurance[n]			Medicaid[n]			Not Covered[n]		
Age	1980	1989	1995	1980	1989	1995	1980	1989	1995
Under 15	75	72	65	10	11	21	13	16	14
15-44	79	77	71	4	4	7	14	18	21
45-64	84	83	80	3	3	5	9	11	12
Race and Ethnicity	%	%	%	%	%	%	%	%	%
White	82	80	75	3	4	9	11	14	16
Black	60	59	53	18	17	25	19	22	20
Hispanic Origin[a]	—	51	47	—	10	20	—	31	32
Income[o]	%	%	%	%	%	%	%	%	%
Less than $14,000	39	35	24	28	27	41	38	37	34
$14,000-$24,999	61	71	56	9	5	14	26	21	28
$25,000-$34,999	79	88	75	3	1	5	15	9	17
$35,000-$49,999	90	92	88	1	1	2	6	6	8
$50,000 or more	94	96	94	1	*	1	4	3	5
Total	79	77	71	6	6	11	13	16	17

—Not Available
*Less than 0.5 percent

[a] Hispanic origin based on self-report; may include persons classified as either white or black according to race.

[o] Family income categories for 1989 and 1993. Family income categories for 1980 are less than $7,000, $7,000-$9,999, $10,000-$14,999, $15,000-$24,999, $25,000 or more.

[n] The sum of the percentages for private insurance, Medicaid, and no coverage may not come to 100 percent because other types of health insurance such as Medicare or military policies do not appear in the table and because persons with both private insurance and Medicaid are counted in both columns.
(Source: National Center for Health Statistics, Health United States, 1996-97 (Hyattsville, Md.: Public Health Service, 1995), p. 269.)

children were covered by Medicaid in 1985, this increased to 60% by 1994.[105] Even with this, the proportion of uninsured children went up from 13% in 1980 to 14% in 1995. Because of a decline in health insurance coverage it is clear that there has been a decline in potential access to health care, particularly for people between the ages of 15 to 44.

When examining realized access to health care we will consider three types of services: 1) hospital admissions, which represent services in response to serious illnesses; 2) physician visits, which correspond to a combination of primary and secondary care; and 3) dental visits, which conform to rarely life threatening conditions, but which still have an impact on people's functional status and quality of life. (See Table 2 in page 57).

The hospital admissions in the U.S. doubled between 1930 and 1953. They increased in that space of time from 6 admissions per hundred persons per year, to 12 admissions.[106] This trend continued until the 1960's and early 1970's as the number of admissions per hundred persons per year reached 14. This was all due to an increase in the standard of living, the beginning of voluntary health insurance, the growth of the legitimacy of the modern hospital as a place to give birth and treat acute illnesses, and the increase in sophisticated medical technology. It was until the mid 1970's that the use of the acute care hospital began to decline. By 1987 the rate of admissions per hundred population had dropped to ten, and by 1993 it was down to nine. The emphasis placed on cost reduction brought about a great change from more expensive inpatient care to the less expensive outpatient one. The whole system of payment began to change as well. The most common fee-for-service arrangement gave way to prospective payments by Medicare, reduced coverage, and benefits with coinsurance payments and deductibles. Medical technology

---

[105]ROWLAND D., LYONS B., EDWARDS J., *"Medicaid: Health Care of the Poor in the Reagan Era,"* Annual Review of Public Health 9 (1988): 427-450.

[106]Statistical data is taken from: ANDERSEN R., ANDERSON O., *"Trends in the Use of Health Services,"* in Handbook of Medical Sociology (3rd ed.), eds. FREEMAN H.E., LEVINE S., and REEDER L.G., Englewood Cliffs, N.J.: Prentice Hall, 1979, pp. 374, 378, 379.; National Center for Health Statistics, Health United States, 1994, Hyattsville, Md.: Public Health Service, 1995, pp. 169, 171, 177, 178, 179, 180.; Dental visit data from National Center for Health Statistics, unpublished data from the National Health Interview Survey, persons aged twenty-five years or older.

Access to Health Care in the U.S.

TABLE 2: PERSONAL HEALTH CARE USE BY INCOME

	From 1928 To 1931[a]	From 1952 To 1953[a]	From 1963 To 1964[a]	1974[a]	1987[o3]	1993[n]
Hospital Admissions (Admissions per 100 persons per year.)						
Low Income®	6	12	14	19	14	14
Middle Income©	6	12	14	14	11	9
High Income[2]	8	11	11	11	8	7
TOTAL	6	12	13	14	10	9
Physician Visits (Visits per person per year)						
Low Income®	2.2	3.7	4.3	5.3	6.8	7.3
Middle Income©	2.5	3.8	4.5	4.8	5.4	5.9
High Income[2]	4.3	6.5	5.1	4.9	5.3	5.9
TOTAL	2.6	4.2	4.5	4.9	5.4	6.0
Dentist Visits (Percentage seeing a dentist within year)						
Bellow poverty□	—	—	—	—	33%	36%
Low Income®	10%	17%	21%	35%	42%	—
At or above poverty□	—	—	—	—	52%	64%
Middle Income©	20%	33%	36%	48%	60%	—
High Income[2]	46%	56%	58%	64%	76%	—
TOTAL	21%	34%	38%	49%	58%	61%

[a]Source: Various surveys, reported in R. Andersen and O. Anderson, "Trends in the Use of Health Services," in Handbook of Medical Sociology (3rd ed.), eds. H.E. Freeman, S. Levine, and L.G. Reeder (Englewood Cliffs, N.J.: Prentice Hall, 1979), pp. 374, 378, 379.

[o]Source: National Center for Health Statistics, Health United States, 1994 (Hyattsville, Md.: Public Health Service, 1995), pp. 171, 179, 180.

[n]Source: National Center for Health Statistics, Health United States, 1994 (Hyattsville, Md.: Public Health Service, 1995), pp. 169, 177, 178.

®Low Income = lowest 15 percent to 27 percent of family income distribution.

©Middle Income = middle 51 percent to 73 percent of family income distribution.

[2]High Income = highest 12 percent to 32 percent of family income distribution.

[3]1989 for dental visits.

□Dental visit data from National Center for Health Statistics, unpublished data from the National Health Interview Survey, persons aged twenty-five years or older.

also began to change so as to provide more services on an outpatient basis.

The visits to physicians also increased tremendously between the 1930's and the early 1950's. The average of the total visits per person per year between 1928 and 1931 was 2.2. By 1953 this number had almost doubled to 4.2. The reasons for this growth were similar to the ones for the increase of hospital admissions. Yet, unlike hospital admissions, physicians visits per person per year continued to increase into the present decade of the 1990's. For example, in 1974 visits per person per year had reached 4.9, and by 1993 it was up to 6.0 visits. The shift from inpatient to outpatient care may account for this divergence between hospital admissions and physician's visits in what relates to realized access to health care.

There is a similar trend in dentist visits for the total U.S. population to the one seen above for physician visits. In 1930 twenty-one percent of the population visited a dentist in the U.S. There was a consistent increase in the proportion of people visiting the dentist in subsequent years. By 1974 the number reached half the population, and by 1993 it was 61%.

When the socio-economic factors of race and income are taken into account in the statistics discussed above, there is a mixed picture as to whether there is equitable access to health care. Since 1980 until the present time, it seems that minorities and low-income people are the least likely to have private insurance. For example, in 1993 seventy-five percent of white people had private insurance while only 51% of the blacks and 49% of people from Hispanic origin had such insurance. (See Table 1 in page 55). While 94% of the population earning $50,000 or more had private health insurance, only 26% of those earning less than $14,000 a year could afford it. Medicaid compensated for part of this inequality, but still 23% of blacks, 34% of Hispanics, and 35% of the low-income people were left uninsured in 1993. Even though the percentage of uninsured among the low-income group has decreased slightly from 1989 to 1993 (38% to 35%), the same is not true for middle-income groups. In the category of people earning between $14,000 and $24,999 the percentage of the uninsured has gone from 21% in 1989 to 27% in 1993. The same pattern holds true for those earning between $25,000 and $34,999. In this category the percentage of uninsured people went up from 9% during 1989 to 14% during 1993. Since 1980 the trend of uninsured in these categories had been going down, but after 1989 they started to go up dramatically again to the same level they were in 1980.

When analyzing equity in the level of hospital admissions during 1928-1931, the highest income group had the highest admission rate. (See Table 2 in page 57) By the early 1950's the rates had equalized. For example, from 1952-1953 the hospital admissions per 100 persons per year were 12 for the low income group, 12 for the middle income group, and 11 for the high income group. After the early 1950's, this began to change again, and for example, by 1987 these numbers had already changed showing 14 for low income group, 11 for the middle income group, and 8 for the high income group. By 1993 the trend was still continuing in the same direction with the numbers being 14 again for the low income group, 9 for the middle income group, and 7 for the high income group. Does this indicate that an inequity exists in favor of the low income group? Hardly so. Studies recently have suggested that the greater hospital use for low-income people can be accounted for by their higher rates of illnesses and disabilities that require hospitalization.[107] The same holds true for blacks as compared to whites. (See Table 3 in the next page). The hospital admission rate per 100 persons per year for whites in 1964 was 11, while for blacks that same year was 8. However by the early 1980's the rate for blacks exceeded that of whites 14 to 12, and it continued to increase into the 1990's. This same pattern which we see in hospitalization rates, can also be seen in physician visits per year. By 1974 the lowest income group was visiting a physician more than the highest income group, but once again the high rate may account for the low-income people's greater need and worse health.

Dental visits document a very clear instance of inequity according to income and race. Even though the proportion of people seeing a dentist has increased in all income groups, still by 1993, of the people living below the poverty level, only 36% saw a dentist compared to 64% of those above the poverty level. Forty-seven percent of blacks saw a dentist, as compared to 64% of whites.

Effective access studies concerning medical services received much attention during the late 1980's due to some major developments happening on the national scene. There was a research program proposed by the Health Care Financing Administration which was called *Effectiveness Initiative,* with the intention of ensuring quality of care for the 30 million people who received Medicare. Part of the idea was to determine which medical practices worked the best, and thus aid in the

---

[107]DAVIS K., ROWLAND D., *"Uninsured and Underserved: Inequities in Health Care in the United States,"* Milbank Quarterly 61 (1983): 149-176.

TABLE 3: PERSONAL HEALTH CARE USE BY RACE

	1964[a]	1981-1983[o]	1987-1989[a,n]	1993[®]
Hospital Admissions (Admissions per 100 persons per year)				
Black[©]	8	14	12	11
White	11	12	10	9
TOTAL	11	12	10	9
Physician Visits (Percentage with physician visit within year)				
Black[©]	58%	75%	75%	79%
White	68%	76%	77%	79%
TOTAL	67%	76%	77%	79%
Dental Visits (Percentage seeing a dentist within year)				
Black[©]	22%	36%	44%	47%
White	45%	53%	60%	64%
TOTAL	43%	50%	58%	61%

[a]*Source:* National Center for Health Statistics, Health United States, 1993 (Hyattsville, Md.: Public Health Service, 1994), pp. 174, 179, 180.

[o]*Source:* National Center for Health Statistics, Health United States, 1988 (Hyattsville, Md.: Public Health Service, 1989), pp. 107, 111.

[n]1989 for dental visits

[®]*Source:* National Center for Health Statistics, Health United States, 1994 (Hyattsville, Md.: Public Health Service, 1995), pp. 172, 178.

[©]For 1964, the total given as "black" actually includes all non-Caucasians.

allocation of Medicare resources.[108] During the same time a program called *Outcomes Research Program* was authorized by Congress to study utilizations and outcomes of medical interventions. These programs tried to deal with the limitations of the research system previously used in which basically mortality rates were used as the outcome variable. Studies like the *Medical Outcomes Study* were undertaken in order to compare the different health care systems, which included traditional fee-for-service plans, independent practice associations, and health maintenance organizations. The results of the study showed that increasing levels of severity of the illness were associated with decreasing levels of functional status and well being, and increasing levels of utilization, which differed greatly among systems of care. The study revealed that financial access was highest in prepaid systems. The fee-for-service plans offered the best organizational access, continuity, and accountability. The health maintenance organizations revealed the highest coordination and the lowest comprehensiveness.[109] This research clearly indicated that there are multiple factors that affect patient outcomes such as patient mix, medical specialty, and system of care. When the characteristics related to patients and physicians are controlled, there is great variability in the quality indicators of primary care.[110]

Regarding efficient access there has been a *Health Insurance Study* where the change in financial incentives and better management of resources was seen as a strategy to reduce inefficiencies.[111] Cost sharing was portrayed as a mechanism to reduce the inappropriate utilization of health services and thus produce more efficient care. The participants in

---

[108] ANDERSEN R.M., RICE T.H., KOMINSKI G.F., *Changing the U.S. Health Care System*, p. 32.

[109] SAFRAN D.G., TARLOV A.R., ROGERS W.H., *"Primary Care Performance in Fee-For-Service and Prepaid Health Care Systems: Results from the Medical Outcomes Study,"* Journal of the American Medical Association 271(1994):1579-1586.

[110] ANDERSEN R.M., RICE T.H., KOMINSKI G.F., *Changing the U.S. Health Care System*, p. 33.

[111] MANNING W.G., LIEBOWITZ A., GOLDBERG G.A., *"A Controlled Trial of the Effect of a Prepaid Group Practice on Use of Services,"* New England Journal of Medicine 310 (1984):1505-1510.

this study were randomly assigned to a group that was offered free health care or to insurance plans that required them to pay part of the costs. A panel of physicians ultimately judged whether the symptoms were minor, and thus not warranting a physician visit, or serious, and thus warranting one. When serious symptoms were considered, there was no difference between the two groups. However, when minor symptoms were under consideration, the rate of utilization was decreased by more than 30% in the cost-sharing group. This study provided evidence that efficient utilization management can be achieved by modifying the behavior of patients through cost sharing. For the most part, health outcomes were not compromised in that way.[112]

To summarize the figures discussed above we quote a statement by the Committee on Monitoring Access to Personal Health Care Services of the Institute of Medicine from 1993 when it said that "there is little evidence of progress over the last decade."[113] True that there have been many advances in areas such as reducing deaths from heart attacks by preventing high blood pressure, improving the statistics related to breast cancer screening, and improving the survival among low birth weight infants through better neonatal care, among other advances, yet, these have been counterbalanced by other illnesses that can be avoided, such as tuberculosis and congenital syphilis, which are being diagnosed in increasing numbers. The growing division between the "haves" and "have-nots" in the American society is particularly disturbing. Advancements and improvements in access to health care which affect the whole population, seem to be slower to come for blacks and other minorities. This Committee from the Institute of Medicine noted that a case can be made that from one-third to one-half of the mortality gap between black and white middle-aged persons can be attributed to access problems.[114]

---

[112]SHAPIRO M.F., WARE J.E., SHERBOURNE C.D., *"Effects of Cost Sharing on Seeking Care for Serious and Minor Symptoms: Results of a Randomized Controlled Trial,"* Annals of Internal Medicine 104 (1986):246-251.

[113]ANDERSEN R.M., RICE T.H., KOMINSKI G.F., *Changing the U.S. Health Care System*, p. 36.

[114]Ibid.

C. A STUDY OF THE FACTORS THAT LIMIT ACCESS TO HEALTH CARE

As it has been shown, there are many different variables that can be used to measure access to health care. These variables are the tools to analyze the problems that have surfaced. There are factors that contribute to the development of these problems. In this section we will address those factors that limit the effectiveness of medical assistance and that affect access to care. There are especially four of them that seem to be very significant. These are: social factors, cultural factors, institutional factors, and geographical factors.

1. Social Factors

There are two main topics that need to be analyzed related to the social factors. The first one is the impact of the socio-economic realities of the population and how these affect access to health care. These socio-economic problems become even greater when we consider the inadequacies of Medicaid. The second topic that needs to be discussed is the problem with the uninsured and the underinsured in the United States.

a. Poverty and the inadequacies of Medicaid

The segregation that can be seen in the United States today in what concerns health care is primarily the function of socio-economic status. It is difficult to attribute to the lack of financial resources the greatest weight, since there are other factors as well that seem to affect, such as race and ethnic background. Since ethnic minorities still comprise a disproportionate share of the nation's poor, these groups are still the primary victims of the disparities seen within the society.[115] Without downplaying the evidence that corroborates the discrepancies that result from racial and ethnic reasons, it is safe to affirm that such discrepancies, at least in part, are a product of the socio-economic status. Some studies have shown that the socio-economic factors are so powerful, that even with universal health insurance, there will still be differences created by the unequal distribution of wealth in society. These studies show that even in countries where there is universal health insurance, there is the same

---

[115]BROOKS D.D., SMITH D.R., ANDERSON R.J., *"Medical Apartheid. An American Perspective,"* Journal of the American Medical Association 266(19):2746, November 20, 1991.

socio-economic status health gradient as seen in the United States, where there is no such insurance. Even within the United Stares there are differences that can be found at the upper levels of the socio-economic hierarchy, and this is another proof of the importance of the socio-economic status. It is assumed that at these levels everybody has some kind of health insurance, yet differences are still found in what relates to access to care depending on the amount of income. A connection has been shown to exist as well between socio-economic status and health-damaging behavior. Those who are lower in the socio-economic scale are placed more at risk to adverse physical and psychological conditions that can have an effect on health.[116] Even when considering people above the poverty level and with a job, there were socio-economic related factors that affected the individual's ability to engage in health-promoting and disease-preventing behaviors. For example, a study based on California bus drivers found out that 60% of those diagnosed with hypertension were found to be untreated or uncontrolled, even while enjoying full access to care, due to the fact that the diuretics prescribed to them brought about a condition that they were incapable to deal with because of the lack of accessible bathrooms during their tightly scheduled bus routes.[117]

The way that the social life is structured has a tremendous impact, and sometimes even causes, the differences that we see in what has been called the "natural lottery." It has been almost 60 years ago that Henry Sigerist in an article entitled *"Social Medicine"* for the Yale Review wrote that "the chief cause of disease is poverty."[118] Today it is evident that class differences contribute to the etiology of disease in a way that it is not easy to dismiss human illness as just a natural component of the human genetic lottery. There is a connection between ill health and poverty. Disease then, can not be seen as just a chance and uncontrollable occurrence for which no one is responsible, but more and more the vicious circle of illness and poverty has become evident in our society. Some are ill because they are poor, some become poor because of ill health.

---

[116]ADLER N.E., BOYCE W.T., FOLKMAN S., SYME S.L., *"Socioeconomic Inequalities in Health. No Easy Solution,"* Journal of the American Medical Association 269(24):3141, June 23-30, 1993.

[117]Ibid.

[118]CHURCHILL L.R., *Rationing Health Care in America*, p. 84. This article by SIGERIST appeared in the *Yale Review* 27(3):462-481, Spring 1938.

Household income has become an independent predictor of access to health services. In a study of 7633 respondents 22 years of age or older which included working-age adults of every age category, poor and nearly poor respondents were more than 3.6 times as likely to lack health insurance as compared to those with higher incomes, yet, low-income adults, with or without medical insurance, were consistently found to have less access to care than those with higher incomes.[119]

In 1987 the uninsured represented 47.5% of those with incomes below the poverty line, 45% of those with an income between the poverty line and 125% of poverty, 36.7% of those with an income that ranged from 125% of poverty to 200% of poverty, 17.8% of those between 200% and 400% of poverty, and 8.8% of those with incomes above 400% of the poverty level.[120]

Many people are denied emergency hospital care because of their inability to pay. In 1983 alone, for example, 200,000 persons were denied treatment because they could not pay the hospital. Many times hospitals justify this inability to offer services by the fact that they have witnessed an alarming increase in the number of indigent patients that are being transferred from private hospitals to them.[121] It has not helped the fact that most hospital closings in recent times have been of the ones providing a disproportionate amount of care to the poor. The closings of small, not-for-profit, rural hospitals, are on the rise. These usually tend to be in non-white areas. For example, among the 81 community hospitals that closed during 1988, there were 11% of them that were public. These served a disproportionate number of the poor and disadvantaged patients.[122]

---

[119]HAYWARD R.A., SHAPIRO M.F., FREEMAN H.E., COREY C.R., *"Inequities in Health Services Among Insured Americans. Do Working-Age Adults Have Less Access to Medical Care Than the Elderly?,"* New England Journal of Medicine 318(23):1509, June 9, 1988.

[120]FRIEDMAN E., *"The Uninsured. From Dilemma to Crisis,"* Journal of the American Medical Association 265(19):2492, May 15, 1991.

[121]DOWELL M.A., *"Hill-Burton: The Unfulfilled Promise,"* Journal of Health Politics, Policy and Law 12(1):154, Spring 1987.

[122]BINDMAN A.B., KEANE D., LURIE N., *"A Public Hospital Closes. Impact on Patients' Access to Care and Health Status,"* Journal of the American Medical Association 264(22):2899, December 12, 1990.

Measures to contain costs and the new competitive health care marketplace, encouraged many hospitals to lower their commitment to provide for uncompensated care to the poor. The economic considerations of whether or not a patient could afford to pay, weighted more than the behavior of hospital administrators, to the point that emergency care was denied. Sometimes when treatment was not denied, huge deposits were required of those who had no insurance.[123] Public hospitals, that for many years had been considered a safety net for the poor, all of a sudden ceased providing much needed services to the poor, and even when providing them, they did so with much less effectiveness and efficiency than in the past. In some studies about patients who had to leave the hospital without receiving treatment in an emergency situation, part of the reason was that they had to deal with long waits, discomfort, transportation difficulties, child care responsibilities, and conflicts with their work schedules.[124]

Even in the case of the elderly population, who are assumed to have uniform benefits because of Medicare, when the actual reception of benefits was studied, it was found to be very irregular. Elderly with a higher income, meaning $15,000 or more, received 60% more services and 45% more hospital care than lower income elderly, meaning those with incomes under $5,000 not covered by Medicaid.[125]

These problems resulting from a low socio-economic status get worse when the program established to offer medical assistance to the poor does not help. As we have already discussed above, Medicaid is a state-level program passed by Congress in 1965. Part of the problem with this kind of insurance legislation is that each state defines the income levels and other standards that decree when someone is eligible for Medicaid. There has always been great diversity among states. Historically, there has been strong resistance from the states to increase

---

[123]DOWELL M.A., *"Hill-Burton: The Unfulfilled Promise,"* Journal of Health Politics, Policy and Law 12(1):153, Spring 1987.

[124]BAKER D.W., STEVENS C.D., BROOK R.H., *"Patients Who Leave a Public Hospital Emergency Department Without Being Seen by a Physician. Causes and Consequences,"* Journal of the American Medical Association 266(8):1089, August 28, 1991.

[125]DAVIS K., *"Inequality and Access to Health Care,"* Milbank Memorial Fund Quarterly 69(2):258, (1991).

local spending for Medicaid funds, even when mandated by Congress.[126] Many times the states set the eligibility standards for the poor far above the official poverty line. The states are also free to restrict the range of services named "optional" and the number of allowable hospital days. Since at times the levels of reimbursement provided by Medicaid are so low, access to most private practitioners is precluded.[127] Medicaid has also been an inadequate safety net for chronically ill and disabled low-income children. The continuity of coverage for those children has been a problem. In 1980, for example, only 67% of all poor children were covered on a continuous basis. There were great disparities among geographic areas and coverage by insurance. In 1983 seven percent of the children considered among the most severely disabled special education students in Rochester, New York, did not have insurance coverage. This percentage among the same group of children in Charlotte, North Carolina, was 32%.[128]

Medicaid is not available to the large segments of the population it was designed to serve. Today there has been a decrease in the federal support of the program and an increase on the part of the states in the restrictions in order to be considered eligible. Less than 50% of the people who live below the poverty level are covered by Medicaid. The working poor and children have been the most affected.[129] Related to children, for example, between 1979 and 1983 poverty among them increased 35% while the children covered by Medicaid increased only by 4%. In the same way, while poverty among women between the ages of 18-40 increased 60%, Medicaid coverage for this group only increased by

---

[126]FRIEDMAN E., *"The Uninsured. From Dilemma to Crisis,"* Journal of the American Medical Association 265(19):2492, May 15, 1991.

[127]BAYER R., CALLAHAN D., CAPLAN A.L., JENNINGS B., *"Toward Justice in Health Care,"* American Journal of Public Health 78(5): 585, May 1988.

[128]BUTLER J.A., ROSENBAUM S., PALFREY J.S., *"Ensuring Access to Health Care for Children with Disabilities,"* New England Journal of Medicine 317(3): 163, July 16, 1987.

[129]STEVENS P.E., *"Who Gets Care? Access to Health Care as an Arena for Nursing Action,"* Scholarly Inquiry for Nursing Practice 6(3): 189, Fall-Winter 1992.

20%.[130]

b. The problem with the uninsured

Some authors have observed that in the United States, the most intractable public problems usually have two important characteristics. The first one is that they occur to a relative minority of the population. The second is that for the most part these problems result from the arrangements to provide substantial benefits to a majority of the population or to a powerful minority.[131] This tendency has resulted in cycles of attention to some problems such as poverty, racial discrimination, poor housing etc. Yet, once it becomes clear that solving these problems involves paying a high cost that the majority is unwilling to pay, then the interest in these problems wanes. At that time "our public ethics do not seem to fit our public problems."[132]

The current patterns in the United States regarding health insurance for the population, do not meet the minimal standards of social justice and fairness in order to promote the common good. The most critical problem is that a large segment of the population lacks health insurance. This creates enormous problems for the whole country. The uninsured and underinsured in the country are the most solid piece of evidence of a system that is clearly unjust and in which great disparities exist between rich and poor; between those who have access to care and those who do not.

It is not easy to find exact statistics regarding the uninsured, since this number tends to change from year to year, yet it is clear the numbers are on the increase. For example, the number of uninsured Americans under age 65 between 1979 and 1984 went from 28.7 million to 35.1 million.[133] This number has continued to grow, and today approximately 40 million Americans lack health insurance at a given time, and 50 to 60

---

[130]DAVIS K., *"Inequality and Access to health Care,"* Milbank Memorial Fund Quarterly 69(2):265, (1991).

[131]BEAUCHAMP D.E., *"Public Health as Social Justice,"* Inquiry 13(1):3, March 1976.

[132]Ibid.

[133]DOWELL M.A., *"Hill-Burton: The Unfulfilled Promise,"* Journal of Health Politics, Policy and Law 12(1):153, Spring 1987.

million people in the country can be said to be without health insurance at some time during the calendar year.[134] In a national survey done in 1982, fifteen percent of the uninsured reported the fact that they had needed medical care but could not get it. Another 16% confessed that they had found it more difficult to get medical care than in previous years.[135] More recent reports say that these people who are uninsured have less access to care, use less care as compared to those with private insurance, cannot obtain some specific services, are twice as likely to be hospitalized for a condition that could have been treated through outpatient care, and have a higher risk of death when in the hospital.[136] Using data from a 1987 study of hospital discharges that included almost 600,000 patients from a national sample, it found that the uninsured had a 44% to a 124% higher risk of in-hospital mortality as compared to the privately insured. The death rate was actually 1.2 to 3.2 times higher among the uninsured than among those with private insurance, even after controlling for their health status upon admission. This means that the uninsured were less likely to receive high-cost or high-discretion treatments.[137]

In terms of age, the breakdown of the uninsured is as follows: Those who are between the ages of 19-24 are the most likely to be uninsured. In 1987, for example, 20.3% of this group were uninsured for the whole year. Another 18.2% were uninsured for part of the year. The next group with a high percentage of uninsured was the one of children under age 18. In this group nearly 25% of them were uninsured either all or part of the year. In the category of people between the ages 25-54 years old, 19.8% were uninsured all or part of 1987. The most disturbing statistic is that in the group between 55-64 years old, there were 13.6% of them uninsured. This is more than one in eight Americans uninsured in a

---

[134]SCHROEDER S.A., *"The Medically Uninsured-Will They Always Be With Us?"* New England Journal of Medicine 334(17): 1130, (1996).

[135]BASHSHUR R.L., HOMAN R.K., SMITH D.G., *"Beyond the Uninsured: Problems in Access to Care,"* Medical Care 32(5):409, May 1994.

[136]SCHROEDER S.A., *"The Medically Uninsured-Will They Always Be With Us?"* New England Journal of Medicine 334(17): 1131, (1996).

[137]DAVIS K., *"Inequality and Access to Health Care,"* Milbank Memorial Fund Quarterly 69(2):266, (1991).

group that probably faces the highest risk of serious illness.[138]

The figures mentioned above basically state that between 14% to 17% of the population, or one of every six to seven Americans, lacks coverage of any sort for health care costs. Most times this is not a choice, but the result of the lack of financial capabilities to purchase insurance, the lack of coverage from public insurance, and the underwriting practices of current private insurance companies. This is a process of selecting which groups will be most profitable to insure and which groups will not. Those groups who will not be profitable to insure, become part of a high risk population, and many times are left out by insurance companies. Roughly 7% of the uninsured are medically uninsurable by the current underwriting practices.[139]

Besides this, there is an additional 17% of the population that is underinsured. This means that these people risk an overwhelming financial burden would they get seriously ill or injured, due to the fact that there are gaps in their coverage, or cost sharing requirements that are higher than what they could manage.[140] The underinsured are most likely to be poor, members of a family without a worker, women and their dependents, or a person with a nongroup health insurance between the ages of 55-65 in fair or poor health. The lack of coverage by Medicaid is also a concern, since studies have shown that a high percentage of Medicaid beneficiaries are covered only for periods of time. For example, using data from the 1977 National Medical Care Expenditure Survey, only 43% of the Medicaid beneficiaries at the beginning of a three-year period were still insured 32 months later.[141]

The problem with the uninsured and the underinsured is the most critical problem the current health care system in the United States has to

---

[138]FRIEDMAN E., *"The Uninsured. From Dilemma to Crisis,"* Journal of the American Medical Association 265(19):2491, May 15, 1991.

[139]BEAUCHAMP T.L., CHILDRESS J.F., *Principles of Biomedical Ethics*, p. 348.

[140]STEVENS P.E., *"Who Gets Care? Access to Health Care as an Arena for Nursing Action,"* Scholarly Inquiry for Nursing Practice 6(3):188, Fall-Winter 1992.

[141]DAVIS K., *"Inequality and Access to Health Care."* Milbank Memorial Fund Quarterly 69(2):262, (1991).

face. Many may claim that in other nations who have universal insurance and are forced to ration health care, the insured must sometimes wait for health care services. In the United States the uninsured can wait forever. It can be said that the U.S. health care system is the best in the world, but if tens of millions of Americans have little or no access to care, the claim rings hollow.

2. Cultural Factors

Just like any social system, health care does not exist apart from the inequities and social problems that exist in the American society, nor is there immunity to these problems in the way that health care is administered. The problems connected to racism, a heterogeneous population with many ethnic minorities, and gender and age differences affect how the system organizes, allocates, and maintains health resources. These cultural factors create problems that cannot be eliminated simply by providing universal health care coverage, since even if such was the case, there would still be plenty of opportunities to discriminate on the basis of economic, educational, labor, medical, and legal structures that emphasize the differences in our society.

Statistics concerning health care in the United States reveal that blacks and other ethnic minorities, those with low income and the poor, and the less educated, benefit substantially less from the health care system than other Americans outside those categories.[142] Comparisons that have been made in order to study the probabilities of having access problems according to socio-demographic realities revealed that certain groups of people show a higher incidence of these problems. Adults between the ages of 18-64, females, single people, widowed, divorced, separated, and members of minority groups were some of those groups of people.[143] It is not the purpose of this section to analyze in detail all these cultural problems, but it will be worthwhile to give some indication of the most pressing ones and how they affect health care delivery in the United States.

Racism is the most pressing cultural issue affecting access to health care. Even when it could be shown that some ethnic minorities are

---

[142] DOUGHERTY C.J., *American Health Care. Realities, Rights, and Reforms*, p.3.

[143] BASHSHUR R.L., HOMAN R.K., SMITH D.G., *"Beyond the Uninsured: Problems in Access to Care,"* Medical Care 32(5): 415, May 1994.

72   Health Care and the Common Good

worse off than the black population in the country,[144] still the ramifications of racism are so extensive, that it has to be the first problem addressed. Despite the improvements that African-Americans have experienced in health care since the 1960's, they still have twice the infant mortality rates than those for whites, and a life expectancy that is six years shorter.[145]

Some recent studies have shown that even when blacks get access to the system, they are less likely to receive some specific therapies and surgical procedures. One of these procedures is the treatment of cardiovascular disease. The findings of these studies raise questions, not only about the quality of care for blacks as compared to that for whites, but also about the quality of communication between doctor and patient. There is a higher incidence of cardiac arrest among blacks than among whites, which points to the need for better access to primary care so that these tragedies could be prevented by timely treatment of hypertension and coronary artery disease.[146] In another related study it was determined that in order to receive a high-technology cardiac service, a patient had to be admitted to an institution that offers such a service. This condition, that may seem so obvious, is not always easily satisfied. Only one in five hospitals in the U.S. offer cardiac catherization, and only 13.1% of all hospitals offer bypass surgery. In this study the purpose was to find out if blacks received fewer high-technology cardiac services such as coronary angiography, bypass surgery, and coronary angioplasty, than white patients because of having less access to hospitals offering those services. In cases in which the nearest hospital did not include one offering such high-technology services, whites were more likely than blacks to travel what it took to get those services in other hospitals which provided them. When the nearest hospital did offer those services, whites were still more

---

[144]A good article on how Hispanics in the country are affected by the lack of access to health care, and how in many categories they are worse off than any other minority, can be found in: GINZBERG E., *"Access to health care for Hispanics,"* Journal of the American Medical Association 265(2): 238-41, January 9, 1991.

[145]Editorial, *"Black-White Disparities in Health Care,"* Journal of the American Medical Association 263(17):2344, May 2, 1990.

[146]AYANIAN J.Z., *"Heart Disease in Black and White,"* New England Journal of Medicine 329(9):656, August 26, 1993.

likely to present themselves to those offering the services.[147]

During a study of patients admitted to the New York state hospitals in 1986, blacks and whites presented themselves equally to hospitals offering high-tech cardiac services when having a heart attack. Yet, when home-to-hospital distances were recorded a clear pattern of racial differences emerged. If they would have been at similar proximity to the hospitals, blacks and whites would not have presented themselves to those hospitals equally. White patients were more likely than blacks, not only to bypass the hospital nearest to them in order to present themselves to hospitals offering the high-tech services, but to present themselves to high-tech centers even when their nearest hospital provided such services.[148]

Death rates caused by preventable and manageable conditions are 77% higher for blacks than for whites, and this is associated with poor access by blacks to existing services as well as preventive services.[149]

In a national survey of almost 15,000 patients who started treatment for end-stage renal disease between the years 1981 and 1985, and thus covered by Medicare,[150] it was found that the likelihood of receiving a kidney transplant was related to race and income, and that the effects of these two factors were independent from each other. Patients who were in institutions that served mostly a white population and that were located in a high-income area were almost twice as likely to receive a kidney transplant as were patients treated at institutions that dealt with

---

[147]BLUSTEIN J., WEITZMAN B.C., *"Access to Hospitals with High-Technology Cardiac Services: How is Race Important?,"* American Journal of Public Health 85(3):345-347, March 1995.

[148]Ibid., p. 348.

[149]STEVENS P.E., *"Who Gets Care? Access to Health Care as an Arena for Nursing Action,"* Scholarly Inquiry for Nursing Practice 6(3): 193, Fall-Winter 1992.

[150]In 1972 the End-Stage Renal Disease Program was passed by Congress as part of the Medicare program, which assured universal access to people suffering from such disease or needing a kidney transplant.

a primarily black population and located in low-income areas.[151]

On a national telephone survey held in 1986 it was discovered that blacks were more likely than whites to say that their physicians did not inquire sufficiently about their symptoms, did not tell them how long it would take for the medicine prescribed to work, did not explain to them the seriousness of their condition, and did not explain the findings of the tests they made.[152]

In the case of the elderly who are covered by Medicare, even though it must be recognized that after Medicare access to care was improved tremendously for the elderly blacks, in the early years of the program African-American beneficiaries were less likely to receive as many benefits as white beneficiaries.[153]

There is evidence that the incidence and mortality rates due to cervical cancer in women is two to three times higher in blacks than in whites. Even when the incidence declined between the years 1975 and 1984, black women continued to have much higher rates. The women least likely to have received a Pap smear were poor, black, and rural residents. The major reason for the inequities was connected to the distribution of health resources, and not to a genetic or biological condition in black women.[154]

This pattern was also true in the case of elderly patients receiving Medicare and Medicaid benefits. In a study of these patients, white Medicare-Medicaid recipients were more likely than black recipients to receive treatment from a physician. In a recent study that selected 32 medical procedures and diagnostic tests usually needed by elderly people, elderly whites were more likely to receive care throughout the year by a 80.4% to a 72.9% among elderly blacks. Whites were more likely as well, to receive 23 of the 32 services studied. Whites were between 2.0 and 3.0 times more likely to undergo bypass surgery than blacks. The same ratio was true for coronary angioplasty and carotid endarterectomy. In contrast

---

[151]Editorial, *"Black-White Disparities in Health Care,"* Journal of the American Medical Association 263(17):2345, May 2, 1990.

[152]Ibid.

[153]DAVIS K., *"Inequality and Access to Health Care,"* Milbank Memorial Fund Quarterly 69(2):258, (1991).

[154]Ibid., pp. 266-267.

to this, blacks were more likely to receive only 7 of the 32 services, but the differences here tended to be small. Three of the seven were ophthalmologic procedures used to treat open-angle glaucoma or proliferative diabetic retinopathy. When area of residence was considered, it still made no great difference in results. Elderly whites were more likely to receive care than blacks whether they had an urban or a rural residence. In urban areas whites received care 81.0% of the times, while blacks had a 72.6% care rate. If it was a rural area, the percentages were again in favor of the elderly whites by a 79.1% to 73.5% margin. The procedure of coronary angioplasty is the most dramatic example of race discrimination. Among the elderly white the use of this procedure was similar regardless of whether the person lived in an urban or rural area. Their rates were 10.1 cases per 10,000 if urban residence and 9.4 per 10,000 if rural residence. For elderly blacks the cases were 4.1 per 10,000 if urban residence, but ten times less, or 0.4 per 10,000, if rural residence.[155]

One more interesting study that took place in the southern progressive state of North Carolina, indicates that hospital discharges tended to show a discriminatory pattern between whites and blacks. There were greater delays in hospital discharges for nonwhite patients since they encountered significant difficulties in finding an alternative placement after being ready for discharge. This placement in most occasions was a nursing home bed. The definition of "delayed discharge" is the time that goes by between when a patient is medically ready to leave the hospital and when he or she is actually discharged. This study looked into the practices of 76 hospitals, and non-white patients experienced much longer discharge delays than white patients. There was no difference in this fact regardless of age, sex, medical condition, family cooperation, or financial preparedness. The only explanation was the preference of nursing home owners for white patients, and the problems created by having to accommodate a black patient in a double room with a white patient who was already a resident in the nursing home.[156]

---

[155]ESCARCE J.J., EPSTEIN K.R., COLBY D.C., SCHWARTZ J.S., *"Racial Differences in the Elderly's Use of Medical Procedures and Diagnostic Tests,"* American Journal of Public Health 83(7):949-951, July 1993.

[156]FALCONE D., BROYLES R., *"Access to Long-Term Care: Race as a Barrier,"* Journal of Health Politics, Policy and Law 19(3):584, 591, Fall 1994.

76   Health Care and the Common Good

Some of the access problems of minority group patients and especially the black population, are caused by the shortage of minority group health professionals. Black physicians see on average 2.5 times as many Medicaid patients as white physicians. There are less than 3% black physicians, while in the U.S., 12% of the population is black.[157]

Another cultural factor affecting access to health care has to do with gender. We have already mentioned how there are higher rates of cervical cancer in black women as compared to whites. This is an issue that affect women as a whole too, since it is a medical problem that affects only women. A similar problem with the overall women population has to do with pre-natal care. It has been shown that a low birth weight is one of the most critical factors affecting the health of a child. In the state of Arizona, for example, between 1982 and 1989 there has been a marked increase in the number of women receiving inadequate pre-natal care. A recent study found that there was a 147% increase in the number of women who had less than five prenatal visits during this time period, and a 277% increase in the number of women who began to receive prenatal care in their last trimester of pregnancy or not at all. A study by the Institute of Medicine found that for every dollar spent on good prenatal care, there is a saving of $3.38 during the first year of a child's life. The study in Arizona, done by the Study Committee on Services to Pregnant Women in 1992, estimated that appropriate prenatal care would have saved the state $7,147,000 during that year alone.[158]

3. Institutional Factors

There are two main topics under this heading that will be discussed. The first one is the influence of the market mentality in health care. The second one is the role of primary care in U.S. health care delivery.

a. Market justice and health care
The growth of a corporate ethos in health care is one of the most

---

[157]HIMMELSTEIN D.U., WOOLHANDLER S., *"Pitfalls of Private Medicine: Health Care in the USA,"* Lancet 2 (8399):392, August 18,1984.

[158]JOHNSON J.L., PRIMAS P.J., COE M.K., *"Factors That Prevent Women of Low Socioeconomic Status From Seeking Prenatal Care,"* Journal of the American Academy of Nurse Practitioners 6(3):106, March 1994.

significant consequences of the changing structure of medical care. While during the 1970's the main talk was about "health care planning," now the talk is about "health care marketing." Everywhere in our society there is a growth of the marketing mentality in health care. Yet, a corporate sector in health care is likely to aggravate the inequalities in access to health care since profit making enterprises are generally not interested in treating those who cannot pay. In the American experience, the dominant model of justice has been market justice. Under such model, people in society are entitled only to those valued ends such as status, income, happiness, etc., that they have acquired by fair rules of entitlement, or in other words, by their own individual efforts, actions, and abilities. Such is believed to be the "American way." In what relates to health care, when care of the sick was mostly done within the family and communal circles, it was not considered a commodity. There was no price in money or a need to produce for a financial exchange. When people who were ill began to resort to physicians, and later to hospitals, or bought a medicine that had been patented instead of preparing their own remedies, they motivated the move from the household to the market. All of a sudden the rules were changed, and the social and economic relations of illness would be altered. There was resistance to this, and that is why the social history of medicine in the 19th century can be considered, both, as the extension of the market mentality, and its restrictions as well.[159]

Applied to health care, the principles of market justice basically say that physicians own their skills and have the right to sell those skills to whoever they please. This can promote in the health care professional an attitude that makes him or her treat the patient as some sort of "thing" to "be repaired." Sometimes this attitude can be unconscious and unintentional.[160]

In essence, as mentioned already, a free market in health care can only lead to the non-coverage or under-coverage of large segments of the population. The reason for this is that the market model is inappropriate for allocating medical resources. In order for a market model to function fairly, every person must be a free and rational agent, capable of making choices in an intelligent manner. Health care is not like any other need.

---

[159]STARR P., *The Social Transformation of American Medicine*, p. 61.

[160]BRUNGS R.A., *"Toward a Theology of Health Care,"* Review for Religious 45:33, Jan-Feb 1986.

The principle used in commerce of *"Let the buyer beware,"* does not have the same use when dealing with medical care. When people are ill or injured, they are usually not in a position to bargain. Their capacity to make judgments can easily be compromised, and choices can be greatly limited. On the other hand, the economic laws of supply and demand do not apply to the health care "market". Most of the times physicians generate their own business and enjoy a privileged and respected position with their patients. Actually, the evidence in what concerns the laws of supply and demand seem to be the reverse in health care. The greater the supply of doctors, the more the demand and the higher the costs of medical services. Physicians are the experts who decide for the most part who needs care, how much care, and what kind of care. Physicians are also bound to each other by fraternal ties and ethical codes which prevent competition. This is exemplified by the traditional prohibition of advertising services.[161] In other markets, an excess supply drives down the prices. Any supplier who refuses to lower the prices, ends up losing customers or having to close down the business. This does not happen in health care because the American situation has developed under the influence of incentives for private decision makers to increase and improve medical services. These incentives are now part of the everyday functioning of health care delivery. With the third party payers provision, people have little incentive to weigh costs, and usually rely on professionals for guidance as to what treatment to follow.[162]

Market justice contains as well a merit criterion for access to medical care. In other words, it functions on an assumption that those who can afford the services are deserving, while the ones who cannot, may not be. This is an acceptance of the economic disparities that exist in society. Even when this is not explicitly stated, there are all kinds of negative assumptions about the indigent under a system dictated by the market. Some level of disparity is always acceptable in any society, perhaps even desirable, but large differences which deprive the poor of access to at least a basic minimum of care should be repugnant to us as we consider what should be morally acceptable. Worse than this is that to allow the market model to take over how medical care is distributed, would destroy the covenant between doctors and society that makes medicine morally

---

[161]CHURCHILL L.R., *Rationing Health Care in America*, p. 77.

[162]STARR P., *The Logic of Health Care Reform: Why and How the President's Plan Will Work*, pp. 23-24.

intelligible.[163]
There are other setbacks that result from the reliance on a market economy. When there are great disparities in income and no entitlement to health care, the provision of insurance, preventive care, and the care of those dependent on others can easily be deferred in favor of purchasing other goods that satisfy other needs thought to be more important. It also may allow for a large number of people to seek for a free ride in the system choosing to wait to get insurance when they get ill, and raising prices and costs for everyone who wants and needs to be insured. We have seen already how the financial considerations raised by a market based system can lead insurance companies to underwriting policies that leave many without insurance. Finally, a market economy has caused the closing down of many hospitals dedicated to serving the poor because of their inability to compete financially. This has also influenced the choice of geographical areas to which doctors are attracted to establish their practice. This certainly should not be determined solely by market forces.

Most recently, some authors have defended the market system as promoting competition which could help in bringing the escalating health costs under control. This is the mentality behind health maintenance organizations and what has come to be called "managed competition." These writers have challenged the public not to take competition and profit seeking to be the same.[164] There will be more about these aspects in chapter two.

b. Role of primary care
Another important institutional factor which affects access to health care is the importance and the role of primary care. It was mentioned above how the market economy model has many consequences in the health care system of the United States. Another consequence that can be mentioned here is the one of encouraging specialization among physicians. There is a very high percentage of specialists among physicians in the U.S. The reasons for this are varied, and certainly one of them is the element of freedom and choice by students of the

---

[163]CHURCHILL L., HAUERWAS S., SMITH H., *"Medical Care for the Poor: Finite Resources, Infinite Need,"* Health Progress 66(10): 34, December 1985.

[164]MENZEL P.T., *Strong Medicine: The Ethical Rationing of Health Care*, p. 132. See also ENTHOVEN A.C., *"Managed Competition: An Agenda for Action,"* Health Affairs 7(3): 25-47, Summer 1988.

profession. Yet it is also true that many doctors are lured to specializations because of the attractiveness of the market, as well as the need, among other things, to earn the financial resources necessary to pay for their student loans. It was shown above how the fragmentation and complexity of the system created by a market mentality, gives way to administrative burdens with grave consequences. This has created a situation in the nation's health care system in which there is very little emphasis on primary care. In other words, there are too many surgeons and too few primary care doctors because the financing system has encouraged doctors to "invest" in surgical training.

The definition of primary care by the Institute of Medicine mentions five characteristics of true primary care which may help us see the importance that it has. These five characteristics are: accessibility, comprehensiveness, coordination, continuity, and accountability.[165] The concern of this institute is to assure access to first-contact care, which should be "readily, efficiently, considerately, and competently ministered wherever one lives or is visiting in the country."[166] It is through this kind of primary care that a system, with unequivocal dedication to provide geographically and temporally accessible care, is created. In many countries of Western Europe and also in Canada, Japan, Australia, and New Zealand, forty to fifty percent of all practitioners are general physicians. Specialists are available upon referral.[167] This shows a commitment to universal access to health care. In the U.S. only 15% of physicians are general practitioners. One interesting fact when comparing the U.S. to all the above-mentioned countries, even though there is a higher standard of living in America, all of those countries have a longer life expectancy and lower infant mortality rates.[168] With the absence of primary care, the hospital becomes the locus of medical care. Many times the hospital is an inappropriate and expensive setting for treatment, especially when physical problems could have been avoided or at least

---

[165]PELLEGRINO E.D., THOMASMA D., *A Philosophical Basis of Medical Practice. Toward a Philosophy and Ethic of the Healing Professions*, p. 234.

[166]Ibid.

[167]DOUGHERTY C.J., *American Health Care. Realities, Rights, and Reforms*, p.13.

[168]Ibid., p. 14.

lessened in severity had they been treated on a more timely fashion at a physician's office. One example of this is seen when looking at the in-hospital mortality rates due to bacterial pneumonia. Patients who were admitted late had a ten times higher rate of mortality. Some of these deaths could have been avoided had there been access to primary care physicians at an earlier stage of the disease.[169]

4. Geographical Factors

One of the factors that at times has become a problem for people trying to get medical care has been the geographical location of the places where health care is offered. For example, in one study made in the state of Michigan, it was found that having a source of care more than 30 minutes away was a problem for a large number of people. Clearly this was not the most common problem discovered by the study, nevertheless 232,500 persons in the state complained about this and mentioned geography as an impediment for them in accessing health care.[170] There are many geographical regions in the country that have been designated as "medically underserved."[171]

Another problem related to the geographical factors has to do with the absence of physicians from areas where there is a large concentration of poor people. These people become geographically isolated. Recent studies have revealed that in the country's largest metropolitan centers there is a ten-fold or greater differential in the proportion of physicians to people between well-to-do areas and low-

---

[169]FLEMING S.T., *"Primary Care, Avoidable Hospitalization and Outcomes of Care: A Literature Review and Methodological Approach,"* Medical Care Research Review 52(1):90, (1995).

[170]BASHSHUR R.L., HOMAN R.K., SMITH D.G., *"Beyond the Uninsured: Problems in Access to Care,"* Medical Care 32(5):414, May 1994.

[171]There are many studies about this. See CARPENTER E.S., *Concepts of Medical Underservice: A Review and Critique* in *Securing Access to Health Care: The Ethical Implications of Differences in the Availability of Health Services, Vol. III.*

income, minority neighborhoods.[172] There are great differences in the nation when these ratios are considered. For example, in the San Francisco Bay Area some hospitals even report physicians applying for the position of head nurse. The patient to physician ratio in the city is approximately 150 to 1. In contrast, in one low income section of the Bay Area the ratio is 8,300 to 1. There are many towns in the American heartland who are still looking to attract one physician.[173]

---

[172]GINZBERG E., OSTOW M., *"Beyond Universal Health Insurance to Effective Health Care,"* Journal of the American Medical Association 265(19):2560, May 15, 1991.

[173]FRIEDMAN E., *"The Weird New Healthcare Boat. Titanic or Good Ship Lollipop?,"* Health Progress 70(1):34, Jan-Feb 1989.

UNIT TWO

THEORIES AND PRINCIPLES INFLUENCING HEALTH CARE DELIVERY IN THE UNITED STATES

This section will deal with the philosophical theories and ideas which have influenced the development of health care delivery in the United States. The aim is to show that the present system in the country has its roots in the ideas and ideals which have shaped the American psyche throughout the decades.

Chapter three will deal with the fundamental questions of rights and obligations, and how to define and interpret these. Chapter four will share some of the answers that have been given based on the main philosophical theories related to health care delivery.

THREE

THE FUNDAMENTAL QUESTION OF RIGHTS AND OBLIGATIONS

When dealing with the topic of access to health care delivery, one of the fundamental tasks is to analyze what sort of claim people have to health care, and how is that claim to be fulfilled. Unavoidably, this quest leads to a discussion about rights, duties, and obligations. If there is no foundation for any claim on health care, there would not be any reason to discuss this in any society. It would be as absurd as to say that we should have a claim on good weather.

This part of the chapter will analyze the whole issue of whether we have a right to health care, and how is this right to be understood. It is important to define what a right is and what it is not, as related to health care. At the same time, it will be important to consider whether using the notion of "rights" would be the best alternative, given the specific reality of the United States.

It is important as well to define the very concept of "health." It is a common confusion in many writings to see a right to health care identified with a right to health. These are two different things.

Finally, this part will analyze the limitations of the claim we have to health care as a right, and how other notions such as responsibilities and obligations play a role in clarifying how health care delivery in a just society is to be understood and implemented.

A. THE CONCEPT OF A RIGHT TO HEALTH CARE

1. Defining the Meaning of "Right"

In the traditional sense, rights in moral philosophy and political theory have always been understood as a serious entitlement that people have to some liberty, service, or good, derived from social rules and institutional roles. The notion of "entitlement" is very important since it is what distinguishes rights from privileges, personal ideals, group ideals, or acts of charity. These rules and roles mentioned above may be more or less explicit ones of law or the vaguer ones of morality. Rights are socially guaranteed because of the duties they entail for others. They can be relinquishable by their possessor and sometimes for good moral reasons. Even though rights are usually binding, they can be overridden by other more important rights or in the case of extreme circumstances.

Rights can be negative, positive, or both. A negative right is the one that guarantees the ability to pursue a course of action or to enjoy a state of affairs. A positive right, on the contrary, is one that allows us to obtain a good, opportunity, or a service.[1]

Rights are also generally distinguished into right *in re,* and right *ad rem.* The first one—a right *in re*—is also called real, and means that it has as its object a specific thing which belongs to the possessor of the right in order that he or she may claim it from any other person who may be retaining it. The second one—a right *ad rem*—denotes that there is a personal obligation directed not to a thing, but to a person from whom the holder of the right can claim the thing.

The topic of human rights was greatly recognized in the world following the French Revolution, since it was one of the battle cries that gave rise to the upheaval. The term was incorporated in many national constitutions since then, including the one of the United States of America. The general content of such a phrase is clear: Human beings, solely by the fact of being human, possess certain fundamental rights that are inalienable. Some of these have been considered to be physical life, including bodily and psychic elements, personal liberty, freedom form want in what concerns means which are indispensable to life, equality before the law, and political freedom to participate in government decisions.

In the United States, "rights language" has also a legal connotation. Once a right is recognized in society, the way to guarantee it is through a legal enactment. These laws become public policy established by the legislatures which bring about patterns of rights that can be enforced by the state. The Constitution of the United States names certain basic human rights such as life, liberty, and the pursuit of happiness. Since health care is not mentioned among these general rights, the prevailing legal view in the country is that there is no constitutional right to health care. This is so even when there is no explicit constitutional constraint for such a right, and solid moral reasons that would support it.

---

[1]BEAUCHAMP T.L., FADEN R.R., *"The Right to Health and the Right to Health Care,"* Journal of Medicine and Philosophy 4(2):120, June 1979.

Generally it is argued that if there are legitimate obligations to provide for something in our society, there are rights involved. Usually these rights are claimed against some person, or some institution, as for example, the state.

Another important element regarding rights is that a legal right, in order to have some meaning, must be enforceable. There needs to be a clear concept of what is being claimed by a right, and upon whom is the claim being made. It cannot be just based on powerful rethorical appeal, but there must be a concrete claim that can be described with other-than-vague terminology, and that is clearly a value to the people who claim the right.

2. Defining the Meaning of "Health"

The study of the definition of "health" is one of the most perplexing and interesting ones since the inception of this term centuries ago. This definition problem is crucial to understanding and determining a health care policy. Etymologically, the word "health" is related to the Anglo-Saxon word from which words like "holiness" and "wholeness" are derived. Its root word denotes completeness. It has been suggested that historically, the first scientific paradigm for health was the development of the machine model of the human body.[2] Following this model, health came to be seen as the perfect working order of a self-propelling machine. The methods used, even today, to determine pathologies and diagnostics which come from this view, consider illness to be a natural and individual reality. The treatment for disease, therefore, is to be accomplished on an individual basis, and through bio-chemo-surgical processes. The social causes of illness and their relevance and implications, are relegated to a category of secondary importance.

Since the early days of medicine there has been a recognition that, at least partially, illness has a social basis. Yet, the greatest boost for what has come to be known as the environmentalist approach to health, came from the mid-19th century publications in England of the Chadwick Report and of the Shattuck Report in the U.S. This approach went beyond the bio-individualist one, and recognized that health comes from a developmental process in which there is interaction between the individual

---

[2] This section follows the outline of KELMAN S., *"The Social Nature of the Definition Problem in Health,"* International Journal of Health Services 5(4): 625-642, 1975.

and his social environment.

Given the machine model mentioned above and the disregard for emotional processes, there is very little accounting in medicine for the evidence on placebo effects and psychosomatic illnesses. These have been dismissed simply as emotional stressors that disrupt the equilibrium of the human body. These emotional and social processes have been relegated to temporary perturbations of a common biological state, and are not considered strong determinants of such a state. The bio-individual school has developed all kinds of germ theories to determine a specific pathology which can be imposed on what could otherwise be considered a complicated dialectic between the organism and socially induced stress. The tension that has developed has to do with whether health is itself determined mainly biologically or socially. Psychologists have begun to recognize the existence of "qualitatively differing cognitive competences," yet, it does not appear that the health care scholarship has recognized the fact that there are "qualitatively differing organismic integrities" as well.[3] The emphasis of science has been cure, rather than prevention, and this has brought about a limited understanding of the diseases that affect humanity and the development of two different and conflicting notions of health. These two notions of health can be described as "experiential health" and "functional health." The first one can be defined as freedom from illness, the capacity of human development and self-discovery, and the transcendence of alienating social circumstances. The second one simply refers to an intrinsic organismic integrity that can only accept and treat the extrinsic causes of disease through drugs or surgery. Experiential health notions recognize that health behavior is primarily socially determined, while functional health notions consider it to be strictly biologically determined. There is a new paradigm emerging in the science of health which recognizes that health behavior in society is socially determined and, in essence, primarily social. Human beings are the basis of the forces of production and the relations of production, and health can only be understood in the concrete context of the particular form of organization of production and the connection between productive forces and relations. If the systems of production dominate over the social organization, it can be expected that society will develop more the notion of functional health, while the notion of experiential health will diminish. In other words, the structural modes of

---

[3]KELMAN S., *"The Social Nature of the Definition Problem in Health,"* International Journal of Health Services 5(4):629, 1975.

production, condition the dominant personality modes. If self-employment is the norm and dominant pattern of a certain society, rugged individualism becomes the socially approved personality mode. When the structures of production become more and more concentrated while self-employment ceased to be the dominant pattern, the so-called "organization man" supplants the rugged individualist. In a capitalist society, health becomes nothing more than the prevailing standoff at a certain point in time between its experiential and functional aspects. In summary, the machine model of the body and the germ theory of disease that goes with it, do not incorporate the emotional, social, and psychosomatic processes into its paradigm of health. The human body is seen as a series of organs that are meant to function harmoniously together to form a single life process. Given contemporary knowledge concerning stress, cancer, and other environmentally-related illnesses, it is understood that health is more than the lack of organismic breakdown, and related to the form of society in which it is studied.

The World Health Organization has come up with perhaps the most widely known definition of health: ". . . a complete state of physical, mental, and social well being, not merely the absence of disease. . ."[4] This definition significantly tied health to a sense of "social well being." Other definitions, such as the one by Rossdale, have echoed similar notions. In his definition, health is "the product of a harmonized relationship between man and his ecology."[5] These two definitions do not incorporate the structural limits to the attainment of such health which is inherently part of a capitalist society, thus both fail to accurately depict health behavior in contemporary American society.

Other less-than-utopian definitions of health have been offered. For example Dubos gives the following, which leaves some terms not clearly specified: "A *modus vivendi* enabling imperfect men to achieve a rewarding and not too painful existence while they cope with an imperfect

---

[4]BRUNGS R.A., *"Toward a Theology of Health Care,"* Review for Religious 45:33-34, Jan-Feb 1986.

[5]KELMAN S., *"The Social Nature of the Definition Problem in Health,"* International Journal of Health Services 5(4):635, 1975. Definition is quoted from the article *"Health in a Sick Society,"* New Left Review 34:82-90, 1965.

world."[6] It is not clear what does he mean by a "rewarding" existence, thus making this definition ahistorical. At the same time, it is not clear how this definition of health differs from other subject matter such as "wealth" or other material goods. Another similar definition is given by Blum when he writes that "health is the state of being in which an individual does the best with the capacities he has, and acts in ways that maximize his capacities."[7] What does "doing the best" mean, remains unclear and abstract.

There are also more functionally-oriented definitions of "health." For example, Parsons defines health as "the state of optimum capacity of an individual for the effective performance of the roles and tasks for which he has been socialized."[8] This definition seems to consider the ability to perform as the only requirement of health. The experience of illness in itself does nothing to mitigate what can be achieved. For Dreitzel, this is not a problem at all, since for him health is institutionally defined as "the capability to help produce the very surplus the owners of the means of production appropriate."[9] This is clearly a definition of functional health, yet it suffers from the fact that its economic determinism does not recognize the dialectical nature of health and the political experiential reality of it.[10]

In the American society today, it can be said that health is the prevailing contradiction between the experiential and functional dimensions. Its normative conception could be defined as the situation in which both are in balance, or in other words, health is the experience of well-being coinciding with the ability to fulfill a social role. This may sound as a very attractive notion of health, yet, this is an indeterminate

---

[6]KELMAN S., *"The Social Nature of the Definition Problem in Health,"* International Journal of Health Services 5(4):635, 1975. Definition is quoted from R. Dubos, *Medicine, Man, and Environment*, New York: Praeger Press, 1968.

[7]BLUM H., *Planning for Health Development and Application of Social Change*, p. 93

[8]PARSONS T., *Patients, Physicians, and Illness*, p. 107.

[9]DREITZEL H.P., *The Social Organization of Health*, pp. v-xvii.

[10]KELMAN S., *"The Social Nature of the Definition Problem in Health,"* International Journal of Health Services 5(4):636, 1975.

construction, and in that sense ahistorical. Analyzing these facts, it would seem that the quest for a settlement of the "dialectic" of health must be based on a form of analysis that would be explicitly historical and that searches for the social conditions needed for the separation of experience from objectification. In other words, the resolution as to what is health, would be based in a form of social organization that would make such conditions possible.[11]

During the time of the Enlightenment in the 18th century, the secularization of thought came about together with the advancement and the compromising of "health." Science began to be seen as a mechanism for improving experiential health and human welfare. The religious metaphors about disease were supplanted by the machine metaphor based on the philosophy of Descartes. Vesalius and Harvey, in their medical and scientific work, saw the human body as a machine—an idea which was affirmed with the growth of mercantilism and the mercantile state. The human body became the analogue of the machine, and was conceived as functioning in a similar fashion. With the rise of science during the mercantilist period, the emancipation and the objectification of the human organism occurred simultaneously. Since science was subordinated to the larger society, health became increasingly subordinated to the mercantilist state and later to production itself.

By the mid-18th century, the self-sufficient village life, with agriculture and artisanship as the primary economic activities of the 17th century, were replaced by a growing ideology of independence, equality, anti-mercantilism, and self-sufficiency, that, together with the increasingly repressive mercantilism of England, brought about the American Revolution. From this came the solidifying of the American state, American capitalism, and the growth of cities as urban manufacturing centers. This led to the period known as Jacksonianism which brought about the rise of the common man and the individualism of the mid-19th century. The popular health movements of this time, such as Thomsonianism, which was mentioned in the first chapter, stressed self-reliance, self-help, prevention, and treatment of the whole person.[12] These popular movements reinforced the notion of experiential health.

---

[11]KELMAN S., *"The Social Nature of the Definition Problem in Health,"* International Journal of Health Services 5(4):637, 1975.

[12]Ibid., p. 638.

In contrast to this development, scientific medicine was mostly an imported commodity. Basically all scientific physicians practicing in the country before 1890 were educated in Europe, and their form of scientific practice was not the norm until the end of the 19th century. Since prior to the Civil War in the mid-19th century the nature of American society was largely agricultural, a functional notion of health was largely non-operational for the white population. The most clear expression of functional health during that time was found in the antebellum southern plantations, specifically in the way they dealt with black slaves. It is interesting and ironical to note that health care was much more systematically available for the slaves than for whites or freed blacks during that time. Health care was basically an investment, or, as was considered at the time, "a maintenance expenditure."[13] There were prepaid contracts arranged with physicians so that slave owners could cover the costs of caring for their slaves. Sometimes entire holdings of slaves would be moved to a safer location in order to evade an epidemic affecting a certain area or locality. Irish workers would be hired sometimes in order to prevent the slaves from working in malaria-infested fields. Once the anticipated cost of health care ceased being financially justified for slave owners, medical care was withheld. Slaves were considered as means of production, and it is not surprising that their mortality rates were lower than freed blacks or lower class whites.[14] There was a clear economic interest from the part of the slave owners, as well as a good measure of paternalistic administration within the plantations, in the maintenance of the slaves as human property as long as this did not exceed their replacement cost or capital value, while there was no similar incentive to extend medical care to lower class whites.

With the end of the Civil War, and the beginning of full scale industrialization, scientific oriented physicians redefined illness clinically rather than experientially, de-emphasizing prevention and self-help, relegating normal health behavior such as childbirth to the category of illness, suppressing midwifery, and alienating notions of experiential health in a way that would last for almost a century until the 1960's.[15]

---

[13]KELMAN S., *"The Social Nature of the Definition Problem in Health,"* International Journal of Health Services 5(4):638, 1975.

[14]Ibid., p. 639.

[15]Ibid.

It is clear that today with the new emphases on managed care and employer-based insurance, the notion of functional health has become the strongest definition guiding health care and trying to become the systematic basis of national health policy. This is especially true in corporate circles. The statement by the Steel Industry Board to President Truman in 1949 concerning the conditions in the steel industry, which was getting ready to face a strike by its workers, is very revealing. It said as follows:

> "Social insurance and pensions should be considered a part of normal business costs to take care of temporary and permanent depreciation in the human "machine" in much the same way as provision is made for depreciation and insurance of plant and machinery."[16]

It is clear from this statement that the functional definition of health was already taking a strong hold of the employer-labor relations. Today a growing number of major corporations are insisting in reestablishing the health care system through employer-sponsored health maintenance organizations. The company becomes equated with the family doctor, and thus institutionalizes a system not unlike in philosophy to that of the southern plantation of old. That is the case concerning the relationship between the company and the individual employee, or in other words, at a micro-level. At a macro-level, this system has a tendency to rationalize the aggregate expenditures in health care by calculating the investment in human capital. This would only create a situation in which people who would not be considered central or who could be easily replaceable in the process of capital accumulation, would experience greater pressure to remain "functionally" healthy. It is evident that this would set back any progress in recognizing experiential health, and would move a functional health definition to the center stage of national health policy. A strictly technical orientation to the problem of health will not be sufficient, since at the very moment we accept such definition, health itself ceases to be the basis for reform and allows itself to be used in order to foster other interests.[17]

---

[16] KELMAN S., *"The Social Nature of the Definition Problem in Health,"* International Journal of Health Services 5(4):639, 1975.

[17] Ibid., p. 640.

3. Balancing the Notion of Rights

A right to health care is commonly understood as a positive right, since it is a right to the positive actions of other persons or entities, and to obtaining social goods or services. In the struggle to justify a positive right to health care in the United States, especially since there is nothing specific in the Constitution about it, the terminology of "social obligation" has been used. In this way a certain level of health care is expected to be provided. Some authors have repudiated the language of "rights" concerning health care because of its relative inflexibility and intractability as compared with that of needs and desires which leads to a societal obligation.[18] The problems with this approach are related to the search of a moral principle or set of principles to justify and describe such obligation.[19]

During the 18th century, the Catholic tradition had developed a position that health care should be provided as an act of charity. The famous Hotel-Dieu Hospital in Paris was established following these ideals. In the period that led to the French Revolution, these ideas were radically challenged. What used to be considered simply as an act of charity became the duty of all, including the authorities.[20] It seems that the French revolutionaries were influenced by the theory of natural rights developed by John Locke. These rights were considered as basic entitlement to the conditions that were thought to be necessary for human existence. It is interesting to note that Locke did include health as a natural right. This view of the French philosopher developed into a notion which said that if one could not provide for his own health, then one was

---

[18]SIEGLER M., *"A Right to Health Care: Ambiguity, Professional Responsibility, and Patient Liberty,"* Journal of Medicine and Philosophy 4(2):149, June 1979.

[19]BEAUCHAMP T.L., FADEN R.R., *"The Right to Health and the Right to Health Care,"* Journal of Medicine and Philosophy 4(2):126, June 1979.

[20]One example of this was the one given by governor Jacques Turgot (1727-1781) while governor of Limousin in the year 1770 when he wrote: *"The relief of men who suffer is the duty of all, and all the authorities will cooperate toward this end."* In this way it was clear that the provision of health care was not simply supererogatory but a matter of strict duty. See MCCULLOUGH L.B., *Justice and Health Care: Historical Perspectives and Precedents,* p. 57.

entitled to the health care necessary as an obligation which was based on the person's right to existence. According to this view neither age, illness, or poverty should be considered as obstacles to adequate health care.[21] In his view, every citizen had a natural right to health care that was logically, morally, and historically prior to the existence of the particular social order. These rights became the basis upon which a society would be considered just or unjust. Failing to provide health care to its citizens was a clear sign of an unjust society.

Even the documents coming from the papacy in the years that followed, as were the social encyclicals *Rerum Novarum* and *Quadragesimo Anno* of Leo XIII and Pius IX respectively, drew upon the notions coming from the philosophy of Locke and his conception of rights while at the same time criticizing the individualism that was part of his conception of human nature. Nevertheless, Pope John XXIII clearly expressed that health care should be a right of every human being based on the dignity inherent in every person. John XXIII did this in his encyclical *Pacem in Terris* when in number 11 he stated that human beings have "the right to bodily integrity and to the means necessary for the proper development of life, particularly food, clothing, shelter, *medical care*[22], rest, and, finally, the necessary social services."

But this notion of "rights" developed by Locke and its interpretation has become part of the problem in the United States. His philosophy was the inversion of the Aristotelian ideal in which society was seen as prior to the individual since for Aristotle the individual person was clearly not self-sufficing. Whereas Aristotle assumed the existence of society and then moved to a consideration of just and virtuous actions of individuals, Locke assumed the existence of the individual person and then proceeded to address the problem as to how to form a just society. The questions of the nature of human beings thus became irrelevant to morals and political philosophy, and instead the notion of rights became the starting point. Human beings could attain the human good alone. This philosophy influenced greatly during the founding years of the United States to the point that the Aristotelian notion of persons being social by nature was replaced by the Lockean notion of man in his state of nature being solitary and individuated. This would have been the worst possible

---

[21]MCCULLOUGH L.B., *Justice and Health Care: Historical Perspectives and Precedents*, p. 57.

[22]Italics are mine.

scenario for Aristotle, nevertheless all of a sudden it became the normative posture in the country.²³ This Lockean individualism tended to emphasize rights to the detriment of duties and obligations. Rights were no longer seen as subordinate to duties and sociality as intrinsic to human nature. Society, democratic institutions, and the rule of law were only meant to offer protection, especially in what concerned the preservation of private property.²⁴

Some authors in recent years have embarked in a project to uncover this difficulty in the way the United States interprets the whole notion of "rights."²⁵ The way that Americans have tended to use the notion of "rights" is both a symptom and a contributing factor to a kind of disorder in the body politic. This way of dealing with "rights" is different from the way rights are interpreted in other liberal democracies, especially in continental Europe. American *rights talk* is set apart by "its starkness and simplicity, its prodigality in bestowing the rights label, its legalistic character, its exaggerated absoluteness, its hyperindividualism, its insularity, and its silence with respect to personal, civic, and collective responsibilities."²⁶ New rights are proclaimed in the country without much consideration to the ends to which they are oriented. There is little consideration about how different rights are connected to one another, to corresponding responsibilities, and to the general welfare of the people. The self is placed at the center of the moral universe. At the same time, nearly every social controversy has been framed as a clash of rights, and the courts of law have become the new "universities" where Americans learn how to survive by defending individual rights. In its silence concerning responsibilities, this *rights talk* "seems to condone acceptance of the benefits of living in a democratic social welfare state, without

---

²³CHURCHILL L., *Rationing Health Care in America*, p. 51.

²⁴TAYLOR C., *Philosophy and the Human Sciences*, p. 293.

²⁵One of these authors is Mary Ann GLENDON in her book *Rights Talk: The Impoverishment of Political Discourse*, The Free Press: New York, 1991.

²⁶GLENDON M.A., *Rights Talk: The Impoverishment of Political Discourse*, p. x.

accepting the corresponding personal and civic obligations."[27] There is a tremendous need when addressing health care concerns in the United States today to include the language of responsibilities, duties, and obligations. In the particular situation of the country, to propose health care as a right, risks the possibility of further confusing the issue by proposing to the public a terminology that is already misunderstood. Evidence of this is that the whole notion of a "right to health care" has been consistently rejected in the country while at the same time there seems to be a general restlessness about the appropriateness of the current health care system.[28] Until the notion of rights can be understood in its proper context, which includes duties and civil obligations, it is very difficult that the population will be capable of understanding what the conversation regarding access to health care is all about. In what relates to health care at this time, Americans can be compared to the person who learns enough of a foreign language to ask for a hotel room or for something to eat, yet remaining unable to fully enter into dialogue with the people of that country. Because of a limited understanding of rights it can be said that the typical American citizen today lacks the full grammar of cooperative living.

In the midst of these limitations, different philosophical currents have tried to address the health care situation in the country. The importance of studying these theories has to do mainly with the issues that

---

[27] GLENDON M.A., *Rights Talk: The Impoverishment of Political Discourse*, p. 14.

[28] Very recently there has been some controversy about the recommendation of a Consumer Bill of Rights by a 34-member presidential advisory commission. This recommendation was officially endorsed by President Clinton on November 20, 1997. The commission took no position as to how the rights to regulate consumer protection in health care matters was to be implemented. There was immediate opposition by certain groups, such as the U.S. Chamber of Commerce and Blue Cross/Blue Shield Association, to any effort that would turn such Bill of Rights to legislation. One thing that was interesting among the reactions to the bill had to do with the lack of willingness by people involved in the process to endorse new "rights." For example, one of the commissioners expressed her opposition in the following way: *"I can't take any more state mandates and I certainly don't want any more federal mandates. The main point I have difficulty with is the word 'rights'."* See MECKLER L., *Panel Endorses "Bill of Rights" for Health Care*, The Times Picayune, November 20, 1997, p. A-20.

have been raised related to how to provide better access to health care in the United States. We now turn to a study of those theories.

FOUR

THE FUNDAMENTAL ANSWERS
BASED ON THE PHILOSOPHICAL FOUNDATIONS
OF AMERICAN HEALTH CARE

This chapter will discuss three major philosophies that can be said to be crucial to an understanding of the ethical debate concerning access to health care. These are utilitarianism, libertarianism, and egalitarianism. There are other schools of thought that have developed, such as contractarianism and communitarianism, yet, these are in some way connected to one of the main three philosophies already mentioned. There are major tensions that have developed among these major schools, which for the most part have been responsible for the actual system of health care in the United States.

The quintessential American belief in individualism and self-reliance, which has led to the notions of limited government and market justice, combined with the notions of maximization of the good for the majority of the population and the belief in equal opportunity for all, has brought about many conflicts as to what should be the content of any right or obligation concerning health care.

These conflicts have dealt with questions such as: What is the role of the state concerning health care? Can health care be treated simply as a commodity? Should there be a basic package of health services offered equally to all in society? Should society allow a two-tiered system of health care? How much can market forces be left unregulated in matters concerning health care? Is rationing health resources inevitable, and if so, how should it take place? These are just some of the conflicts that the different philosophies have brought about, and the answers to these questions in themselves have much to say about the ultimate way in which health care is treated in the American context.

It is necessary to take a close look at each one of these philosophies, their origins in American history, their most important tenets, the health care issues each one has raised, and how modern thinkers who have been influential in the United States have embraced such philosophies in an effort to solve problems related to health care.

A. ORIGINS OF AMERICAN THOUGHT BEFORE MODERN THEORIES

The United States of America came into existence under a series of special events that gave birth to a very unique republic. Even today there are very strong influences that have prevailed through time in order to preserve this uniqueness. The student of American society may ask, for example, why is there no socialism in America, or at least no sizeable socialist party? Why have trade unions been weak compared to other democracies? Why has the country preserved mainly a two-party system instead of a multi-party system with radical parties?

There is no question about the fact that the American people have developed a unique character and personality full of special qualities, ranging from unusual moderation to creedal passion. This sections will uncover some of the major influences that have molded American thought and the personality of its people.

Some authors have suggested that what makes the United States truly different and special is the deeply embedded belief that liberty and equality can be mutually reinforcing. In other words, the cultures of individualism and egalitarianism can co-exist.[29] Equal opportunity and equal results can be made compatible. As a matter of fact, and unlike other western democracies, American egalitarians have historically allied themselves with individualism instead of the hierarchy in the state.

This has been evidently manifested in the way philosophical thought has developed in America since the founding fathers' days. The libertarian tendencies of self-reliance and the frontier spirit have co-existed with the notion of equal opportunity for all in a way that has not kept either one of these notions out of the equation of a functional system of government. These very diverse philosophies have combined to provide a fruitfulness that cannot be matched. They have also contributed in providing a national character that is easy to recognize. One author has expressed this idea in this way:

---

[29]WILDAVSKY A., *"Resolved, That Individualism and Egalitarianism be Made Compatible in America: Political-Cultural Roots of Exceptionalism,"* in *Is America Different?*, edited by Byron E. Shafer, p. 118-119.

The Fundamental Answers Based on the Philosophical Foundations 101

> America is about possibilities, not certainties. You can (but you don't have to) get rich. America is about promises. Here class divisions do exist but they don't have to matter. Because in America, competition can be compatible with equality, there is the promise of classlessness.[30]

This distinctive character in American thought reflects first of all the differences between the men an women who came to America during its colonial history, and those who stayed home. In the first place we have the puritanism of the early settlers. It is important to mention it in such terms instead of simply referring to the "puritans," since this name was related, not simply to a people who settled New England, but primarily to the religious movement that originated in England in the middle of the sixteenth century.[31] The name comes from the fact that these people were a group of Protestants who wanted to "purify" the Church of England from the ceremonial and authoritative elements of the Roman Church, and decided to separate themselves from the English Church due to the slow progress it was making in regards to this purification. By 1634 there were some 10,000 people who had emigrated and began the foundations of the different Puritan colonies in the New World.[32] The goal of the Puritan ideal was to set up a "city of God" which would make the lifestyle, based on the apostolic way, a reality for all the world to see. These religious ideals came from the Calvinist tendencies they spoused, in which the weakness and the depravity in man was transformed by a God who saved by freely bestowing unearned grace.

But the decrees of God were not completely arbitrary. He had made a covenant with humanity by which those elected by Him had a right by contract to receive such grace. The government of the Church was, because of this, to be somewhat democratic. Rationality should not be considered the exclusive domain of theologians and religious authorities, but laymen and scholars could use this rational logic too. This reliance on human reason—on pragmatic or utilitarian foundations which came from

---

[30] WILDAVSKY A., *"Resolved, That Individualism and Egalitarianism be Made Compatible in America: Political-Cultural Roots of Exceptionalism,"* in *Is America Different?*, edited by Byron E. Shafer, p. 128.

[31] MACKINNON B., (ed.), *American Philosophy: A Historical Anthology*, p. 3.

[32] Ibid.

old puritan values—would become the order of the day among men like Franklin, Paine, Allen, Priestley, Jefferson, Rush, Cooper, and Palmer.[33] Human nature was God's art work, thus the Puritans interpreted natural law as part of the divine order, and the social obligations that came from this were seen as divine law.[34]

There was a deeply humanistic element of Puritanism in the teaching on Christian humility. When the Puritan saw a prisoner walking to the gallows, he would exclaim: *"There, but for the grace of God, go I."*[35] This showed a sympathetic understanding for the weaknesses of human nature, which saw sin as something that happened to a person, and was not simply the result of deliberate choice.

There were many immigrants as well that came to the land fleeing from the scourges of oppression and class persecution. Their experience was part of a great adventure that forced them to sever ties with their past. Economic motives also became a main reason why people came to America. The main problems for those pioneers was the one of conquering the land. In the words of a student of American thought:

> The arduous work of clearing forests, opening mines, cultivating fields, building cities, roads, bridges, and harbors, which in Europe had taken many long centuries, was, because of the character of the people, their inventiveness, training and use of machinery, performed here by less numerous people and in much less time.[36]

These people had been released from the feudal restraints of ownership, and now had the opportunity to possess land of their own. Many times they had to go through many difficulties in order to accomplish this, which included taking the land from the native American settlers by treaty or battle, the struggle through trackless forests in order to find these lands, working the land with only a few rustic tools, and

---

[33] MUELDER W.G., SEARS L., *The Development of American Philosophy*, p. 65.

[34] MACKINNON B., ed., *American Philosophy: A Historical Anthology*, p. 4.

[35] COHEN M.R., *American Thought*, p.25.

[36] Ibid., p.21.

dying because of the daily struggle with the elements and the lack of food and water. These experiences shaped the American spirit.

Some elements that began to surface in the American character because of the frontier experience were the competitive drive for favorable land, the need to kill in order to stay alive, the quick resort to pure strength in order to survive, and the toughness that came from the absence of law and order throughout the transition involved in the occupation of the new lands. The "get-rich-quickly" mentality was fostered by the dramatic changes that could take place in someone's life in a very short period of time. A little luck could turn all things literally into gold.

The frontier experience also brought the good traits of energetic activity and dignified manual labor. The independent, self-reliant farmer is still today a symbol of those positive qualities.

The strenuous activities connected with the expansion of the territory generated an atmosphere in which the enterprising spirit of humanity grew more readily. The very life of the community was bound to economic enterprise, and thus, those who struggled by exploiting nature and its resources, usually received not only material reward, but also great prestige and honor in society.[37]

This struggle to bring the wilderness under control made the practical-minded entrepreneur, who had little time for leisure and no interest in other cultures, the ideal person who everyone should imitate. This developed into a worship of business, which is not simply connected to the financial elements, as many times is misinterpreted by other cultures who try to describe this American trait, but is rather connected to a worship of the active life. This is very far removed from the old world attitude which saw man's wealth as connected to the exemption from the need to engage in socially productive labor. This tendency in conjunction with the ideas of laissez-faire capitalism, which sought to minimize the role of government in economic affairs, would later gravitate back to the teachings of people like Adam Smith, who had favored free trade and opposed controls by the government which would affect the laws of supply and demand.[38]

It is an interesting coincidence that 1776—the year of the American Declaration of Independence—coincides with the publication

---

[37]COHEN M.R., *American Thought*, p.21.

[38]GROB G.N., BILLIAS G.A., *Interpretation of American History: Patterns and Perspectives*, Vol. I., p. 64.

of Adam Smith's *Wealth of Nations*. Both of these are known as significant documents of the liberal philosophy of the Enlightenment. Reason and human rights are fundamental categories in both, and they represent an attempt to abolish all privileges and restrictions on manufacturing and exports.[39] Adam Smith is responsible for the beginning of scientific thought concerning economics. He argued that the wealth of nations is primarily a product of goods exchanged freely, without government intervention. His arguments emphasized the advantages of division of labor and free trade. These arguments are consistently cast in materialistic terms, and the wealth of nations in his treatise is restricted to material goods. In this as well it can be said that Calvinism was a major source of inspiration.[40] The typical concept about government was a pessimistic one of total corruption, and religion became an antidote to government by promoting the individualistic notion of the "elect." When faced with the problem of developing the concepts for a national economy, the founding fathers showed tremendous respect for the ideas of Adam Smith.[41]

The spirit of the frontier has had a definite impact in the social and political traditions of the United States. The frontier man tended to live in isolation on the fringes of civilization, and bound by few administrative regulations. He recognized a type of law which was the spontaneous outgrowth of certain basic needs of social order and security. He developed a natural distrust of an intrusive government, and became quite impatient with the slow administration of justice which came about from executive governmental action. Many times he took justice upon his own hands, instead of leaving matters to the courts of law. Actually, it could be said that trials in court became almost a form of entertainment in which the people had a part to play, but the decrees of the court did not necessarily hold a priority over the summary justice of lynchings and revenge.

Even to this day, the American farmer, in the absence of a feudal tradition in agriculture, seems at times more progressive than the city man. But the farmers' slogans come from the old American philosophy of natural rights and not from the more modern ideas of social theory.

---

[39]COHEN M.R., *American Thought*, p. 87.

[40]Ibid., p. 88.

[41]Ibid.

It was under all these varied influences that the main values and ideals of the American society came into existence. It can be said that even to this day there is a tremendous philosophical struggle to bring together the notions of freedom and individualistic action and the strong belief in the welfare of all without exception. These struggles were once more called to the fore with the development of the major modern philosophical theories, when once again the social policies enacted in the United States had to deal with how to accommodate the different tendencies supporting freedom and equity as ideals that could be proposed and searched for together. The resulting philosophical solutions, as we will see, have not always been optimal, nor has there been acceptable solutions achieved when dealing with health care.

B. THE UTILITARIAN PHILOSOPHY

1. Main Tenets of Utilitarianism

Utilitarianism is a philosophical theory that emphasizes the greatest happiness for the greatest number. Concerning society, it seeks to maximize public utility. The utilitarian concept of justice requires that allocation of resources be applied in such a way that the overall gain in utility that results from any kind of expenditure is maximized.

There are two kinds of utilitarianism. Act utilitarianism defines rightness with respect to particular acts. An act is only right if it maximizes utility. The other kind of utilitarianism is Rule utilitarianism, which defines rights with respect to rules of action and makes the rightness or wrongness of particular acts depend upon the rules under which those acts fall. A rule is right only if general compliance with that rule, or set of rules of which it is part, maximizes utility. A particular action is right only if it falls under such a rule. Rule utilitarianism mandates the greatest utility in social policy. If other factors are held to be equal, rule utilitarianism will lean toward the distribution of resources that will create equal satisfaction of basic needs. These would include equal access to health care services for basic medical needs.

Both of these types of utilitarianism fall under either classic or average utilitarian theory. The first one defines the rightness of acts or rules as a maximization of aggregate utility. In other words, this means the utility of the whole. Average utilitarianism defines the rightness or wrongness as the maximization of the per capita utility.[42] The distinction between rule and act utilitarianism is important since the former must include an account of when institutions are just. Some utilitarian thinkers state that the principles of justice are important and are the most basic moral principles since the utility attached to following them is great.[43] That is why they could be enforced if necessary.

Related to health care, utilitarianism purports that the expenditures used for medical care must produce the maximum possible gain in utility. This objective is reached when the gain that results from the allocation of extra resources is the same in all the directions possible.[44] This criterion has been called Pareto-optimality, named after Vilfredo Pareto, the Italian theorist who developed the concept. Another way of explaining the concept is by recognizing the point at which a policy will not be viable because it is hurting too many groups. This would require to distribute resources in such a way that every allocation will be most efficiently applied.[45] When this Pareto-optimality is not reached, according to utilitarian philosophy, planners can be held responsible for the death and disease that has resulted from this unnecessarily. If the most cost-effective services were given priority, more lives could have been saved, and disease prevented or cured. Utilitarian theory might go further than this in order to mandate equalization of all health care. This could be conceivable if three considerations are kept in mind: First, beyond the satisfaction of the basic health care needs, there would have to be less confidence in the assertion that a dollar is of more value to the less well-off. There is no way that society could guarantee entitlement to equal satisfaction based on the desires of the rich since this would be subsidizing Faustian insatiability, to the detriment of more pressing needs. Second, it is clear that non-egalitarian incentives have worked in American

---

[42]BUCHANAN A., *"Justice: A Philosophical Review."* SHELP E.(ed.), Justice and Health Care, p. 4.

[43]Ibid., p. 5.

[44]VAN DER WILT G.J., *"Cost-effectiveness Analysis of Health Care Services, and Concepts of Distributive Justice,"* Health Care Analysis 2(4):297, November 1994.

[45]RHODES R.P., *Health Care: Politics, Policy, and Distributive Justice. The Ironic Triumph*, p. 57.

capitalism increasing the amount of wealth in society. It would seem to work against the notion of greater utility to obstruct those incentives that have brought so much wealth since they have helped to create resources that in turn have allowed for more satisfaction of basic needs. Finally, a commitment to strictly equal satisfaction of health care needs, even if only basic needs, cannot maximize utility, since basic may mean very different things to different people. Some "basic needs" may be too expensive for any society to afford.[46]

2. Issues Raised by Utilitarianism Concerning Health Care

There are many issues that have come up in health care that can be said to have their origins in utilitarianism. The role of rationing, the market and managed care, and diagnosis-related groups (DRG's) among others, have all been subjects related to ways of maximizing utility in health care matters. A discussion of these issues follows.

a. Rationing health care

The notion of rationing health care comes from the realization that we cannot afford to do everything we are capable of doing for everyone, due to the fact that, in medical matters, there tends to be an unlimited demand for services while there is a limited supply. Some authors claim that, even before there was any formal development of notions related to rationing, the U.S. system was already promoting certain types of rationing techniques.[47] Patient allocation to hospital facilities, for example, is often considered a form of rationing, in the sense that it has to take into account particular situations in time, as well as hospital capacity and availability. However, when rationing is mentioned today, there are more clear and well defined notions that have come about. What was unthinkable in the early 1960's, has now become a compelling reality. Rationing for health care resources is being taken seriously today, and it means that not every person will have complete access to the best level of

---

[46]DOUGHERTY C.J., *American Health Care. Realities, Rights, and Reforms*, pp. 46-47.

[47]KISSICK W.L., *Medicine's Dilemmas. Infinite Needs Versus Finite Resources*, p. 48.

health care available as part of official policy.[48] This involves leaving some people without particular forms of health care that might be beneficial to them. It may be only temporarily but most probably against the patient's wishes. Regardless of the per capita spending on health care, which in the U.S. is more than in any other country in the world, still many will not be able to obtain certain types of health care services that would be beneficial.

Health care rationing starts off with the legitimate concern of rising health care costs. It later finds them uncontrollable by any means except rationing, and then comes to the conclusion that physicians, and as a matter of fact the whole health care providing system, must act as guardians of society's resources. This approach will conserve tests, treatments, operations, hospitalizations, and other services. Costs will be reduced by eliminating what is believed to be unnecessary care. This is the only way that the maximizing of health care benefits, and not the waste of resources, can come about.

For many, universal health care is neither feasible nor plausible without some form of rationing. Yet, the very notion of rationing evokes an idea that seems almost offensive to the picture of the United States as a rich and powerful nation. Rationing goes against the notion that the country can afford whatever it takes, to do whatever it wants. Without a system of universal health insurance in the country, rationing is seen as the logical outcome based on reason and restraint.[49] Rationed care has become the way to define what decent care is all about since maximal care is impossible for all.

One initiative that has concretely dealt with the problem of rationing has evolved in the state of Oregon. It has received much notoriety as one of great national importance.[50] Faced with growing costs and demands for more efficient and fairer access to health care, the Oregon legislature passed the Basic Health Services Act on July 1989. The state used a combination of technical and economic considerations, while tempering them with expressed public values, to set up a system of

---

[48]KISSICK W.L., *Medicine's Dilemmas. Infinite Needs Versus Finite Resources*, p. 58.

[49]CALLAHAN D., *"Symbols, Rationality, and Justice: Rationing Health Care,"* American Journal of Law and Medicine 18(1-2):1-2, 1992.

[50]Ibid., p. 9.

health care priorities. The long term goal is universal health care in Oregon, yet the way to achieve that was by providing health care coverage to everyone who falls below the federal poverty line instead of eliminating some people altogether in order to give unlimited care to those who qualify. The plan also included provisions for those above the poverty level by requiring workplace-based coverage for all employees and an all-payers' high-risk insurance pool. The Oregon plan limited services by establishing a priority list. Work began on such a list by organizing community discussions on health care policy and especially on the kind of priority setting the people wanted. This gave the public a chance to become better educated on the issues.[51] The act also created the Oregon Health Services Commission (OHSC), which was in charge of producing the list of priority services that would define the idea of basic decent minimum of health coverage by Medicaid.[52] This twelve-member health service commission, which consisted of five primary care physicians, a social worker, a nurse, and five consumers, ranked medical services according to their benefits, including what they called "quality of life" and "compassion," and their possibilities of curing the illness.[53] The Oregon legislature is in charge of establishing a budget to fund health care and decide the percentage of available assets coming from tax revenue that can be used for health care among other needs such as education, environment, etc. Citizens of the state of Oregon have been forced through these measures to develop an overall health policy and to decide how much money to allocate for health care.

The Oregon plan, and rationing in general, are not without critics. Some authors consider that rationing is often presented as enhancing fairness and social justice, and as the guarantor that all consumers have access to essential products. Yet, health care rationing as discussed today would deny the poor and near-poor of care, while penalizing the middle class, and not affecting the rich class at all. They claim this is so since

---

[51]CALLAHAN D., *"Symbols, Rationality, and Justice: Rationing Health Care,"* American Journal of Law and Medicine 18(1-2):11, 1992.

[52]BEAUCHAMP T.L., CHILDRESS J.F., *Principles of Biomedical Ethics,* p. 367.

[53]DUFFY T.P., *"Rationing Health Care: Its Impact and Implications for Hematology-Oncology,"* Yale Journal of Biology and Medicine 65(2):76, March-April 1992.

health care rationing usually takes place through the refusal to reimburse for certain treatments and not through the rationing of an actual service. In other words, the rich who can pay for the service, will not be affected whatsoever by the rationing. Only the people unable to pay, will. When the Oregon plan, for example, decided to include bone marrow transplants as one of the rationed treatments, they cut reimbursements for those on Medicaid. Those who could pay the bill out of their own pockets, or move to a neighboring state, could undergo the transplant.[54] Rationing in this way only serves to extend the prevailing class structure to health care matters. Rationing will only help in extending the reach of the already existing class structure in health care.

Others directly criticized the Oregon approach, since it would rank procedures according to their benefit. This way it would cut off payments for those below a line established according to the available funds. This crude process of ranking fails to take the patient's prognosis into account, and thus would result in the system at times denying care to patients with a chance of recovery while approving care for others with very little or no possibility of recovery. The Oregon plan calls for a system that regulates specific clinical situations, and thus includes a highly intrusive level of control by the state.[55]

b. Managed care and the market

Another kind of critique has to do with the belief that a free market and open competition as the American way, would do much more to advance better and more just health care without the constraints that by definition would have to be placed by rationing. These critics assert that this value of free market and competition is much more embedded in the American psyche than any other value, and that with the lack of the high sense of responsibility for each other which exists in other countries such as Great Britain and Canada, the U.S. is better off holding on to a market

---

[54]ETZIONI A., *"Health Care Rationing: A Critical Evaluation,"* Health Affairs 10(2):94, Summer 1991.

[55]STARR P., *The Logic of Health Care Reform: Why and How the President's Plan Will Work*, p. 46.

model.⁵⁶

There is no question about the increasing involvement of management in health care matters. The current trend signals that the market mentality which prevails in the United States will continue to grow. Even though doctors will always be at the center of action and concern for health care issues, there is no question that today in many cases more and more doctors are being placed on the sidelines. Their clinical autonomy has been placed at risk because of managed care.

The market tries to tackle the same problem that was mentioned above concerning rationing, but it does it in a different way. Cost-benefit analysis becomes the key tool to determine which health services are to be practiced at specific moments. By this method, health outcomes, including continued life itself, are converted to monetary equivalents. Some other authors have favored what is called cost-effectiveness analysis, which differs from the first one in that it calculates the cost of alternative health initiatives in financial terms instead of individual health outcomes.⁵⁷

For the market approach to succeed, there must be competition present. As we have already seen in chapter one, most health care markets depart substantially from competitive conditions. Sometimes this happens inevitably and sometimes as a result of deliberate public or private policy. The interference on the market comes from the methods of financing health services that have developed over the years. A great deal of health care is paid for either by private insurance or the government, or in other words, by third party payers rather than the consumer of health care. There is little incentive for the consumer to shop around for lower or comparative prices, to question whether a particular medication or procedure is actually needed, or to ask whether there is a less expensive alternative. In many cases physicians are paid by a third party on a fee-for-service basis, thus he or she has a personal financial incentive to provide repeated care. Finally, both physicians and hospitals are reimbursed for services by third parties on the basis of reasonable costs. If either physician or hospitals can gain acceptance for higher fees, they

---

⁵⁶DUFFY T.P., *"Rationing Health Care: Its Impact and Implications for Hematology-Oncology,"* Yale Journal of Biology and Medicine 65(2):75-76, March-April 1992.

⁵⁷KILNER J.F., *Health-care resources, allocation of. Encyclopedia of Bioethics,* Volume 2, (Revised Edition), Warren Thomas REICH, Editor in Chief, p. 1071.

can increase revenues. As long as the reimbursements are on a reasonable basis in respect to the cost, there is no incentive to lower the costs or to seek a less expensive alternative.

Managed care has been an attempt to improve the function of the market, not by controlling prices directly, but by focusing on the limits of quantities through price incentives as well as by the indirect effect of competitive forces on prices. These policies may stress the role of the physician in the decision to utilize services or the role of the consumer in the same decision. This decision, regardless of whether it is influenced by the provider or the consumer, determines the quality as well as the kind of service utilized.

One example of an organization that attempts to stimulate competition by emphasizing the physician as the decision maker or gatekeeper is what is known as a health maintenance organization or HMO. These organizations have jettisoned the old style medical practice, into something entirely new. Doctors become gatekeepers while patients become "covered lives." Managers, who are removed from the actual patient, decide who gets a certain treatment and who does not.[58]

HMO's have their origins in 1970, when the Nixon administration was looking for some distinct approaches to deal with health care problems. It developed pre-paid plans as a central part of the national health policy. A Minnesota pediatric neurologist, with the name of Paul Ellwood, coined the term "health maintenance organization."[59] HMO's assume the role of insurers and providers, with the consumer paying a fee that is predetermined, for which he will receive health care. The providers become the risk bearers who are obligated to render the needed services. If the costs are greater than the income of the predetermined fee, the providers suffer financially. If the costs are less than the income, then the providers benefit.

The existence of such prepaid group practices, such as HMO's, has established the possibility of fair economic competition. In this way the problems related to cost, access, and quality of care have been dealt with by maximizing benefits, or in other words, through a utilitarian

---

[58]LARSON E., *"The Soul of an HMO,"* Time Magazine, January 22, 1996, p. 45.

[59]STARR P., *The Logic of Health Care Reform: Why and How the President's Plan Will Work*, p.35.

solution.[60]

Competition is an important element of managed care, as was mentioned above. The experience in the U.S. with successful models of competition among health care plans has suggested that the tools are available to allow sponsors to use competition to achieve a degree of efficiency and equity for their populations which would be reasonable. Some experts believe that if there was multiple choice available and alternative delivery systems established in every community, there would be competition not only in prices, but also in other aspects which have to do with convenient access to care, emphasis on health-maintenance and prevention, and other consumer-related benefits.[61] Economists have been reviewing in recent years the differences between regulation and the market, and have seen that regulation has had its systematic failures also. In a world that is not perfect, perhaps the market can be a viable solution if its failings are corrected.[62]

Most recently the term that has been used to express these matters has been managed competition. Its essence is the use of available tools to structure cost-conscious consumer choice in a system that considers the consumers as well, and not only the health plans and the sponsors. People who defend managed competition claim that the reason that the market has failed in health care is because health risks or expected medical costs have been distributed unevenly among the different plans. In that way discrimination against the sick in the form of under service and underwriting practices has been encouraged. This has produced in extreme cases the cancellation of coverage which has brought about widespread lack of coverage especially among those who need the most

---

[60]GOLDFIELD N., *"Why We Cannot Agree on the Direction of Health Reform: An Exploration of American Values,"* Physician Executive 18(4):18, July-August 1992.

[61]ENTHOVEN A.C., *Health Plan. The Only Practical Solution to the Soaring Cost of Medical Care*, pp. 91-92.

[62]Charles Schultze, for example, has proposed what he has called "the command and control techniques of government bureaucracy," by which he means that we should make public use of private interest and correct the problems of the market instead of substituting it with regulation. Cf. ENTHOVEN A.C., *Health Plan. The Only Practical Solution to the Soaring Cost of Medical Care*, p. 70.

health care.⁶³

Managed competition then refers to an approach to regulating the competition that occurs among plans. Not all of the plans need to be based on managed care. If managed competition is designed correctly, it would inhibit the growth of some managed care plans that enroll only healthy beneficiaries. The rules of managed competition have the purpose of overcoming discrimination and the lack of informed choices among the citizens.⁶⁴

There are conflicts that come up as a result of managed care. Even when it seems to be true that managed care has been able to provide quality care at lower than fee-for-service arrangements, mainly due to a low rate of hospitalization among members, there may be a great deal of self-selectivity at work. By this we mean that persons who join a managed care plan tend to be cost-conscious themselves and low utilizers of services. If this is true, then it would be unlikely that such numbers would be maintained once the majority of the population is induced to join one of the managed care organizations.⁶⁵ Recently there has been much attention paid to this, and the statistics seem to confirm that HMO's profits are shrinking fast precisely because of this.⁶⁶

Also, when considering managed care, it has been pointed out that while financial arrangements vary a great deal, plans that offer doctors incentives to control referrals, can create a conflict between the

---

⁶³ENTHOVEN A.C., *"Managed Competition: An Agenda for Action,"* Health Affairs 7(3):28-29, Summer 1988.

⁶⁴STARR P., *The Logic of Health Care Reform: Why and How the President's Plan Will Work,* p. xl, 49.

⁶⁵CARNEY K.,*"Cost Containment and Justice,"* in SHELP E., (ed.), Justice and Health Care, Volume 8, p. 175, 1981.

⁶⁶One recent article states that nearly 80 million Americans are enrolled in a health maintenance organization or another managed care plan. This is double the number of only five years ago. See HAMMONDS K.H., *Hit Where It Hurts: Why HMO Profits Are Shrinking Fast,* Business Week, October 27, 1997, pp. 42-43. Another recent article which puts the number of people enrolled in HMO's to be approximately 70 million, says that since 1993 this number has increased 50% and so have the complaints about rationing of procedures and a narrower choice of doctors. See DICKERSON J.F., *Dr. Clinton Scrubs Up,* Time, December 8, 1997, p. 48.

physician's interests and the patient's. Even when it is true that a fee-for-service arrangement is in no way exempted from such a dilemma, since many times a general practitioner may hesitate to refer a patient to a specialist due to the risk of that patient never coming back to him or her again, in the case of managed care it is clear that there will be a direct financial reward for the physician coming from the non-referral since there has been a pre-paid sum already agreed upon.

Finally, managed care has affected the area of disease prevention. In the U.S. there is a distinction between "identified" and "statistical" lives. The first refers to those lives that have actually been accounted for among those affected by certain illnesses and how they have responded to treatment. The second type of lives, refers to those who are not actual cases, or in other words, those statistics that have not come to pass, since effective preventive care was instituted in time to prevent them from happening. The American society places little value on statistical lives and prefers to deal with the identified ones. This view fails to see that statistical lives considers people who may be alive and apparently well now, but are at risk of future injury, illness, disease, or death.

It has been shown that prevention is much more important and significant in reducing morbidity and mortality than any therapeutic and custodial service. Very few insurance plans in the U.S. pay for routine preventive care, while at the same time the increase in government payments for curative care has not been matched by public health expenditures. Because of this, preventive health care is inadequate for all groups in the U.S., and accounts for only 2.3% of all health expenditures. It has been estimated that a moderately effective preventive plan could save up to 400,000 lives, or the equivalent of 6 million person-years of life, and at the same time save more than 6% of total health expenditures every year.[67] A well known study concluded that if there was better control of fewer than ten risk factors in the country, it could prevent between 40 and 70 percent of all premature deaths, one third of all cases of acute illness, and two-thirds of all illnesses considered as chronic.[68]

---

[67]HIMMELSTEIN D.U., WOOLHANDLER S., *"Pitfalls of Private Medicine: Health Care in the USA."* Lancet 2 (8399):393, August 18,1984.

[68]The study was done by MCGINNIS and reported in an article entitled *"National Priorities in Disease Prevention,"* Issues in Science and Technology 5:46-52, 1989. Cf. BLANK R.H., *"Rationing Medicine: Hard Choices in the 1990's."* American Journal of Gastroenterology 87(9):1077, September 1992.

Even though prevention could be considered in a utilitarian way, or as a set of priority rules for restructuring existing market rules in order to maximally protect the public, in reality the market forces guided by utilitarian considerations have been about the most powerful ones to preclude the establishment of good preventive measures in the U.S.

c. Diagnosis-related groups

The implementation in 1983 of what became known as diagnosis-related groups or DRG's, represents a clear example of a utilitarian solution to the problem of rapidly increasing health care costs which were intended to maintain an equitable level of care provided to all Medicare patients. This was an initiative by Congress to replace Medicare's previous arrangement to reimburse hospitals.

DRG's are basically connected to pricing lists for medical treatment that are prepaid by Medicare or Medicaid after considering such factors as age, sex, and other variables which help in obtaining an average cost for a typical set of tests or procedures. DRG programs assign in advance a fixed sum of money or a fixed number of days of hospitalization to more than 400 disease categories.[69] To give just one illustrative example, DRG #346 is the amount of money attributed to the treatment of prostate cancer for those who are 70 years of age and older. DRG #347 is for the same problem in patients who are under the age of 70. These numbers vary because of the factors mentioned above and the possibility of full recovery.

One dilemma posed by such an approach to health care is the conflict that develops between optimization of results and equality of access. For example, in the case of prostate cancer we can assume that the treatment of the younger patient will produce more efficient results in life-days per dollar spent. Optimizing results would seem to require that we shift the resources given to DRG #346 and invest them in DRG #347. The fact that the same illness is divided between age groups signals the reality that, when faced with limited resources, maximizing utility will be emphasized. Some authors have tried to interpret DRG's on other philosophical grounds, for example egalitarian ones, yet it is clear that the egalitarian mold does not blend with the notion of DRG's as well as the

---

[69]PELLEGRINO E.D., THOMASMA D.C., *For the Patient's Good. The Restoration of Beneficence in Health Care*, p. 176.

The Fundamental Answers Based on the Philosophical Foundations 117

utilitarian one. For example, if an egalitarian notion is used, and we would consider again the same example with prostate cancer, then it would mean that more resources should go to DRG #346 in order for the older patients to benefit equally when in comparison to their younger fellow patients.[70]

There are many problems related to DRG's. It seems that the DRG system does not provide incentives to reduce unnecessary hospital admissions. Since the hospitals are the ones affected by the system's measures and not the doctors, it gives the latter ones no incentives for cost containment.

There is also a problem with determining what is "necessary" in order to provide quality care for a particular patient. The DRG's system is one based on average lengths of stay in the hospital for each disease. Since no two diseases manifest themselves in the same way in every patient, some may suffer due to such differences. Instead of treating individual patients, DRG's foster the treatment of an abstract disease entity. In this way the original aim of quality care is at least partially compromised. This compromising of quality care has been experienced by the fact that patients are being discharged quicker and sicker, and also by the lack of extra funds for cases that fall outside the statistical projections.[71] Empirical studies have revealed that many elderly patients have been discharged from hospitals before effective, optimal, and even necessary care was provided. This was done so as to comply with the DRG limits.[72]

Another problem related to DRG's has been the practice of placing limits on the number of physician contacts per patient and even, at times, limits on lifetime medical expenditures. Such limits, imposed in such arbitrary ways, can only promote shifting the burden of medical care to the patient or to hospitals and physicians who would be forced to provide uncompensated care.

---

[70]RHODES R.P., *Health Care: Politics, Policy, and Distributive Justice. The Ironic Triumph*, p. 33.

[71]PELLEGRINO E.D., THOMASMA D.C., *For the Patient's Good. The Restoration of Beneficence in Health Care*, p. 178.

[72]BAYER R., CALLAHAN D., CAPLAN A.L., JENNINGS B., *"Toward Justice in Health Care,"* American Journal of Public Health 78(5): 586, May 1988.

d. The presidential commission

A presidential commission was formed in the mid-seventies in order to study some issues related to health care delivery in the U.S. The whole question of whether there is a right to health care was discussed. The commission bore the long name of the *President's Commission for the Study of Ethical Problems in Medicine and Biomedical and Behavioral Research*, and in its 1983 report called *Securing Access to Health Care*, framed the ethical standard for the evaluation of the health care system in terms of what was called "adequacy." The Commission members felt that by incorporating this term instead of the language of "rights," they were providing a term of art that would take into account the professional consensus, while at the same time incorporate the broadly supported cultural standards regarding what the health care system ought to provide to citizens in need. This commission explicitly rejected the rights-oriented language, while affirming the community's ethical obligation to provide equitable access to an "adequate" level of medical care. When emphasizing the primacy of access to health care, they did this by using a utilitarian argument in favor of such perspective. For the Commission, the level of care to be provided would be determined by the level of resources devoted to producing it. The allocations should reflect the costs and benefits of the care given to the people. They wanted a broad picture of what should be considered as personal benefits achieved through health care, which would include the improvement in the individual's functioning, quality of life, and the peace of mind that comes from adequate health care. Social benefits should be seen also in a broad sense, which would include a strengthening of the sense of community and the idea that no one in need of health care would be left without it.[73]

3. Modern Utilitarian Thinkers and a Critique of Their Main Ideas

a. John Stuart Mill

John Stuart Mill in the last chapter of his book *Utilitarianism*, makes an effort to resolve what he considers the only real difficulty in the utilitarian theory of morals by treating extensively the connection between

---

[73]President's Commission for the Study of Ethical Problems in Medicine and Biomedical and Behavioral Research, *Securing Access to Health Care*, p. 36.

utility and justice.[74] He concludes that justice does not constitute a moral obligation separate from utility considerations. Justice is involved in the very meaning of utility. Of all the ambiguous and conflicting ideas of justice, "social utility alone can decide the preference."[75] Justice grounded in utility is the most sacred and binding part of all morality.[76]

Relevant to this discussion is Mill's understanding of equality. This is a significant element of justice, but, as justice itself, is subordinated to the principle of utility. Says Mills: "All persons are deemed to have a right to equality of treatment, except when some recognized social expediency requires the reverse. And hence all social inequalities which have ceased to be considered expedient, assume the character not of simple inexpediency, but of injustice."[77]

This utilitarian thinking envisages individuals in the aggregate, and takes the administrative view of society at large; thus moral obligation is tied to the general welfare. Maximization of aggregate happiness is the moral duty, with no sense of intrinsic rightness or wrongness. The value of life itself might succumb to utility. Individuals are seen as means to an end.

b. Joseph Fletcher

Joseph Fletcher offers one of the best examples of utilitarianism as applied to health care. He is an act-utilitarian to the core who believes that distributive justice is the key question for biomedical ethics, and who argues forcefully and directly that the utilitarian approach to the difficult problems of distributive justice is the only plausible answer given the realities of contemporary society. Those realities in his opinion are limited resources, insatiable demands, the highly social dimension of the ethics of health care today, the accountability of legislators, the role of reason, and the competing factors of numbers and values involved.

Fletcher sees ethics as the business of rational critical reflection, involving choices between competing values. He believes that the task of

---

[74]MILL J.S., *Utilitarianism,* in ROBSON J.M. (ed.), *John Stuart Mill*, pp. 225-228.

[75]Ibid.

[76]Ibid., p. 222.

[77]Ibid., pp. 226, 239.

the just man and the legislature is to select that course which realizes the greatest good for the greatest number. He believes human acts are fundamentally justified by consequences. No act is of itself good or evil; rather it depends solely on the balance of the results. He says it himself in his 1979 work *Humanhood: Essays in Biomedical Ethics*: "In short, everything depends on the consequences. This singular general or formal principle or highest good, can be labeled as general utility or happiness or the good of persons or agapism or human welfare."[78]

Fletcher perceives rules and reason as incompatible, and declares that human beings must live by one or the other. "The fundamental ethical question is whether we are to live and act by rules or by reason."[79] He opts for reason and believes that human choice in each act is guided by the principle of utility.

Fletcher uses the all-inclusive definition of health given by the World Health Organization, discussed in the beginning of this chapter, to state that the essence of bioethical decisions revolves around the questions: ". . .what, of what can be done, should be done; what, of what should be done, can we afford; and what, of what we can afford, are we willing to pay?"[80]

For Fletcher, at the heart of the problem of distributive justice is how to allocate resources. He proposes what he calls "ethimetrics." He has this to say:

> Just as others have coined the term "econometrics" for mathematics and quantification methods applied to economic data, I suggest that "ethimetrics" can be used for ethical analysis seeking distributive justice. It is a good label for applying statistical terms of amount and probability to macromoral problems, even down to such levels as allocating funds between developing an acceptable artificial heart and meeting the needs for patients in renal failure. To be ethical requires knowledge and careful calculation; because loving concern is the same as justice—it has to be distributed.[81]

---

[78]FLETCHER J., *Humanhood: Essays in Biomedical Ethics*, p. 32.

[79]Ibid., p. 5.

[80]Ibid., p. 8.

[81]Ibid., p. 51.

Fletcher's ethics is compatible with his vision of man whom he perceives as "caught in a tight web of radical interconnectivity," and thus for him ethics is essentially social.[82] In this tight web, society is faced with problems and dilemmas which are virtually unresolvable, but all we can do is the best for the most.

Realizing the ethical issue at stake is the private versus the common interest, and anticipating the objection of those who think of man as an end in himself and not merely a means to be used for the satisfaction of others, Fletcher rebuts by explaining that "to sacrifice the one for the many is to sacrifice the one for the many ones. The greatest number is not an abstraction; it is the sum of real, particular and personal individuals."[83]

Fletcher believes it is necessary to understand the nature of human beings; who or what they are if society is to resolve its problems. Therefore, he develops an inventory of humanhood that will provide the necessary "criteria for humanness to supply the parameters of quality judgments and selections."[84] Fletcher's task is to establish criteria for personhood, rather than human life, that is, personal status deserving of legal protection, for not all human are persons. Man does not have a fixed, substantive nature, but rather a history. He then proceeds to his task of developing "for the purposes of biomedical ethics," a profile of man which consists of fifteen positive and five negative propositions, the "sine qua non, the indispensable trait or criterion is mind, what we call *cerebration*."[85]

The implications of this are profound, since those who do not meet this inventory do not have the same claim upon society as those who do. Fletcher can with impunity state definitely that "idiots are not humans;" or that in terms of fetal life, for example, "pregnancy when wanted is a healthy process and when not wanted is (. . .) a venereal disease."[86]

---

[82] FLETCHER J., *Humanhood: Essays in Biomedical Ethics*, p. 46.

[83] Ibid., p. 51.

[84] Ibid., p. 19.

[85] Ibid., p. 20.

[86] Ibid., pp. 22, 138.

In order to achieve his goal, Fletcher develops stipulative definitions about man, his nature, and relationships in society. Arguing against a fixed, substantive nature, he nonetheless states that the *"sine qua non"* is the mind, without which there is no full humanhood or personal status. This very assertion moves Fletcher toward the notion of an essential substantive nature which he disclaims.

Another problem with Fletcher's position is the implication that rules are incompatible with reason. In Fletcher's presentation, one must choose either, but such a choice eliminates the possibility of the other. The implication that can be drawn from this is that rules result in unreasonable people and that for reasonable people, rules have no place or function. This goes against, not only intuition, but concrete life experience.

Incredibly, while acknowledging that ethics is the business of rational, critical reflection, Fletcher would assign the task of making moral decisions to the computer, which is neither rational nor reflective. He says: "Artificial intelligence is the only answer to the magnitude of human relations in a technological world of runaway material production and human reproduction."[87]

c. *Tom Beauchamp*

Another example is the rule-utilitarianism of Tom Beauchamp. He denies any natural or constitutional right to health care and begins a search for what he asserts is the necessary criterion for justifying any level of right to health care: a moral principle requiring a social obligation to provide some level of health care.

His search shifts for what he considers essential: a moral principle sufficient to show there is a social obligation to provide some level of health care. His immediate problem is to discover such a principle, but there are difficulties in the conviction that one cannot justify practical matters of great complexity by highly abstract moral principles. In his mind, it is impossible to apply general principles of justice to social policy. He thus abandons the search for an appropriate moral principle, and moves from a purely philosophical framework to a more appropriate one, a mechanism rooted in utilitarianism, namely, cost-benefit analysis.

In a 1979 article with R. Faden, Beauchamp, while relying heavily on cost-benefit analysis, qualifies his approach with the statement

---

[87]FLETCHER J., *Humanhood: Essays in Biomedical Ethics*, pp. 12, 47.

that "it does not follow from our arguments that there is no social obligation whatsoever to provide health care goods and services. It follows only that one must restrict, by careful argument, the scope of any claim made to a right to health care."[88] He further notes that "it is hard to imagine that we are not obligated by a string of moral principles such as beneficence, non-maleficence, and justice to provide a decent minimum of health care."[89] He contends that utility could support a decent minimum of health care.

Many theorists agree that efficiency is an important consideration for accountable policy makers, who should certainly prefer it to inefficiency. However, where it becomes the only value upheld in a theory, other values can be violated or negated, not the least important of which can be equality, respect for persons, and justice itself. There would be merit in a one-principled theory, where costs and benefits could be measured, weighted and balanced, if other values were not sacrificed in the process. But it is questionable whether the relative ease and simplicity of cost-benefit analysis, typifying the utilitarian approach, qualify it as the best possible choice available. When utility is used as the only principle, with no concern for the shape of the distribution of benefits and burdens to individuals, it yields results unacceptable to any society which upholds the principles of equality, justice, and respect for persons.

C. THE LIBERTARIAN PHILOSOPHY

1. Main Tenets of Libertarianism

The philosophy of libertarianism emphasizes personal freedom as its core. Human beings as rational agents, are entitled to freedom from measures that violate their rights of individual liberty. The fundamental right of every person is to have his rational agency respected. People also have a corresponding duty not to interfere with the liberty of others. This is to be so, regardless of the consequences.

Libertarians emphasize negative rights over positive ones. Positive rights of access are unjustified demands against someone else's liberty or property. According to this point of view, people must be free

---

[88] BEAUCHAMP T.L., FADEN R.R., *"The Right to Health and the Right to Health Care,"* Journal of Medicine and Philosophy 4(2):128, June 1979.

[89] Ibid.

to pursue their own life plans, which include their economic livelihood. The fundamental rights are liberty rights of noninterference. Persons have inherent rights to life, liberty, and property. The role of government is only to prevent others from interfering with those pursuits, to see that those rights are not violated, and, if they are, to secure just compensation to the person whose rights were infringed upon. No one should be forced to give up part of what he or she has earned to pay for other people's needs. The lack of capacity by some people to purchase necessary things is unfortunate but not unfair. There are many situations in life that certainly can be categorized as unfortunate, but that does not mean that they are unfair. For a libertarian is impossible to determine the fairness of an unfortunate situation, especially if it entails determining an obligation on the part of others to take care of the unfortunate event.[90]

That is why, for libertarians, it is important to establish ownership of property first. There can be no right to what is not personally owned. Individuals have a property right to whatever material holdings they achieve if their actions conform to two main principles: 1) the principle of justice in initial acquisition and 2) the principle of justice in transfer.[91] The first principle deals with the ways in which individuals can come to own things without acting in violation of anyone else's rights. This follows the ideas of John Locke as to how one can make natural objects one's own: by mixing one's labor with them and improving them in the process. Some libertarian authors claim that one can do this as long as one's appropriation of the object does not worsen the conditions of others in significant ways, or there is an appropriate compensation to those whose condition is worsened by the appropriation.[92]

The second principle refers to the fact that one person may justly transfer his legitimate holdings to another person through an act of sale, trade, gift, or bequest. The person receiving those holdings is entitled to those goods so long as the one from whom the goods were acquired was

---

[90]BOUCHARD C.E., *"Healthcare Reform's Moral, Spiritual Issues. The Problems Are Not Just Political,"* Health Progress, May-June 1996, p.58.

[91]BUCHANAN A., *"Justice: A Philosophical Review,"* in SHELP E.E., (ed.), *Justice and Health Care,* D. Reidel Publishing Co. Dordrecht: Holland 1981, Vol. 8, p. 11.

[92]Ibid. These ideas come mainly from Robert Nozick, whom we will discuss in detail later.

entitled to the transferred holdings. In other words, a distribution of goods is just if and only if it comes from another just distribution done through legitimate means.[93]

Once this principle of legitimate transfer of holdings is recognized and enforced, the attempt to force anyone to contribute any part of his or her legitimate holdings in order to favor the welfare of others, is a clear violation of that person's property rights. This is true regardless if the action is undertaken by private individuals or the state itself. For libertarians, only the minimal state can be compatible with such principles. Any existing holding that did not come about through the just steps specified above, can be liable to a principle of rectification of past injustices. This would mean that if it could be shown that any present possession of resources resulted from injustices in their original acquisition or in the history of their subsequent transfers to persons or institutions, it would be incumbent upon the government to rectify those past injustices. In the case that individuals who suffered the injustices could not be identified, a systemic compensation might be appropriate.[94]

2. Issues Raised by Libertarianism Concerning Health Care

There are two main problems that must be studied when considering the effects of a libertarian philosophy on access to health care. The first one has to do with the role of government, and the second one with the acceptance of health care as a market commodity. We will take a look at each of these problems individually.

a. The role of government

Libertarians believe in a limited role of government, but, as was seen above, there is a legitimate role of the state, especially if rectifications need to take place. This acceptance by libertarians of some degree of governmental involvement opens the door to the whole issue of specifying the beneficial and non-beneficial elements brought about by the involvement of the state. This debate has raised very important issues

---

[93]BUCHANAN A., *"Justice: A Philosophical Review,"* in SHELP E.E., (ed.), *Justice and Health Care*, D. Reidel Publishing Co. Dordrecht: Holland 1981, Vol. 8, p. 11.

[94]DOUGHERTY C., *American Health Care. Realities, Rights, and Reforms*, pp. 33-34.

concerning health care. When the balance of the consequences that would entitle citizens to some level of health care is a favorable one, the negative claims of libertarianism concerning government involvement would have to be especially strong in order to overrule the recognition of the desirability of such involvement. There are social costs that are paid as a consequence of governmental growth and bureaucracy, not the least of which would be the reduction of a healthy degree of individuality. Yet, there are other factors that would certainly merit the weighing in of increased involvement by the state.

Libertarians rely on their philosophy to state that health care providers own their trade just as anyone else would own some personal property. Because of that reason, they have a right to use their profession as they wish, expecting remuneration for their services. When someone cannot pay for health services, it is an unfortunate situation, yet it does not give rise to an unfair situation. Such people should rely strictly on the charitable impulses of the community and on available public clinics and hospitals established specifically to provide services to the poor and uninsured. With the growth and development in the health care industry, though, the question has been raised as to what to do when private philanthropy and local governments alone cannot provide for the foundations of an adequate health care system. Just like a minimum of material resources are an absolute necessity for human life if persons are to be recognized as members of the human community, it can be said that the same applies to a certain level of health care. Unless there is an absolute scarcity of such resources, the community has an obligation to help fulfill such basic needs. When charity and local government help is not enough to fulfill the communal obligation, this obligation does not cease to exist. Even if the scheme developed involves the limiting of governmental involvement, still it must consider some extent of governmental rules and incentives to achieve the necessary objectives.[95]

The inability of accomplishing the fulfillment of societal obligations through charity or local governments brings up another issue. This can be explained by what is called the principle of subsidiary function. This principle states that, just as it is gravely wrong to take away from individuals what they can accomplish by their own initiative and industry, it would be as wrong and a disturbance of the right order to assign to a greater and higher association what lesser and subordinate

---

[95]PAULY M. et al., *"A Plan for 'Responsible National Health Insurance',"* Health Affairs, Spring 1991, p. 6.

organizations can do. Still, this principle implies that when the lesser or subordinate organization does not have the capacity to accomplish what is needed, then it follows that there is a legitimate role of the greater and higher organization. Libertarians would claim that the state will work more freely, powerfully, and effectively when given those things that belong to it alone. As we saw already those things that belong to the state alone according to the libertarian philosophy would be to guarantee the ability of persons to pursue their life plans, to see that individual rights are not violated, and to enforce rectifying actions in case of any violations of such rights. Nevertheless, when the lesser organizations come up short of fulfilling the social obligation to provide certain basic needs, there is a legitimate role of government to not only direct, watch, urge, or restrain action, but to assume the social obligation as its own.[96]

Libertarians have contributed to the debate on health care as well by bringing forth the serious consideration of how much government involvement is necessary in relation to medical assistance. Actually, this question can be posed differently. It could be phrased as: Is it absolutely necessary that the government be involved in health care providing? As we saw above, the state has an obligation to participate in the societal response to problems related to health care for the citizens, but it does not have the sole responsibility for this or even the principal responsibility.[97] Concerning health care, it is conceivable to develop a systemic argument that is not statist. In other words, it is possible to have a coordinated systematic social response to the need for health care, but this does not automatically mean that it must be through a state-sponsored program.[98] It is a possibility for the state to be considered the final guarantor that such an obligation will be fulfilled, and also to be available to collaborate with other agencies which may become the principal means by which the social obligation is met. In other words, the fulfillment of the societal obligation to offer help so that all people can take care of the basic needs they have, can be accomplished through different designs of reform in which the government does not need to be the principal agent. Related to health care

---

[96]*Quadragesimo Anno,* n. 79 in CARLEN C., *The Papal Encyclicals,* p. 428.

[97]HEHIR J.B., *"Policy Arguments in a Public Church: Catholic Social Ethics and Bioethics."* Journal of Medicine and Philosophy 17(3):361, June 1992.

[98]Ibid.

it means that it is not necessary for the government to run the health care system in the country, since there could be multiple plans in which consumers could have a choice.[99] There are many models for structuring a health care system, and clearly, government regulated is not necessarily the same as government operated.[100]

Some countries, in response to the rising costs of health care, have utilized the device called global budgeting. This is an annually negotiated cap on total expenditures in health care. Even when this type of device is used, it does not imply a governmental takeover of health care policies and finances. Global budgeting is compatible with a private health plan. In the German system, for example, global budgeting negotiations take place among nongovernmental groups who are responsible for setting the annual cap. With global budgeting there is no need for detailed, centralized budget decisions. It simply calls for the setting of budget ceilings which eventually may paradoxically result in less government regulation. These caps provide an assurance to government, employers, and the public that total health care expenditures in the country will remain within a predetermined limit. This may make it less likely that they would pursue the kind of micro regulation of health care that we see taking place in the United States today.[101]

b. Health care as a market commodity

Libertarians consider health care as a market commodity. Services related to health are like any other commercial products that are meant to be bought and sold. In their view, as we have seen, there is no entitlement to health care. Individuals seeking health care must pay for what they "buy," and the lack of ability to pay in no way should be considered the basis for provision of such services free of charge. There is no problem if charity is the basis for providing the needed services, but there is no obligation to provide without cost what is considered the property of another human being.

---

[99]STARR P., *The Logic of Health Care Reform: Why and How the President's Plan Will Work*, p. 69.

[100]DOUGHERTY C.J., *American Health Care. Realities, Rights, and Reforms*, p. 60.

[101]STARR P., *The Logic of Health Care Reform: Why and How the President's Plan Will Work*, p. 43.

There are many issues raised the moment health care is considered simply as a commodity. Obviously, one of the first ones is the fact that physicians are entitled to a financial compensation for their services. Throughout the history of health care in the United States, the most prevalent form of compensation for physicians has been the fee-for-service arrangement. It is only in recent times that other forms of payment methods have become more prevalent. Historically, though, doctors in the past have opposed the corporate enterprise in medical practice not only for the sake of preserving their autonomy as physicians, but also because they wanted to prevent the emergence of a third party that would act as an intermediary between patient and doctor which would keep for itself the profits available from the medical practice. In the Code of Ethics that the American Medical Association adopted back in 1934, it was clearly stated that it was unprofessional for a physician to allow a direct profit to be made from his practice. This did not mean that the AMA felt that it was wrong for physicians to make a profit from their work. What the AMA was opposed to was the possibility for an investor to make a return from the doctor's work. The idea was to prevent the possibility of capital formation through medical care, other than the one doctors accumulated. If there was any need for capital that doctors could not provide, it would have to come freely from the community, instead of from investors seeking a profit.[102]

From the above example, it is clear that from the very beginning of the considerations of health care as a profit-making enterprise, there were serious debates that argued against treating health care merely as a commodity from which a profit could be made, but as a primary social responsibility. When health expenditures are privatized in an exclusive way, it carries with this the assumption that medical care is like any other commodity.[103] Even if it was the case that health care could be considered unlike other commodities, or for example, as a precious commodity, this language of "commodity" would still be miles away from the consideration of health care as a community good which should be provided as a response to a societal obligation.

---

[102]STARR P., *The Social Transformation of American Medicine*, p. 215.

[103]BAYER R., CALLAHAN D., CAPLAN A.L., JENNINGS B., *"Toward Justice in Health Care,"* American Journal of Public Health 78(5): 588, May 1988.

Another aspect of health care considered simply as a commodity, has to do with what happens in the relationship between physician and patient when the profit motive is primary. Some authors have referred to the role of the physician in modern times as a "gatekeeper." Usually it has to do with what is called "negative gatekeeping," which is meant to help reducing medical costs by motivating physicians to promote efficient and effective access to health care. But this arrangement may also work in the other direction. In positive gatekeeping a doctor is constrained to increase rather than to decrease the access to services. The purpose in this is enhancing profits. Those who can pay for medical services are provided them on demand, regardless of medical need. The physician in this kind of relationship becomes basically a salesperson or an independent entrepreneur or the hired hand for investors who have no connection with the traditions of ethics in the medical field.[104] With the positive gatekeeping role, the physician uses his or her de facto position as gatekeeper to his own financial advantage or to that of his employer. The physician who is given the possibility of acting in such a way, begins to think of his relationship with the patient not as one based on a covenant of trust, but as a type of business relationship based on contracts. Ethics cease to be important as a matter of obligation or virtue and become a mere legality. Following the libertarian philosophy, medical knowledge becomes the doctor's private property to be sold to whoever he chooses, at whatever price, under whatever conditions he requires. Thus the patient becomes primarily a source of income, and his or her dependence, anxiety, ignorance, and vulnerability in time of sickness are exploited for profit.[105] Patients generally rely on professionals for guidance on treatment and other critical decisions affecting costs, and are usually not aware of what is behind some decisions which affect them.

When health care is treated as a commodity, according to the tenets of libertarianism, true liberty is confused with autonomy. The whole notion of autonomy tends to emphasize people's isolation from others. The tendency here is to prevent a more relational understanding of freedom which includes the notion of "freedom for" as much as the one of "freedom from." In other words, when the assumptions of the libertarian concerning health care are adopted, there is an erosion in the

---

[104]PELLEGRINO E.D., THOMASMA D.C., *For the Patient's Good. The Restoration of Beneficence in Health Care,* pp. 176-177, 180.

[105]Ibid., p. 180.

understanding of freedom as a facilitating agent for helping others, by emphasizing freedom from the interference of others.[106]

One more problem has to do with the motivation that the notion of health care as a commodity offers prospective doctors to specialize. The "for profit" incentive becomes a decisive factor in professional orientation and choices of medical students. There are too many surgeons in the United States and too few primary physicians.

The capitalist organization of the current health care system in the United States encourages the structuring of health facilities as commercial enterprises. There are financial incentives mixed with the physical assets, the distribution of specialists, and even the patterns of medical practices accepted in society and by medical organizations. Some of the physical assets, by which we mean diagnosis related machines and other equipment, have become key components in the survival of certain health care institutions. Since there is a cost attached to the machines, many times the equipment is used only when the patient can pay for its cost. It is known that one of the reasons why there is too little breast cancer screening in America, is because there are too many mammography machines. As one author has stated: "Only in America are poor women denied a mammogram because there is too much equipment!"[107]

3. Modern Libertarian Thinkers and a Critique of Their Main Ideas

a. Robert Nozick

In his book *Anarchy, State, and Utopia*, Robert Nozick develops his libertarian philosophy. This book written in 1974 is mainly a reaction to John Rawls' *A Theory of Justice*, which we will discuss in depth later. Actually Nozick asserts in his book that one must currently work within Rawls' theory or explain and justify why not.[108]

For Nozick, persons are highly individualistic. Since for him there is no such reality as a social entity, social obligations originate only

---

[106]KILNER J.F., *Health-care resources, allocation of.* Encyclopedia of Bioethics, Vol 2 (Revised Edition), W.T. REICH, (Editor in Chief.) Simon & Schuster, New York, 1995, p. 1069.

[107]STARR P., *The Logic of Health Care Reform: Why and How the President's Plan Will Work*, p. 26.

[108]NOZICK R., *Anarchy, State, and Utopia*, p. 183.

by contractual relationship. By placing the individual in the very center of his theory, Nozick argues for a very narrow state function of protecting all citizens against theft, violence, fraud, and the non-enforcement of contracts.

Nozick develops a theory of entitlement trying to explain his conception of justice. For him there is no need for a principle of distributive justice in his entitlement theory because there is no central distributive function in a society composed of free individuals. The only legitimate distribution that can take place is the one effected by the voluntary exchange of free, rational, and separate individuals, whose ultimate meaning in life is shaping their own destiny.

The notion of justice for Nozick is related to process. When the process of acquiring and transferring goods is legitimate, then justice is achieved. Justice has nothing to do with the amount of the distribution of goods which takes place among the members of society, nor with the end results. The only thing that matters is how the distribution takes place. The resulting pattern of distribution is not important. Justice is then determined by the legitimacy of the procedure by which goods are distributed. The common sense notions of desert and need are not taken into consideration.

Nozick is a strong defender of the right to acquire and transfer property, yet, this right is not an absolute one since it must consider the condition of others qualified by the Lockean proviso. This is the notion discussed before in which an individual acquires property rights in a previously unknown object by mixing his own labor with it, and thus enhancing the value of the object and entitling the individual to property rights in the object. An individual is limited in acquisition by the notion that there must be enough available and as good left in common for others.[109] Nozick explains that the idea behind such proviso is to insure that the situation of others is not worsened. For him this is not a case of property rights being denied, but of such rights being overridden to prevent catastrophe.

For Nozick, people are entitled to their natural endowments based on the claims they have to their natural assets. If they are entitled to natural assets, then they have to be entitled as well to anything that flows from them. In this way, people's holdings flow from their natural assets. Based on this, Nozick concludes that people are entitled to their holdings.

---

[109]NOZICK R., *Anarchy, State, and Utopia*, p. 27.

If they are entitled to something, then they ought to have it, and this overrides any presumption of equality there may be about holdings. Nozick considers natural assets as belonging to the individual.

Nozick's notion that every individual is entitled to his natural endowments can be challenged. If the history of the advantages and disadvantages to which an individual is born could be traced, often it would be found that society itself bears much of the responsibility for them. Even if this was not the case, it can be said that Nozick's absolute theory of entitlement tends to destroy the very respect for every individual that he tries to uphold. This is so since it reduces life to the survival of the fittest, in which the strong with legitimate holdings completely overpower the weak with minimal holdings. This does nothing to foster a common sense notion of justice, and everything to promote a kind of "law of the jungle."

Nozick assumes that all individuals have an equal right to compete in the marketplace of acquisition and transfer. The truth is that the inequalities among individuals as they attempt to compete, many times preclude the possibility of a fair outcome. Nozick seems to give legal justification to such inequalities. His theory is too single-minded, with rights as the only source of morality. His single-principle theory of liberty, has only one single criterion for distributive justice: past actions. His theory is too simplistic and totally ignorant of the complex realities of social life where other values such as equality, merit, and need are held to be important as well.

Since Nozick gives no consideration to need or desert, the only relevant difference between those who receive health care and those who do not, is the availability of funds. Since liberty is the dominant value, physicians are free to render service as they choose. Consumers are free to purchase such services or not, like any commodity in the market. This market is controlled by the laws of supply and demand.

b. Robert Sade

Robert Sade is another libertarian that, like Nozick, champions the cause of liberty especially as it relates to health care. In his famous article entitled *Medical Care as a Right: A Refutation,* written in 1977, he traces the concept of right, which defines a freedom of action, to man's moral nature. Sade begins and ends with a strong defense of absolute liberty. There is no semblance of need to be found in Sade's strong defense of freedom. There is nothing that can interfere with the autonomy of the individual, and particularly of the physician.

The primary right for Sade, without which there can be no others, is the right to one's own life. This implies three other corollaries: ". . . the right to select the values that one deems necessary to sustain one's own life; the right to exercise one's own judgment of the best course of action to achieve chosen values; and the right to dispose of those values, once gained, in any way one chooses, without coercion by other men."[110]

Sade's article is full of value and virtue language in which he extolls the properties of man's mind, the development of capabilities to sustain his own life, and his freedom to exchange with other men the things he produces. In all this, he defends a very limited role of government.

Health care is a service provided by physicians to those who can purchase it, and not a right or privilege. He does not attribute any importance or recognition to the fact that the need for health care differs from the desire for commodities in the market, nor he shows any concern for those without the means to purchase medical care. The liberty of one man is far more important than the life of another, who even though possessing the same liberty, does not have the means or the ability to exercise it effectively.

Sade goes as far as to call the concept of health care as a right immoral because it denies the most fundamental of all rights, which is the right of a man to his own life and the freedom of action to support it.[111] By such a right to health care, a patient would own the services of the physician, subjugating the whole medical profession, and forcing doctors to become servants of the state. Sade finds this completely contradictory in a country like the United States, which was founded on the principles of life and liberty.

He tries to refute what he considers fallacies that follow from the notion of health care as a right by stating that health care is an individual and not a community or social concern; evidence suggests that free enterprise works more effectively than state medicine; medical care does not lie outside the economic laws; and that if physicians were forced to design a health care system in which they did not believe, they would provide the "sanction of the victim."[112]

---

[110]SADE R., *Medical Care as a Right: A Refutation*, p. 573.

[111]Ibid., p. 574.

[112]Ibid., pp. 575-576.

It is ironical that Sade concludes his article by pleading for the upholding of personal values such as integrity, honesty, and self-esteem. These are the values, according to him, through which the physician can achieve his most important professional values and the absolute priority of the welfare of his patients.[113] When he says this, Sade fails to mention the fact that his notion of patient is very selective. In other words, the patient for Sade is the one the physician chooses to serve and the one with the financial ability to pay for the service. Nowhere he mentions the welfare of many of the poor patients who fall through the cracks.

Sade's libertarian notion of medical care is almost completely illusory. There is no way that someone can act with complete freedom in pursuing his or her rights while at the same time disregarding the consequences of those afflicted by such actions. If society is going to be stable and just, it must require some restrictions on such absolute freedoms.

For Sade, the physician's autonomy is to be protected at all costs, yet others do not have the same right. For the ones who are sick, there is no freedom to choose or not. They only have the unpredictable need, which if not met, such person cannot possibly pursue any other life goal. Health care is not simply a commodity in the market to be selected by individuals according to desire, but the very condition necessary to exercise the autonomy that Sade cherishes so much. Sade's protection of his own autonomy can effectively diminish the exercise of the autonomy of others. These inconsistencies are totally against the universalism considered as one of the main requirements for any solid ethical theory.

c. H. Tristram Engelhardt

Another libertarian is H. Tristram Engelhardt who in his 1981 article entitled *Health Care Allocations: Responses to the Unjust, the Unfortunate, and the Undesirable,* dealt with some important issues regarding health care. Engelhardt believes that before considering the allocation of health care resources among those in want, one must first inquire the reasons and to what extent health care should have a priority over other goods. He believes that to do this one must first ask when are these resources to be provided. For Engelhardt there is no definite answer to these questions. They depend on different views of moral excellence and character that will compete for our attention in the face of human

---

[113]SADE R., *Medical Care as a Right: A Refutation,* p. 576.

finitude.[114] It depends on how we choose among those views that will determine which health care allocations are proper. As long as freedom functions as a side constraint, and as long as the moral community is based on respect for freedom and not force, individual persons will have the possibility of holding private entitlements. There may be disagreements as to the way goods should be distributed, including the distribution of goods related to medical care. When this happens, namely that there is a lack of a shared common intuition of what the good life is, this view will be created and not discovered. To create such view there is a need to distinguish between needs and desires. Engelhardt explains it as the distinction between the unfair and the unfortunate.[115] Illness is an unfortunate occurrence, but, to what extent is it also unfair so that some would be obligated to share their resources to relieve the sufferings of others? In all circumstances one needs to anticipate with a certain tolerance the subversive nature of freedom. There is no right or wrong answer, but only different ways to fashion the good life as created by the community in question.

Engelhardt's ideas are self-defeating in the sense that, in trying to protect the freedom of people to use their resources to purchase health care and other desirable goods, it effectively ensures that those with insufficient resources will not have the freedom to obtain health care. His ideas ignore the possibility that the present distribution of general resources is in itself unfair. It also relies in the appropriateness of a free market approach in regards to health care. There is no possibility for a free market to function properly unless individuals are capable of understanding the costs and benefits of the available medical options and be willing to trade health, or even life, for money. This obviously would be absurd and misguided. Engelhardt's whole understanding of liberty, ends up emphasizing solely autonomy, which itself emphasizes people's separateness from one another.

---

[114]ENGELHARDT H.T., *Health Care Allocations: Responses to the Unjust, the Unfortunate, and the Undesirable*, p. 134.

[115]Ibid.

D. THE EGALITARIAN PHILOSOPHY

1. Main Tenets of Egalitarianism

Egalitarian philosophy embraces the notion of equality. The theories based on this way of thinking emphasize equal access to the goods in life that every rational person values. This is usually claimed invoking the material criteria of need and equality. The goal of an egalitarian society is to confer equal rights to all.

Egalitarians believe that the value of the human person is intrinsic. This means that it is not dependent on external relationships. The value ascribed to a person is not relative or dependent on the value given by others, or the attributes of beauty, usefulness or price that can be attached to an individual. The value of persons comes from within. The logical consequence of this pattern of thinking is the declaration that as human beings we are fundamentally equal.[116] Egalitarianism promotes as the ultimate basis of all human rights the equal moral standing of all persons. The primary right of every human being is to be accorded this standing.

Respect for the person requires a right to equality of opportunity. This means that there should be equal rights to personal liberty, to the ability to build and execute a reasonable life plan, and to share in the control of the policies and institutions whose role is to shape society and people's lives. Political and interpersonal freedom should be guaranteed by these rights.

Egalitarianism, when applied to health care issues, would require that if anyone within society has an opportunity to receive a health service, then everyone who shares the same type and degree of health need must be given an equally effective opportunity of receiving such health service. Since as persons we are all equally subject to the possibility of pain, suffering, disability and death at any time, it is not necessary to take into account the consequences, to realize the obligation to provide equal opportunity for everyone. We all have the same basic need when it comes to health care. It is based upon ill health and the prevention of ill health. The provision of health care rests only on this need, unlike other goods such as education or culture which require a certain level of ability and interest among the recipients. By preventing ill health in an individual

---

[116]DOUGHERTY C.J., *American Health Care. Realities, Rights, and Reforms*, pp. 52-54.

person, it can be said that there is also a protection of all people living in society. Never is this seen more clearly, than when society has to deal with an epidemic.

Ill health is not an uncommon reality. It is something that often happens to people throughout their lives, and it usually has effects that go beyond the individual person.

As good as it sounds in theory, egalitarianism is not problem free. One major problem is that persons have unequal needs when it comes to health care. There is a dilemma that is created between procedural equality in treatment versus substantive equality in result. People may be equally free to purchase health care in the market, but may lack the financial and private resources to afford even the most basic health care. In such a case, procedural equality would mask the existence of avoidable human suffering, which is clearly incompatible with the substantive moral mandate of egalitarianism to respect persons. Many times in the U.S. society today, the purchase of necessary health care is deferred in favor of other goods and services that satisfy other more pressing needs. When early, economical, and effective preventive treatment is delayed, usually it results in urgent, more expensive, and less successful treatment later.[117] When this happens, the health care system as a whole tends to be misused, and the emergency room plays the role of the unavailable primary care. Many health care needs simply go unmet. An egalitarian approach to health care makes sense if considered in a similar way as freedom from assault in a just society. This negative right of any civilized society requires large outlays of social resources. There are clearly unequal needs in that area as well; even more than in health care. Some citizens may never have recourse to the police and judiciary, while others may have to recur to them more than they would like. Yet, the investment of society in matters of police safety and protection are so much a matter of fundamental human rights that they are not left totally to the market.

In a sense, the provision of health care is a form of social protection. In both of these cases it is clear that substantive egalitarianism makes more sense than the procedural one. Just as it would not make any sense to provide equal police surveillance in low-crime and high-crime areas, or equal remedial reading courses for all students, whether they needed them or not, so it would not make sense to provide procedurally

---

[117]DOUGHERTY C.J., *American Health Care. Realities, Rights, and Reforms*, p. 58.

equal health care for all, regardless of health status.[118] Each case will require unequal treatment based upon unequal needs in order to approach equality of results for all.

Egalitarianism does not offer a very clear notion as to what constitutes the necessities that society has to ensure for everyone. Its argument justifying the provision of basic needs, lacks also a clear connection with a justification of which way to secure the resources necessary to provide for such needs. For example, different arguments have been developed to justify the collection of resources, such as what is known as the "tax-as-rent" argument, which legitimizes taxes on the population based on the common ownership of natural resources. In other words, if we can agree that the formation of property ultimately involves the use of unowned natural resources, and that the poor ought to have certain necessities they cannot purchase themselves, then there is nothing wrong with confiscating part of other people's property through taxation since there is some part that comes from those unowned natural resources.[119]

Another relevant argument that has been developed is the "caring argument." This one stresses the benefits that everyone gets from guaranteed health care regardless of ability to pay. No one in society would like to see people dying in the streets because of their lack of financial resources. Almost everyone would contribute to prevent this from happening. Looking at it this way it could be said that an egalitarian distribution of health care creates social solidarity and the feeling of community that goes beyond monetary value to provide a sense of social bond. In the words of an author who favors an egalitarian approach: "If health care is not part of the social glue that holds us together, what is?"[120]

2. Issues Raised by Egalitarianism Concerning Health Care

In this section there are two important issues that need to be discussed when considering the influence of an egalitarian philosophy in

---

[118]DOUGHERTY C.J., *American Health Care. Realities, Rights, and Reforms*, p. 60.

[119]MENZEL P.T., *Strong Medicine: The Ethical Rationing of Health Care*, p. 121.

[120]Ibid.

health care. First of all is the consensus that has developed to provide a basic minimum of health care to everyone. The second issue has to do with the problems of a two-tiered system that would result from such a provision.

a. A basic minimum of health care

When we take a look at the main tenets of egalitarianism as they relate to health care, one thing is clear: There are limited health care resources that, in order to be distributed in a way that would bring about substantive equity in results, must be limited in some fashion. This has developed into an emerging consensus in the health care community that the role of health care is to provide an equal and fair decent minimum of assistance.[121] Some authors, while claiming that this notion is not unjust in principle, still believe that the system that comes about from this notion would be unjust in the United States. This is so because, they contend, there is a common appreciation in America of the importance of health care which has carried the people beyond this arrangement. The question for other authors is whether the notion of equal access to health care is as strong in the American tradition as other notions such as a decent basic minimum of health care or free market principles.[122]

The problems arise when one tries to deal with the specifics of what constitutes a decent, fair minimum in health care. Most authors will acknowledge that in order to determine this basic minimum there is a need to balance or maintain such virtues as freedom, variety, and flexibility while at the same time being consistent with sound ethical judgments. Under this approach, the search for a fair, basic, decent minimum would focus on humane rather than technologically oriented health care.[123] The only way that a positive right to health care would be considered then,

---

[121]McCULLOUGH L.B., *Justice and Health Care: Historical Perspectives and Precedents,"* In SHELP, E.E. (ed.), Justice and Health Care, p. 53.

[122]See the opinion of Michael Walzer in BEAUCHAMP T.L., CHILDRESS J.F., *Principles of Biomedical Ethics,* p. 338.

[123]For a study of this issue see the discussion of Gene OUTKA'S 1974 article entitled *Social Justice and Equal Access to Health Care,* and Charles FRIED'S 1976 article entitled *Equality and Rights in Medical Care,* in CHILDRESS J.F., *"A Right to Health Care?,"* Journal of Medicine and Philosophy 4(2):132-147, June 1979.

would be as just a right to a fair share of the community's scarce resources. Obviously the problem being dealt with here is whether society can fairly, consistently, and without ambiguity devise a policy that would recognize the right or the obligation to provide primary care without creating a right to exotic and costly forms of health care. Until there is a definition of what society means by a decent minimum, such a model risks remaining simply as purely programmatic. Some authors believe this is the greatest problem confronting health care in the United States today.[124]

As time has passed, it has been possible to trace a continuous enrichment of our understanding of the ingredients necessary to establish a basic minimum of health care. Such care would have to include in a plausible way some reference to medical need. It would have to be rooted in notions of health care that would be commonly accepted by most people as things that they seek for in adequate medical care. Still, it is clear that even when reaching those commonly accepted notions, such standards cannot be used exclusively, and must allow for flexibility in dealing with the innumerable borderline cases that would arise. Also a decent minimum of average health care has to include a way to judge the efficacy, or lack of efficacy, of certain available treatments to meet those needs. In other words, there must be a system of determining what works and what does not work. From this step it is obvious that the next one is to consider the relative costs and benefits of certain treatments in order to determine if there is a "good return," so to speak, on the money spent. There would be a consideration of reasonable limits as a result of such an approach.

b. A multi-tiered system of health care

The formulation which considers the possibility and desirability of a basic minimum of health care has often implied a willingness to tolerate differential levels of care in which poor and dependent people would have access to a range of health services that differed in quality and kind from those available to individuals who could pay for them or have private insurance protection. In other words, a multi-tiered system of health care would be one that would offer a basic package, or minimum, of services that would be the same for every person, but if individual persons would like to purchase other services not included in the basic minimum but available in the market, they could do so.

---

[124]BEAUCHAMP T.L., CHILDRESS J.F., *Principles of Biomedical Ethics*, p. 357.

Some authors are very skeptical that a system that promotes the notion of a basic minimum of health care can offer a solution to inequalities in access to health care, and refrain from defending it.[125] In their discussion about their concern for the poor and universal access to health care, the American Roman Catholic bishops have voiced strong support for measures that would ensure true universal access to health care and rapid steps to improve the health care services given to the poor and unserved. Yet, at the same time, they have clearly opposed a two-tiered health care system since, to them, separate health care coverage for the poor would result in poor health care. They suggest that linking the health care of the poor and working class families to that of those with greater financial resources is the best assurance of comprehensive benefits and quality care.[126] A two or more-tiered system of health care among citizens of the same country has the tendency to leave the less-advantaged citizens with a lower-quality health care and more restricted services. To some extent this is happening already in the United States since the Medicaid program in many respects, despite its promise of broad benefits, has become a dumping ground for those without financial means, as we saw in the first chapter.[127] The basis for receiving important medical services that others cannot afford, should not be ability to pay. This should be the basis for how much individuals pay for their health care protection and not the determinant of what kind of health care certain individuals receive. Some recent writers have claimed that today there seem to be three, and not two tiers of care being provided in the United States: Standard care for the insured, partial care for people in Medicaid, and emergency care only for approximately 37 million Americans who have no health insurance.[128]

---

[125]For a good discussion of the issue see BAYER R., CALLAHAN D., CAPLAN A.L., JENNINGS B., *"Toward Justice in Health Care,"* American Journal of Public Health 78(5): 583-8, May 1988.

[126]U.S. ROMAN CATHOLIC BISHOPS, *Resolution on Health Care Reform,* Origins 23(7):100-101, July 1, 1993.

[127]BROCK D.W., DANIELS N., *"Ethical Foundations of the Clinton Administration's Proposed Health Care System,"* Journal of the American Medical Association 271(15): 1192, April 20, 1994.

[128]BERNARDIN J.L. Cardinal, *"The Consistent Ethic of Life and Health Care Systems,"* Linacre 52:340, November 1985.

The Fundamental Answers Based on the Philosophical Foundations 143

There are two kinds of egalitarian arguments directly related to health care. A primary health care argument says that all health services should be considered special in some way, and that this fact should force everyone to be an egalitarian when it comes to health care. This does not necessarily apply in the same way to other social goods.

But there is a secondary health care argument which is directly connected with the notion of a two-tiered system. This argument says that there should be a distinction between basic and non-basic categories of care. The problem is that, since these two levels are usually connected to each other causally, there is a risk of failing to deliver the basic level equitably.[129]

Most authors who support a two or multi-tiered system of health care, base their arguments on the fact that such a system offers the greatest possibility of satisfying the different theories of justice. For example, they see that a theory such as Rawls', that promotes fair equality of opportunity, is not incompatible with a multi-tiered health care system. Even when it comes to libertarianism, which endorses universal access to health care if it can be achieved through voluntary agreements and contributions, a two-tiered system could still be compatible and offer some common ground by having society ensure equitable access to the first level of care in a voluntary fashion.[130] Still, the problems that such a system would present, as we have seen, far outweigh any attempts to present it as the only possible compromise.

3. Modern Egalitarian Thinkers and a Critique of Their Main Ideas

a. Gene Outka

For Gene Outka equality is the primary principle to be applied in the distribution of medical care. This should be based on the equal regard owed to each person and expressed in the notion of equal access. He uses

---

[129]DANIELS N., *"Equity of Access to Health Care: Some Conceptual and Ethical Issues,"* Milbank Memorial Fund Quarterly - Health and Society 60(1):75, Winter 1982.

[130]See discussion of the positive elements of a two-tiered system of health care in BEAUCHAMP T.L., CHILDRESS J.F., *Principles of Biomedical Ethics,* pp. 353-355, and in DANIELS N., *"Equity of Access to Health Care: Some Conceptual and Ethical Issues,"* Milbank Memorial Fund Quarterly - Health and Society 60(1):73-75, Winter 1982.

illness as the ground for health care, and the level of sickness as the only relevant difference. In this way he examines the usually acknowledged material principles of justice and opts for the principle of need, in support of the formal principle which defends similar treatment for similar cases, to justify his *prima facie* case for comprehensive health services for all. In his 1978 article entitled *Social Justice and Equal Access to Health Care,* he does not define what might be included in comprehensive services, although he makes reference to the whole spectrum of health services.[131] According to Outka, the principle of merit as applied to health care is ill-suited, because it is a grading conception relating to desert, and, for the most part, ill health is undeserved and beyond one's power to control or predict. We are all equally and randomly susceptible to disease. Keeping this in mind, to distribute health care on the basis of merit or desert is clearly unfair. To him, marketplace medicine which would be based on supply and demand, and supported by the principle of liberty, would also be inappropriate because of the overriding importance of health needs. The conception that best approximates a satisfactory notion of justice in health care to him, would be the one of similar treatment for similar cases, supported by the material principle of need. In other words, need is seen as the relevant difference. Outka makes an important distinction between equal consideration and equal treatment. He opts for the first one, which requires treatment as an equal based on need. He claims that equal treatment could result in an unjust distribution. He summarizes his position by saying: "In short, all persons should have equal access, as needed, without financial, geographic or other barriers, to the whole spectrum of health services."[132]

Outka's thinking and ideas could be criticized in several ways. His defense of the egalitarian goal of assurance of comprehensive health services for every person is an ideal which if not qualified and if carried to fruition could result in a disproportionate amount of society's resources to health services. Therefore he tempers equality with utility in the sense of bringing in the notion of efficiency. When the goal of equal access collides with the reality of finite resources, it is fine to discriminate by the categories of illnesses rather than by socio-economic criteria. Thus he

---

[131] OUTKA G., *"Social Justice and Equal Access to Health Care,"* in *Contemporary Issues in Bioethics,* (eds.) BEAUCHAMP T. and WALTERS L.R., p. 359.

[132] Ibid.

disagrees with a pure utility notion, but accepts one that would be consistent with his basic principles.[133] Outka selects the principles of autonomy, interpreted as respect for individuals, equality as equal regard, need as the relevant difference, and a limited application of utility to support his proposal for a just distribution of scarce medical resources in the shape of equal access.

One interpretation of Outka's thought can be that he believes that all should have equal access based on the need to a qualified level of care which a society is willing to support. One problem that could surface is that such a level could be minimal and meet very few needs, while Outka argues that the whole spectrum of health services should be available to all. Outka acknowledges that any notion of comprehensive benefits to which persons should have equal access is subject to practical restrictions which will vary from society to society, depending on the available resources at any given time.[134]

b. Robert Veatch

Robert Veatch gives priority in his writings to the principle of equality. According to his view, everyone should have access to whatever health care is necessary to provide for a level of access—or even health itself—equal to that of others.[135] He uses respect for persons as the base of his theory, and identifies ill health as the ground for health care. To him, the level of illness should be the only relevant difference when it comes to providing medical care. His conclusion is that implementing the principle of equality may at times necessitate the delivery of inequalities in health care. Justice requires a priority ordering of health goods and services so that they are made available to the people who are sickest insofar as health care can improve their health. In his 1981 book, *A Theory of Medical Ethics,* Veatch describes his notion of egalitarian justice. To him, everyone must end up over a lifetime with an equal

---

[133]OUTKA G., *"Social Justice and Equal Access to Health Care,"* in *Contemporary Issues in Bioethics,* (eds.) BEAUCHAMP T. and WALTERS L.R., p. 359.

[134]Ibid.

[135]KILNER J.F., *Health-care resources, allocation of.* Encyclopedia of Bioethics, Volume 2, (Revised Edition), Warren Thomas REICH, Editor in Chief, p. 1069.

amount of net welfare or have a chance for that welfare.[136]

Health care is different as compared to other human needs in the sense that it varies among individuals, but Veatch does not support the opinion that health care is discontinuous with other social goods. He argues that health care is not more basic than shelter or food; all being essential to human survival at least up to some minimum level for subsistence.[137] He recognizes that individuals have the right to remain sick and cannot be forced to avail themselves of the opportunity to seek care, but those individuals who can be shown to be directly responsible for their own ill health would assume some responsibility for the cost of health care.

Veatch employs in his analysis the level of another person's health as a standard. The problem arises when one asks how is this standard to be determined and by whom? Is a health index to be established reflecting the average evolving from measuring the sickest and the healthiest members of society? These levels could be altered, lowering the level of the healthiest members and raising the level of the sickest. This approach would resemble the aggregate approach of the utilitarians. Veatch acknowledges the possibility that the health of all could fall below optimal levels, but if this becomes necessary to raise the level of health of the worst off, it would be required as far as justice is concerned. The assumption is that a ranking order of health can be made.

The system developed by Veatch is one in which the welfare of each individual takes absolute priority over any notion of the common good or the social entity as a community. Veatch does not ignore the existence of a moral community, yet it is the individual members who get consideration regardless of the effects on the community as such. The welfare of the community is at least potentially sacrificed to the good of all the individuals. Veatch does not allow sufficiently for the real differences among men in spite of their shared humanity.

c. *Bernard Williams*

Another modern egalitarian ethicist is Bernard Williams. He believes that the enterprise of trying to reduce our conflicts and the attempt to legislate to remove moral uncertainty by the development of a philosophical ethical theory is a misguided one. In his 1979 article

---

[136]VEATCH R., *A Theory of Medical Ethics*, p. 265.

[137]Ibid., p. 271.

Conflict of Values, Williams affirms that since conflict is not a logical affliction of our thought, it must be a mistake to regard a need to eliminate conflict as a purely rational demand of the kind that applies to a theoretical system. Since it is not a purely rational demand, he argues that the need to reduce conflict and to rationalize our moral thinking has a more social and personal basis.[138] The public order must be adequately related to private sentiment. All individuals have projects and certain ideals which humanize them and give significance to life.[139]

In his 1971 article entitled *The Idea of Equality,* Williams wrestled with two major conceptions: equality of respect and equality of opportunity. He supports both of these notions, and attempted to ground them at the same time, even when these are two notions that tend to militate and pull against each other. Both relate to different aspects of equality, but, according to Williams, one cannot be abandoned in favor of the other. He attempted to preserve the maximum of each one without impinging unduly on the other.

He began the article by trying to ground the notion of equal respect owed each person in consideration of the common humanity each one shares with others and the moral capabilities of human beings. While this notion may not offer sufficient grounding by itself for promoting equal respect, nevertheless, it is not trivial. Individual human beings do in fact share common traits, such as the ability to communicate, the use of tools, common life in society, and experience of pain and affection.[140]

Having developed the ground for respect owed to each, Williams linked this with the concept of equality in two ways: first, he pointed out the existing social and political inequalities among individuals and the need to go behind the titles and abstract individuals from the structures of inequality by taking the human point of view. This would consider not only their function in society but their life goals and purposes; and secondly, the fact that an individual's awareness that his role in society results, at least in part, from social arrangements, and is either enhanced or diminished by them has an impact on political equality and requires that

---

[138]WILLIAMS B., *"Conflict of Values,"* in *The Idea of Freedom,* (ed.) Alan Ryan, pp. 230-231.

[139]HAKSAR V., *Equality, Liberty and Perfectionism,* p. 121.

[140]WILLIAMS B., *The Idea of Equality,* in *Justice and Equality,* (ed.) Hugo A. BEDAU, p. 120.

the ideal of a hierarchical society be abandoned.

The second aspect of equality, namely equality of opportunity, was considered by Williams under the notion of equality in unequal circumstances and the distribution of goods in situations where such inequalities are relevant. While many argue that the concept of justice or fairness is more appropriate in such contexts, Williams claimed that there is some basis for the concept of equality even in these cases.[141] The notion leads Williams, not to argue for absolute equality of access to or distribution of goods, but rather to the right of equality of opportunity and to the functioning of that right.

Williams differentiated between two types of inequalities and the goods demanded by them. These are inequality of need and inequality of merit. Both of them require relevant reasons, but they differ in what constitutes relevance. In the case of need, there is a presumption that those having the need do, in fact, desire the needed goods and that a particular need in itself constitutes a reason for receiving the good in question. In the case of merit, though, there is a difference since not all have the ability to merit the good, yet necessarily desire it, while some may desire the good without the ability and the effort required to merit it.

Williams argued for equality of opportunity in relation to the allocation on the basis of merit of certain goods, that are generally desired by people, that are earned, but which are limited by nature, or require that certain conditions be met. This is not merely a pro-forma equality of opportunity, which is more verbal than real, but one which is genuine and truly operative. According to Williams "this notion requires that a limited good shall in fact be allocated on grounds which do not *a priori* exclude any section of those who desire it."[142] He expands on this thought when he says:

> A system of allocation will fall short of equality of opportunity if the allocation of the good in question in fact works out unequally or disproportionately between different sections of society, if the unsuccessful sections are under a disadvantage which could be removed by further reform

---

[141] WILLIAMS B., *The Idea of Equality*, in *Justice and Equality*, (ed.) Hugo A. BEDAU, p. 127.

[142] Ibid., p. 131.

The Fundamental Answers Based on the Philosophical Foundations **149**

or social action.[143]

When the different pulls of the varying notions of equality are recognized, there is a temptation to abandon one of the notions—the one of respect or the one of opportunity. Williams says that this would be a serious mistake:

> A highly rational and efficient application of the idea of equal opportunity, unmitigated by other considerations, could lead to a quite inhuman society . . . if it worked . . . which is unlikely. An ideal of equality of respect that made no contact with such things as the economic needs of society for certain skills and human desire for some sorts of prestige, would be condemned to a futile Utopianism and to having no rational effect on the distribution of goods, positions and power that would inevitably proceed.[144]

Williams said that particular needs in themselves constitute sufficient reason for receiving the good in question. One such need is for health care. He claimed in the article that we have a situation in which those whose needs are the same are not receiving the same treatment, though the needs are the ground of the treatment. This is an irrational situation.[145]

Williams does not provide a complete ethical theory. He does not define a health care system that could evolve from the principles he develops. His notion about the desires of individuals as the basis for owing respect offers particular problems, since there are other notions which would explain this better as for example the notion of the individual as a center of freedom and self-determination with intrinsic dignity. The notion of desires and projects could be criticized on the basis that it is possible that something other than these could give primary motivation to life. Beliefs, love, and even self preservation can be mentioned as examples, just to name a few.

Williams is concerned with conditions of inequality for which the individual cannot be held responsible. For the sake of consistency, this

---

[143]WILLIAMS B., *The Idea of Equality*, in *Justice and Equality*, (ed.) Hugo A. BEDAU, p. 133.

[144]Ibid., pp. 136-137.

[145]Ibid., p. 128.

would require that he would hold that inequalities resulting from behavior for which a person could be held accountable, would not give rise to the same claim.

d. John Rawls

To conclude this section on egalitarianism, and actually to do the same for this whole chapter, it is important to consider the philosophical work of John Rawls. We have intentionally left Rawls for the end of this section since his contribution to the theme of justice, and his attempt to develop a theory to promote it, carries special significance.

There are a few things that would be important to mention before we discuss directly his ideas. First of all, it is difficult to categorize him within any of the above-mentioned philosophical systems. Usually Rawls has been described as a Contractarian, or in other words from the tradition based on the "social contract." He argues that justice might be conceived of as roughly what everyone would agree to be the rules of society. These rules would not necessarily guarantee each person an equal share of everything. What they would do, under certain conditions as we will see, is assure that the worst-off in society (who might turn out to be you) would not be in a really terrible position.

Secondly, Rawls does not discuss health care needs directly in his theory of justice. Some authors think that perhaps, due to the unique aspects of health care, he deliberately leaves consideration of this theme out of his theory.[146]

Finally, it is clear that contractarians would not risk inadequate access to health care since health care is definitely a centrally important primary social good, comparable to freedom and the social bases of self respect. Because of this, they would clearly reject a utilitarian distribution, since maximizing total or average health care would not guarantee each person the necessary or even minimal health care. Rawls solution in this matter, as we will see, is to guarantee each member of society, no matter his position or background, an equal right to the most extensive health services the society allows. Since Rawls theory in many respects is strongly egalitarian, we will include him in this section, knowing well that part of our critique of Rawls will deal with the inegalitarian aspects of his theory.

---

[146]DANIELS N., *"Rights to Health Care and Distributive Justice: Programmatic Worries,"* Journal of Medicine and Philosophy 4(2):181, June 1979.

With painstaking effort, Rawls attempts to devise a detailed theory of justice that could offer a critique and an alternative to utilitarianism. In his main work entitled *A Theory of Justice,* written in 1971, there are many different components that blend together in his theory: a deontological approach, the already mentioned social contract theory, a rights-based theory, Kantian influence, pure procedural justice, and a hypothetical situation.

His theory is grounded in his perception of and assumptions about man and social relationships. His starting point is the notion of equality predicated on the equal moral worth of persons, and equal distribution of social goods based on the fact that it is not reasonable for a person under what he calls the veil of ignorance to expect more than an equal share nor to agree to less.[147] However, scarcity is a reality, and claims on available resources conflict because of the different conceptions of good which human beings pursue. He also recognizes that natural contingencies, which in Rawls' mind are not deserved, create inequalities which he believes are inevitable. Such contingencies cannot ground a conception of justice in a well-ordered society. Therefore, principles of justice are necessary in order to regulate inequalities and to adjust the profound and long lasting effects of social, natural, and historical contingencies particularly since these contingencies combined with inequalities generate tendencies that, when left to themselves, are sharply at odds with the freedom and equality appropriate for a well-ordered society.[148]

Abandoning the teleological approach of maximizing the good, Rawls moves to the model of the social contract in the Lockean tradition, which he believes offers a system of justice far superior to that of utilitarianism. His greatest concern is to present a system that would be acceptable for the distribution of rights and duties, benefits and burdens to members of a well-ordered society that nullifies the accidents of natural contingencies. Therefore, the basic structure of society that determines such distribution, rather than individual transactions, is the primary subject of justice, for this structure has profound influence on the members of society as well as in shaping their aspirations and desires.

---

[147]RAWLS J., *A Theory of Justice,* p. 150.

[148]RAWLS J., *"A Kantian Conception of Equality,"* Cambridge Review 96:2225, p. 95, February 1975.

152　　　　Health Care and the Common Good

Rawls uses the social contract model to arrive at principles on which to establish a just society. These are principles that persons who are free and rational, and with a concern to further their own interests, would accept in an initial position of equality as defining the fundamental terms of their association. Such principles would regulate all further agreements, specify appropriate social cooperation and the form of government. This way of regarding the principles of justice, Rawls calls justice as fairness.[149]

This notion of justice as fairness consists of two parts: An interpretation of the initial situation, including the problems of the choice posed there, and a set of principles which, it is argued, would be agreed to. Such principles would be justified by the fact that they would be chosen by free, equal, rational persons in an original situation of fairness. In such a way, Rawls theory is essentially one of rational choice. He develops, in order to accomplish this, a hypothetical situation of the individual under a veil of ignorance. This is what he has to say: "Among the essential features of this situation is that no one knows his place in society, his class position, or social status, nor does anyone know his fortune in the distribution of natural assets and abilities, his intelligence, strength and the like."[150]

About half way through his book *A Theory of Justice,* Rawls presents his third and final formulation of his related principles: "First Principle: Each person is to have an equal right to the most extensive total system of equal basic liberties compatible with a similar system of liberty for all. Second Principle: Social and economic inequalities are to be arranged so that they are both: a) to the greater benefit of the least advantaged (also called the maximin rule), consistent with the joint savings principle (which provides for fair investment in the interests of future generations), and b) attached to offices and positions open to all under conditions of fair equality of opportunity."[151]

Rawls supplements these principles with two priority rules and a general conception. The first rule indicates a lexical ordering of the principles whereby liberty can be restricted only for the sake of liberty. The second rule provides that the second principle is lexically prior to that of efficiency and to that of maximizing the sum of advantages, and fair

---

[149]RAWLS J., *A Theory of Justice,* p. 11.

[150]Ibid., p. 12.

[151]Ibid., pp. 302-303.

The Fundamental Answers Based on the Philosophical Foundations 153

opportunity (b) is prior to the difference principle (a).[152]

The general conception of justice reads as follows: "All social primary goods—liberty and opportunity, income and wealth, and the bases of self respect—are to be distributed equally unless an unequal distribution of any or all of these goods is to the advantage of the least favored."[153] The standard ultimately chosen by Rawls in the two principles reflects strong Kantian, as well as egalitarian, influence. Justice as fairness relates two principles which are liberty, as of equal basic liberties of citizenship, and equality, as in the social and economic arrangements unless inequalities are justified.

Rawls acknowledges that social and economic goods vary in the natural lottery. Some people are more advantaged than others in terms of family background and economic stability. This is inevitable and any effort at redistribution would impinge on the integrity of the person. However, using equality as the starting point of a just society, Rawls develops the second principle in which he attempts to reconcile the notion of equality with the natural contingent advantages enjoyed by some in the society, and to preclude the possibility that these advantages will be used to exploit the less-favored members. The natural distribution of these goods is a fact, neither just nor unjust. However, the way in which institutions deal with this fact can result in the accomplishment of justice or injustice.

The first part of the second principle, which is usually referred to as the difference principle, regulates the distribution of social and economic goods. Each is entitled to a fair share of these goods, but this is not interpreted to mean an equal division among the members. Inequalities are permitted if justified. And how can they be justified? Starting from the concept of an equal distribution of wealth and income, Rawls argues that inequalities which work to the benefit of all, especially the least advantaged, are allowed.[154] Such inequalities can provide incentives for greater productivity, from which all can profit.

There are some elements of this process that are on somewhat shaky ground. The index of primary social goods, for example, might be considered arbitrary and omits some goods that might be included, such

---

[152]RAWLS J., *A Theory of Justice*, pp. 302-303.

[153]Ibid., p. 303.

[154]Ibid., p. 151.

as health care. The predominant concern is with the least advantaged—which are difficult to identify in a complex society—almost to the exclusion of the rights and needs of other members of society. The maximin rule, for example, in situations of uncertainty can bring about results that are counter-intuitive. Let us assume the following choice of situations relating to the unequal distribution of a particular social good. In situation "A" the more advantaged gain 80 units while the less advantaged gain 5; in situation "B" the more advantaged gain 1000 units whereas the less advantaged gain 10 units. Following the maximin rule in which alternative choices are ranked by their worst possible outcomes and the best of the worst possible outcomes is chosen, situation "B" would be chosen, even though the disparity in the distribution is far greater than in situation "A", with the better off realizing a significant gain, balanced by a slightly smaller gain for the less advantaged. Many would view this conclusion reached under Rawls' notion of justice as ethically unacceptable.

The whole notion of Rawls ideal observer has been greatly criticized as well. The sort of individualism that is exemplified in such a notion is antithetical to any communal or social reality. In this ideal observer under the veil of ignorance it is believed by Rawls that every judgment must be applicable to all people because it does not recognize any morally relevant differences grounded in social life. This figure of the ideal observer ignores some of the most important dimensions of ethics, drawing deeply from modern individualism and distorting both the social and personal elements. This theory does not have sufficient place for the social dimension of life. Following traditions that are skeptical to all social ties, this notion perpetuates the American preoccupation with individualism.

Rawls shares with Nozick the same point of departure, which assumes the plurality and distinctness of persons, or separate existences. Both assume that the task is the formation of society, and the task of justice is one of inventing rules by which society will be properly ordered. Rawls' vision is certainly more egalitarian, but their tacit agreement is more important than their divergent conclusions. Each one of them considers social relationships as a choice, an option, and a convenience. Choices to enter a social arrangement presume no previous relatedness among human beings, no web of social nurture or sustenance. As human beings we are in our essential nature, isolated selves, on our own, and we may either choose to be social or remain in our individual state of nature. In the words of a contemporary author: "Rawls has forgotten that moral awareness starts in the middle, in the midst of relationships, and the first task is not to reconstruct a mythic beginning but to describe accurately what we find in the present."[155]

In summary, it is evident that all the theories discussed above attempt to offer *the* solution for the problems that health care in the United States is facing. All of them, in one way or another, focus on the problems related to access to the health care system. None of the theories, though, deals with the health care issues in a way that the social dimensions of the problem are addressed. To do this, the whole notion of societal obligation regarding health care would have to be developed, thus, as has been mentioned above, there would be a need to show on what principle or principles this obligation is based. To spell out these principles is the scope and purpose of the next section.

---

[155] CHURCHILL L.R., *Rationing Health Care in America,* p. 58.

UNIT THREE

A CATHOLIC THEORY OF JUSTICE

The aim of this section is to develop a theory of justice based upon Catholic principles that would show the bases of a societal obligation to provide universal access to health care. These can be later applied to the present health care delivery system in the United States. In order to do this it is important first of all to clearly state that by saying "Catholic principles" there is no intention of ignoring the fact that the principles to be discussed have a much richer and broader historical past than what is denoted by the term "Catholic." The Catholic tradition has incorporated elements of philosophical theories such as the Aristotelian via St. Thomas Aquinas, and has been influenced at certain points by others, such as the philosophy of John Locke on property. At the same time we would like to acknowledge that the Catholic Church, as will be shown, has been one of the institutions responsible for continuously bringing up these principles and challenging the national community to address the health care problems in a systemic way and not simply superficially.

To develop a theory of justice that would rely on Catholic principles and appeal to the national community in matters of health care delivery there is a need to discuss two very important concepts: the common good and distributive justice. We will show how general justice, or "legal" justice, in Thomist terminology, is not absolutely self-sufficient. Its regulation of relations between individual persons is mediated through the common good. That mediation is then made concrete or, in other words, applied, through the implementation of distributive justice.

This unit will expound on the two principles of the common good and distributive justice by showing for each one, first, the historical development of each principle; secondly, the teaching of the Catholic Church's magisterium on the subject through the main official documents of the Church; and thirdly, the present day debate concerning each topic. In other words, chapter five will be dedicated to the principle of the common good, chapter six to the principle of distributive justice, and chapter seven, which will be the final chapter of this unit, will deal with a proposal of what a Catholic theory of justice would look like by utilizing the principles just introduced.

FIVE

THE COMMON GOOD

A. A HISTORICAL SURVEY OF THE COMMON GOOD

Plato addressed the notion of the common good in his political theory, which he developed in close connection with his ethics. For the Greek mentality, life was essentially communal. It was lived out in the city-state and could not be conceived apart from the *polis*. No human being could be perfectly good unless in some way connected to the state. It was only in and through society that the good life was even possible for man, and for Plato, society meant the city-state.[1]

Thus for Plato the common good was identified with the virtue of citizenry. For him the *polis* had primacy over the citizen since it was the first one that was divinely sanctioned by Hermes' gifts of justice and reverence. An individual human being had dignity and worth only by living as part of a political community recognized as being intrinsically just. This type of society based on just laws, namely a society like Athens, was natural for Plato. Thus the common good was the virtuous life of the whole community as carried out by the state.

Aristotle had a dynamic conception of nature. For him all things were in motion, only resting when they attained their aim. All things had natural tendencies toward something, and this "something" was what Aristotle called "the good." In the thought of Aristotle the mind was led to conceive of the common good as the end of a tendency or purpose. The common good was the fulfillment unto which our human society tends. Wisdom was needed to discern such point of satisfaction. To live well meant to aim at that point for oneself and for the community.[2] In other words, for Aristotle, every human activity, every human question, every human custom aimed at some good since "the good" or "a good" was

---

[1] COPLESTON F., *A History of Philosophy*, Vol. I, Part I, p. 249.

[2] NOVAK M., *Free Persons and the Common Good*, p. 22.

precisely that at which human beings typically aimed. Due to human nature, all persons had certain aims and goals that made them move by nature to an specific *telos*. Aristotle argued against identifying such good with money, honor, or pleasure. He gave the good the name of *eudaimonia* but then did not develop clearly what was the content of such good. It was through the virtues that human beings accomplished the good, and the lack of virtues would only help in frustrating the motion to an specific end.

In his most important ethical work, the *Nicomachean Ethics,* there is a magisterial and unique tendency of the writer to speak as more than merely the voice of one person. Whether the book was written and dedicated by Aristotle to his son Nicomachus, or whether this last one was the real author, as some have claimed, consistently the questions are posed as "What do *we* say?" instead of "What do *I* say?" Who is this "we" in whose name Aristotle writes? In his answers the great philosopher was not trying to invent an account of the virtues but to articulate an account of what was already assumed to be a part of the thought of an educated Athenian citizen. He expressed himself in the rational voice of the best citizen of the best city state, since it was in the unique political form in which the virtues of human living were best exhibited.[3] Political society existed for the sake of noble actions and not of mere companionship.[4]

Aristotle did not limit himself to mention the common good as the fulfillment toward which human society tended. For him there was a primacy of the common good that had to be taken into account. Even when the end was the same for the individual and the state, still the good of the state was a greater and more complete good, both to attain and to preserve. This was the focus of the study of politics: the common good. What is clear is that this did not mean that the individual was only a means or an instrument of the community. Aristotle was not a materialist since he had a very clear sense of the divine and spiritual elements in the person. He could stress simultaneously the roles of the flesh, the senses, and the human passions. The human person was a unity and not a duality, as others had tended to express. The human person was for him a "reasoning

---

[3] MACINTYRE A., *After Virtue: A Study in Moral Theology,* pp. 147-8.

[4] *The Politics,* Bk. 3, Ch. 9 in MCKEON R., *The Basic Works of Aristotle,* pp. 1188-89.

animal," and "embodied spirit."[5]

For Aristotle the *polis*, or the political association, aimed at the highest, most comprehensive good. In his book on *Politics* he said:

> Any *polis* which is truly so called, and is not merely one in name, must devote itself to the end of encouraging goodness. Otherwise, a political association sinks into a mere alliance, which only differs in space from other forms of alliances where the members live apart; and the law is only a convention (...) and has no real power to make the citizens good and just.[6]

A little later in the same chapter he added: "The end of the state is the good life, and [the institutions of social life] are means to that end."[7] It is only as participants in political association that human beings could realize their nature and fulfill their highest ends.

Cicero spoke of the commonwealth as the "people's affair."[8] The people to him was not any group of human beings brought together in any sort of way but "an assemblage of people in large numbers associated in agreement with respect to justice and a partnership for the common good."[9] In his work *On the Commonwealth*, Cicero put on the lips of Scipio—the most distinguished Roman citizen of his time—that the original cause of this coming together of human beings was "not so much weakness, as a kind of social instinct natural to man, [since] human kind is not solitary, nor do its members live lives of isolated roving; but it is so constituted that, even if it possessed the greatest plenty of material comforts, [it would nevertheless be impelled by its nature to live in social

---

[5] NOVAK M., *Free Persons and the Common Good*, p. 23.

[6] *The Politics*, Bk. 3, Ch. 9 in MCKEON R., *The Basic Works of Aristotle*, p. 1188.

[7] Ibid., p. 1189.

[8] CICERO, *On the Commonwealth*, (Sabine/Smith translation, 1929), p. 129.

[9] CICERO, *On the Commonwealth*, 1, 25, 39. Cfr. HOLLENBACH D., *The Common Good Revisited*, Theological Studies 50: 80, 1989.

groups.]"[10] Speaking about the republic of Rome as it existed fifty years before the beginnings of Christianity, Cicero had already concluded that it was through their own faults and not by accident that they no longer had the substance of a commonwealth but only the apparent form of one. It had long betrayed the true notion of what a commonwealth should be.

Four centuries later Augustine in his work *The City of God*, which was written against the background of the barbarian invasion of the Roman Empire, discussed the definition of a people or a commonwealth given by Cicero through Scipio. In response to the accusation that the expansion of the Christian faith had brought about the downfall of the empire, he took the sensible approach of asking about the conditions that had to be present in order for a republic or a people to exist at all. In Book II he acknowledged this Scipionic definition and then promised that later on in his book he would demonstrate that according to this definition of Cicero, there was never a true people in Rome, and thus, Rome was never a state or commonwealth. This was so, continued Augustine following Cicero's mentality, since true justice never had a place in Rome, and Scipio and Cicero had made an agreement about justice as an essential condition to the existence of a state or a people. For Augustine himself these ideas deserved some corrections. Even though he was critically trying to defend Christianity against those who blamed it as the cause of the downfall of the empire, he was not blind to see that to claim that Rome was never a republic, was extreme. So he added that if a more feasible definition of a republic was accepted, it could be granted that there was a republic of some kind in Rome, even when it had been much better administered by ancient Romans than by their modern counterparts.[11]

It is in book XIX where Augustine fulfilled his promise to return to this topic of the Scipionic definitions, and acknowledged the fact that clearly there were problems in the Roman empire. He expressed it as follows:

> A republic cannot be administered without justice. Where, therefore, there is no true justice there can be no assemblage of men associated by a common acknowledgment of right, and therefore there can

---

[10]CICERO, *On the Commonwealth*, (Sabine/Smith translation, 1929), p. 129.

[11]ST. AUGUSTINE, *The City of God*, 2, 21. Cfr. DEANE H.A., *The Political and Social Ideas of St. Augustine*, p. 118.

be no people, as defined by Scipio or Cicero; and if no people, then no weal of the people, but only some promiscuous multitude unworthy of the name of people. Consequently . . . most certainly it follows that there is no republic where there is no justice.[12]

Augustine argued that *de facto* consensus on a notion of justice was necessary but not sufficient in order to create a true republic. For this to happen there had to be a social and cultural agreement among the people that would be centered on what was truly just, namely the common good. For Augustine this was only fully possible in *the city of God*. Actually for Augustine to make civil society the bearer of all of our hopes for happiness and fulfillment was a kind of idolatry.

His revised definition of a *res publica* was the following: "a people is an assemblage of reasonable beings bound together by a common agreement as to the objects of their love."[13] Following this definition it can be said that the quality of life of human beings associated in a community or republic would be directly proportional to the qualities of the loves they shared in common. There would be a superiority of societies united by great and noble loves and dedicated to standards of justice over those with lower goals and cultural values.

It must be stated that Augustine did not identify civil society with Babylon nor the Church with the city of God. There were elements of the city of God in all dimensions of civil society and in the political community as well.

The first work specifically on the common good in Europe appeared at the turn of the fourteenth century in Florence. It was written by Remigio de'Girolami and entitled *De bono communi*. This work took a different perspective from the more accepted principle which stated that the commonwealth remained subordinate to the person's supernatural destiny, even when in the natural order it was prior to the individual. Remigio de'Girolami's thesis was that Christian virtue required before anything else that the person be a good citizen. This approximated more than anybody else before him, Aristotle's position on public virtue. By doing this, Remigio did not intend to establish a secular state, but, on the

---

[12] ST. AUGUSTINE, *The City of God*, 19, 21. Cfr. DEANE H.A., *The Political and Social Ideas of St. Augustine*, p. 119.

[13] Ibid., 19, 24. Cfr. HOLLENBACH D., *The Common Good Revisited*, Theological Studies 50: 83, 1989.

contrary, to convey that only in a Christian community could civil society find the spiritual support it needed for its survival.[14] He differed from Aristotle in that Remigio conceived the common good as the well-being of a spiritual mystical body rather than the realization of an immanently human potential as expressed by the Philosopher.

For Thomas Aquinas a concern for the common good of the political community was a constitutive element of Christian virtue as such. In the case of Augustine and his contemporaries, a doomed empire offered little opportunity for the practice of civic virtue. In Thomas' time, the notion of a Christian republic was as far on its way to earthly realization as it would ever be in history. In his *Summa Theologiae* Aquinas gave three meanings to the common good. It was first applied to a "quasi-collective group or organic whole; second, to a political and juridical community; and third, to God because of his comprehensive final causality."[15] For Thomas, the full common good was God's own self. Human beings achieved their ultimate fulfillment, their good, only by being united with God, a bond that united them to one another and indeed with the whole created order.[16] The common good as applied to a political and juridical community was the proper interest of political philosophy. This would be defined as the good estate of the state's civil community, responsibly shared by those who belong to it, namely citizens.[17]

For Thomas the capacity for community was a positive perfection of personality. The dignity of the human person could be realized only in community, and a genuine community could exist only where the dignity of persons was secured. In other words, for him personhood and community were mutually implicating realities. But there was a second factor that formed part of Thomas' understanding as well. As finite and limited persons, human beings had needs and deficiencies. He could see

---

[14]DUPRÉ L., *The Common Good and the Open Society*, p. 173, in DOUGLAS R.B., HOLLENBACH D. (eds.), *Catholicism and Liberalism: Contributions to American Public Philosophy*, Cambridge University Press, 1994.

[15]Words of Thomas Gilby, O.P. as quoted in NOVAK M., *Free Persons and the Common Good*, pp. 26-7.

[16]ST. THOMAS AQUINAS, *Summa Theologiae* I-II, q.19, a. 10.

[17]These topics are covered by Aquinas in his commentaries on Aristotle's Ethics and Politics, and also in the I-II, qq. 90-97.

that there was a need of other persons and the larger society in order to thrive or even to exist at all. These needs included not only material goods as food and shelter, but also higher goods such as moral and intellectual education. This two-fold foundation of the social dimension of human beings was the basis for his understanding of the analogical nature of the common good.[18]

There can be no doubt about the importance which Thomas attributed to the consideration of the intrinsic order and the "common good" of the cosmos. He established this principally to demonstrate the existence of divine providence against the Greco-Arabian tendencies towards necessitarianism. Nevertheless, when he compared the intellectual substance with the universe, he clearly stated that intellectual creatures, even though like all creatures, were ordained to the perfection of the created whole, were willed and governed for their own sakes. A human person was not a mere cog in the machinery of the world, and God took care of each one for his or her own sake. This in no way prevented each human creature from being related, first to God, and then to the order of creation of which he or she was the most noble constitutive part. In this way Thomas established the doctrine of the primacy of the common good in what related to the practical order in the life of the state. It was when considering this primacy, that the distinction between the private and common good could be found. Aquinas took every opportunity to repeat the saying of Aristotle that the good of the whole was "more divine" than the goods of the parts.[19] The heated debates that have come about due to discrepancies in interpretations of Aquinas,[20] in no way obscure Thomas' belief that spiritual beings related first and foremost to God rather than to the common good immanent in the universe. But for human beings, this

---

[18]HOLLENBACH D., *The Common Good Revisited*, Theological Studies 50:86, 1989.

[19]MARITAIN J., *The Person and the Common Good*, pp. 18-19.

[20]The issue reemerged in a dispute between two factions of Thomists during the 1940's. One position, led by Charles De Koninck, claimed that Thomas granted the common good a primacy over individual goods. On the other side I.T. Eschmann, O.P., strongly defended a position that the common good, though superior to any particular good pursued by the individual and though a *bonum honestum* in its own right, must nevertheless remain subordinate to the *summum bonum* of contemplation which, by its very nature, is individual.

transcendent Good was itself a common one. This highest of goods should not be pursued individually but in community, since it was precisely through the immanent common good of civil society that individuals acquired the virtues necessary to pursue the transcendent Good, whom we call God.[21]

In what relates to the common good, both Augustine and Aquinas had as their premise the true nature of human beings. In their writings it was clear that to deny this nature was equivalent to negate a proper consideration of the connection of human beings to society as a whole.

At the beginning of what is considered as the modern times, Thomas Hobbes (1588-1679) attempted in his work *Leviathan,* published in 1651, a systematic answer to the problems posed by the social changes of his time and the rise of the mathematical sciences. It was a brilliant attempt to conceptualize the developing form of association called the nation state. Influenced by the teachings of Galileo, Hobbes tried to reduce civil society to its simplest elements, and explained political behavior in terms of an underlying mechanical ground-plan. What emerged from this was a justification of government based on a crude naturalistic ethical theory deduced from the human desire for peace and self-preservation. In this system, human beings were like natural machines, while the *Leviathan* was an artificial one. The government in a commonwealth was meant to remedy a human nature that had a tendency to lead to anarchy unless laws were established. Laws did not develop naturally since it was authority backed by force that made a law. Organized society was united by a common power meant to "defend [humans] from the invasion of foreigners, and the injuries of one another, and thereby to secure them in such sort, as that by their own industry, and by the fruits of the earth, they may nourish themselves and live contentedly."[22]

For Hobbes a common power did not mean the same thing as a common good or something more than the aggregate sum of private goods. Actually for Hobbes, the nature of man being what it was, "the setting forth of public land, or of any certain revenue for the commonwealth,

---

[21]DUPRÉ L., *The Common Good and the Open Society,* pp. 174-5, in DOUGLAS R.B., HOLLENBACH D. (eds.), *Catholicism and Liberalism: Contributions to American Public Philosophy,* Cambridge University Press, 1994.

[22]HOBBES T., *Leviathan.*, I, 17. Edited by OAKESHOTT, M. p. 132.

[was] in vain, and [tended] to the dissolution of government. . ."²³

John Locke (1632-1704) saw the common good as definable in terms of the private good. The source of value in society for him was private. Human labor was mixed with a particular object in a way that gave value to the object and made it the private good of a person. He acknowledged that God gave the world to human beings in common, and no human being had an original exclusive private dominion over the common fruits of the world. Nevertheless, every human being had a "property" in his own "person". The labor and work of his hands was proper to that person. Anything that a person removed from the state that nature had provided, by mixing his labor with it, became the property of that person. Locke had one limiting condition on how much a human being could make his or her own. For him, the same law of nature that gave the possibility of private property, also placed boundaries on that property, so that it would be no more than what a person could use before it could spoil. Whatever could or would reach such a stage of decay, belonged to others.²⁴

Thoughts like this may have motivated some modern authors to challenge the notion which said that Locke was a philosopher of atomistic individualism who considered merely private interests. They claim that his philosophy was more concerned with rights and not merely self-interest. This last notion represents in their minds a degradation of the politics of Locke and of the political theory behind the founding of the United States.²⁵ Whether this is a viable defense of Locke is debatable.

---

²³HOBBES T., *Leviathan.*, II, 24. Edited by OAKESHOTT, M. p. 187.

²⁴LOCKE J., *An Essay Concerning the True Original Extent and End of Civil Government,* Chapter V, in *Great Books of the Western World,* edited by HUTCHINS, ROBERT MAYNARD Vol. 35, pp. 30-31.

²⁵One of these authors is Michael Novak who argues that "Locke's political teaching is not one of self-interest but one of rights." For him "Lockean politics include a conception of the common good and a conception of civil society as more than an aggregate of atomistic individuals. His understanding of human nature exhibits a profound appreciation of human sociality, and families and churches play crucial roles in Lockean civil society. Locke teaches not a narrowly calculating selfishness but a set of decent moral virtues. Locke refers repeatedly to the common good in his Second Treatise. For him, the body politic is to be thought of as a whole, in whose name individuals may be obliged by law to sacrifice their own interests." Quoted from NOVAK M., *Free Persons and the*

What is certain is that Locke believed that the source of value in society was private and never coming from a collective understanding. Any common possession is simply waiting until someone could claim it as private while observing the Lockean restriction. The only reason for surplus goods to revert to being a common possessions was in order that someone else could claim them.

During the period of the Enlightenment the notion of the common good began to change dramatically since society began to be regarded merely as contractual rather than responding to the true nature of humanity. The ends of society were said to be determined by self interest.

For Jeremy Bentham (1748-1832) the meaning of the common good was derived from a notion of private interest. As he developed his utilitarian philosophy influenced by David Hume, he had this to say about the notion of community:

> The interest of the community is one of the most general expressions that can occur in the phraseology of morals: no wonder that the meaning of it is often lost. When it has a meaning, it is this. The community is a fictitious *body,* composed of the individual persons who are considered as constituting as it were its *members.* The interest of the community then is, what?—the sum of the interests of the several members who compose it.
> It is in vain to talk of the interest of the community, without understanding what is the interest of the individual. A thing is said to promote the interest, or to be *for* the interest, of an individual, when it tends to add to the sum total of his pleasures: or, what comes to the same thing, to diminish the sum total of his pains.[26]

By the middle of the eighteenth century the notion of the common good was modeled completely on that of the private good, meaning by this mostly the material goods that human beings could accumulate. Adam Smith (1723-1790) published his most important work *The Wealth of Nations* in 1776. It had taken him ten years to write the book which is better described as the work that summarized a new European consciousness. In it he assumes that there was a natural order in the universe which made all individuals strive for self-interest and in such a way contribute to the social good. Government was superfluous except to

---

Common Good, p. 163.

[26]BENTHAM J., *The Principles of Morals and Legislation,* Chap. I, IV, V., p. 3.

preserve order and to perform routine functions. The best government was the one who governed the least, just as the best economic policy was the one that arouse from the spontaneity and unhindered actions of individuals. He was reacting to the strong controls of feudalism and mercantilist structures and the need to remove these constraints.[27]

The Wealth of Nations dealt with the topics having to do with the public interest in economic terms. He based his differentiation of people in any society by the way they made their income. In the conclusion of the first book he mentioned that there were three "great, original and constituent orders of every civilized society, from whose revenue that of every other order is ultimately derived."[28] The first group was the landowners. Their interest was strictly and inseparably connected with the general interest of the whole society. They received rent pay for their land which created a situation of ease and security for them which often would make them ignore and understand the consequences of a public regulation.

The second group was the laborers who lived and worked for wages. Their interest as well was connected with the interests of society. Their wages were high when the demand for their labor increased or when the quantity of people hired during the year increased. When society declined, it brought laborers even below its level of decline.

The third group was the employers who hired the laborers. They were the ones who lived by profit. Yet the rate of profit does not rise with the prosperity of the society. On the contrary, it tends to be naturally low in rich countries and very high in poor ones. This was why the interest of this third order was not connected like the first two to the general interest of society. The interest of dealers could be different and even opposite to that of the general public. Adam Smith warned the public that any legislative proposal which originated with the profit makers should be looked upon with suspicion since their interest was usually in deceiving and even oppressing the public.[29] Adam Smith did not see the common good as the sum total of private interests, he could see moral persuasion as the only way to solve the injustices that could result from the consideration of private interests as priority.

---

[27]SMITH A., *An Inquiry Into the Nature and Causes of The Wealth of Nations,* (Edited by CANNAN E.), pp. vii-x.

[28]Ibid., p. 248.

[29]Ibid., pp. 248-50.

B. THE COMMON GOOD IN THE MAGISTERIUM OF THE CATHOLIC CHURCH

The New Catholic Encyclopedia declares that "[i]t is simply impossible to define the common good in a final way irrespective of the changing social conditions."[30] This is clearly so, especially in this pluralistic age where there is a differentiation among modern institutions which have been assigned their own proper autonomy. This was not the case during the medieval period in which the church was not adequately differentiated from the state. Thus when we discuss the modern social teaching of the magisterium of the Church concerning the common good, it is important to realize that we are dealing with a concept which has a pre-modern origin, and that has experienced a constant evolution according to the changing social conditions.[31]

In this section we will examine the most important documents of the magisterium of the Catholic Church, as a way of tracing the understanding of the common good developed through the magisterial teaching.

The term "common good" is used quite often in the official documents of the magisterium. In them one can see an evolution in the conception of the term as well as an adjustment to the different historical times. The documents of the magisterium show an interesting development of the meaning of the term and what it involves. Unlike approaches that begin and often end with an emphasis on the individual, the common good is fundamentally social and institutional in its focus. Its emphasis is on human dependence and interdependence. However, this should not be seen as some kind of religious analogue to a utilitarian calculus. The common good is the set of social conditions necessary to facilitate the complete realization of human beings—elements which individualism is both unable to account for in theory and likely to neglect in practice. The documents of the magisterium of the Church help us to foresee what it would take to apply the realities signified by such notions and ideas to current day problems, and offer the reader some background for the present day debate concerning the notion of the common good, which we will examine in the next section. We will first consider the

---

[30]*The New Catholic Encyclopedia*, Vol. IV, "Common Good" by NEMETZ A., p. 19.

[31]NOVAK M., *Free Persons and the Common Good*, p. 26.

Catholic Church documents themselves not trying to present an in-depth vision of each document, but a summary that shows how the notion of the common good is explained and utilized by them.

We will divide the documents into five categories. These will be 1) the classic texts of the magisterium, namely the encyclicals *Rerum Novarum* (1891) and *Quadragesimo Anno* (1931); 2) the transition in Catholic social thought as manifested by the encyclicals *Mater et Magistra* (1961) and *Pacem in Terris* (1963); 3) the Second Vatican Council and post-conciliar teaching, namely the constitution *Gaudium et Spes* (1965), the encyclicals *Populorum Progressio* (1967) and *Octogesima Adveniens* (1971), and the Synod document *Justice in the World* (1971); 4) the social teaching of John Paul II as manifested in his encyclicals *Laborem Exercens* (1981), *Sollicitudo Rei Socialis* (1987), and *Centesimus Annus* (1991); and 5) the document *Economic Justice for All* (1986), of the National Conference of Catholic Bishops of the United States.

1. The Classic Texts

When studying the common good in the first of the great modern documents of Catholic social teaching, the encyclical *Rerum Novarum* of Leo XIII, and then the usages of the same term by Pius XI in *Quadragesimo Anno,* there is a clear development. When this term is used it is often done in an adversarial way. Both popes are combating theories that in their minds place too much emphasis on the individual. Because of this, both popes use the term "common good" under a variety of meanings and contexts. However, in virtually every case, they both use the term to emphasize the social dimension of the human condition.

a. Rerum Novarum

The social encyclical *Rerum Novarum* of 1891 gave expression to very important topics concerning the social question. Partially it came as a response to the pluralization of the world in the nineteenth century. The great achievement of this encyclical by Leo XIII was to draw the attention of the public to the issues related to workers, which up to that time had been dealt with only by individual representatives and particular interest groups within the Church. The encyclical was hesitant to propose specific solutions in what concerned issues such as working hours or forms of social insurance. This was so because of the discussions being carried out within the worker's movement which had several divergent trends.

The encyclical was seen as an attempt to bring together the different factions under guidelines that could be accepted by everyone because of their generality and abstraction.[32]

In *Rerum Novarum*, Leo XIII makes a call to all human beings to call in for help from without. By this he meant that the human person is better off by claiming the advantage offered by society. There is a natural impulse which unites human beings in civil society and makes them band together in associations of citizens which he called "lesser societies." These are not the same as the society which constitutes the state since the first ones are more concerned with the *private* advantage of the associates, while the latter is concerned with the interests of all in general.[33] There is a natural right of human beings to enter into private particular societies which cannot be prohibited by the state, yet there are times when the law can interfere to prevent associations when their purposes are clearly bad, unjust, or dangerous to the state because they do not promote the good of all in general, namely the common good.[34]

b. Quadragesimo Anno

With *Quadragesimo Anno*, written forty years later in 1931, Pius XI, considering the social changes of his time, readdressed the norms of the common good. Pius recalled the principles of just distribution that had been developed by Leo in safeguarding the common good of all, and then went on to add his own contribution. The riches that result from social developments must be distributed among individual persons and classes in a way that the common good of all society or community will be safeguarded.[35]

In achieving order in society there is a need for unity to arise from the apt arrangement of a plurality of objects. Social order, if it is to be genuine, requires the various members of society to be joined together

---

[32]COLEMAN J., BAUM G., (eds), *Rerum Novarum: A Hundred Years of Catholic Social Teaching*, pp. 14-15.

[33]*Rerum Novarum*, n. 37 in O'BRIEN D.J., SHANNON T.A., *Catholic Social Thought: The Documentary Heritage*, p. 33.

[34]Ibid., n. 38.

[35]*Quadragesimo Anno*, n. 57 in O'BRIEN D.J., SHANNON T.A., *Catholic Social Thought: The Documentary Heritage*, p. 55.

in a common bond. This bond can be accomplished in two ways: 1) by the common effort of employers and employees of the same group to produce certain goods or provide certain services, and 2) by the common good that all groups should come together in support of. In any association, the common interest of the whole group has to predominate, and among these interests the most important one is the directing of all the group's activities to the common good.[36]

At the time of Pius XI, industrial capitalism had affected the social sphere in a way that the unbridled ambition for domination had succeeded the desire for gain. Because of this, there had been a downgrading of the effectiveness of the state, which should have been concerned with imparting justice and securing the common good. The challenge that emerged from this, in the mind of the pope, was that the public institutions of the nations were to act in such a way that they made all human society conform to the requirements of the common good. Only in this way would the economic system, which was a crucial part of the social life, be restored to right order.[37]

2. The Transition in Catholic Social Thought

a. Mater et Magistra

Issued on May 15, 1961, less than two years before his death, *Mater et Magistra* was the first clear sign of a major change in the character of the pontificate of John XXIII. This encyclical considered the main social problem of the day to be the need for securing a greater balance and perspective in the economic life. The state cannot remain aloof to economic matters. It must do all in its power to promote the production of sufficient supplies of goods that are necessary for the practice of virtue.[38]

For John XXIII the purpose of the state was the realization of the common good in the temporal order. This had to include the economic

---

[36]*Quadragesimo Anno,* ns. 84-85, in O'BRIEN D.J., SHANNON T.A., *Catholic Social Thought: The Documentary Heritage,* p. 61.

[37]Ibid., n. 110, p. 66.

[38]*Mater et Magistra,* n. 20 in The Staff of the Pope Speaks Magazine [Commentaries by CRONIN J.F., et al.] *The Encyclicals and Other Messages of John XXIII,* p. 255.

activity of its citizens. This common good which should be facilitated by the state should include the production of sufficient goods for the practice of virtue, the safeguarding of all the citizens, especially the weaker in society, and the betterment of the living conditions of the workers.[39] Private citizens and public authorities must work together in order that the roles assigned to them fit in with these requirements of the common good. This is so since for John XXIII individual human beings are necessarily the foundation, the cause and the end of every social institution, "for men are by nature social beings."[40]

In *Mater et Magistra* there is a definition of the common good which states that it "embraces the sum total of those conditions of social living, whereby men are enabled more fully and more readily to achieve their own perfection."[41] According to some authors, this definition was helpful in solving a long standing debate over whether the common good referred to a collection of goods or an organizational context in which human beings could flourish. Clearly the pope's definition embraces this latter one.[42] It is important that the common good be considered in light of the whole human society and not just the national dimension. In order to secure this the competitive striving of peoples in the world should be free of bad faith, there should be the fostering of harmony in economic affairs and friendly and beneficial cooperation, and provide effective aid to underdeveloped countries.[43]

b. Pacem in Terris

This encyclical, which was written in 1963 and less than two months before John XXIII's death, was not announced prior to its publication. When it came out on Holy Thursday 1963 it was as unexpected as it was welcomed by the faithful. In a time of nuclear

---

[39]*Mater et Magistra*, n. 20 in O'BRIEN D.J., SHANNON T.A., *Catholic Social Thought: The Documentary Heritage*, p. 87.

[40]Ibid., n. 219, p. 120.

[41]Ibid., n. 65, p. 94.

[42]WEBER W., *Society and State as a Problem for the Church*, p. 240.

[43]*Mater et Magistra*, n. 80 in D.J. O'BRIEN D.J., SHANNON T.A., *Catholic Social Thought: The Documentary Heritage*, p. 97.

uncertainties and world tensions, this encyclical on peace struck a cord that was familiar in both east and west.

The encyclical promoted an active solidarity among nations in order to join plans and efforts whenever one individual government could not achieve its goals. Civil authorities in any given nation, after all, existed, not to confine the people to particular borders, but to protect above all else the common good of the whole human family.[44]

The common good is so intimately bound with human nature that it cannot exist fully unless the human person is considered, and the essential nature and realization of the common good is kept in mind. All the members of the state should be entitled to share in the common good. There should not be any preferences whatsoever. If anything, considerations of justice and equity could require that the civil government paid more attention to the poor and marginated. Quoting Leo XIII and his encyclical *Immortale Dei*, the pope reminded the faithful that the civil authorities must not be subservient to the advantage of any one or a few individuals, since they were established for the common good of all.[45] The common good of all is called to embrace the total of those conditions of social living through which human beings are enabled to reach their own integral perfection in a fuller and easier way. Even when in this life humankind is subject to many limitations, and will never achieve perfect happiness, nonetheless, the common good must be procured by ways and means that can positively contribute to the attainment of eternal salvation.[46]

3. The Second Vatican Council and Post-Conciliar Teaching

a. Gaudium et Spes

The Pastoral Constitution on the Church in the Modern World or *Gaudium et Spes,* dealt, as stated by its title, with "the joys and hopes, the griefs and the anxieties of the men and women of the time." This is certainly the best known and most controversial document of Vatican II. It truly became the symbol for the major changes happening in Catholic

---

[44]*Pacem in Terris*, ns. 98-99 in O'BRIEN D.J., SHANNON T.A., *Catholic Social Thought: The Documentary Heritage,* p. 147.

[45]Ibid., n. 56, p. 140.

[46]Ibid., ns. 55-59.

social thought. The constitution significantly modifies the Church's traditional stance to modern society by presenting a more positive concept of the world than the one found in nineteenth century writings. There is a deep awareness in the document of the profound changes happening in the world and the problems related to the secularization of society. It is the only document of the Council that had its origins in a suggestion from the council floor.

Gaudium et Spes continued to clarify and expand the notion of the common good and the relationship between it and the state. All citizens have a simultaneous right and duty to vote freely in the interest of advancing the common good. Among the duties of all citizens, one which is highlighted is the one of furnishing the commonwealth with the material and spiritual services required for the common good. The authorities have to be mindful of the lawful activity of the family, social and cultural groups, as well as other intermediate bodies and institutions, but the exercise of certain rights by citizens could be temporarily curtailed in favor of the common good.[47] These should be restored as soon as possible after the emergency passes.

b. *Populorum Progressio*

This encyclical written in 1967 offered an economic interpretation of the origins of war and, more importantly, proposed economic justice as the most certain way to achieve peace in the world. Unrestricted private property, free trade, and the profit motive were all rejected as solutions to the problems having to do with the world economy. Paul VI attempted with this encyclical to provide leadership during those transitional years in Catholicism as well as a sense of continuity with the past.

Some authors have suggested that with *Populorum Progressio* the Church became truly catholic, in the sense of acknowledging a universal and planetary understanding of the world. It was a novel synthesis of the ten commandments which called the world to feed the hungry, care for the health of all peoples, educate all humanity, and bring freedom to the enslaved. The pope provided humanity with a vision of what could be called a "common human culture" which human beings have not created

---

[47]*Gaudium et Spes*, n. 75 in O'BRIEN D.J., SHANNON T.A., *Catholic Social Thought: The Documentary Heritage*, p. 217.

but are called to recognize.[48]

The encyclical strongly manifested the believe that there is a common good for humankind. In the mind of Paul VI, the common good demands two important things. The first one is the understanding that the whole of creation was made for humanity. Because of this, men and women have a responsibility to develop this creation and to perfect it for their use. The goods that were created by God should be sufficient, on a reasonable basis, for all. There is a clear assumption by the pope that certain things in creation have been given in common for the use of all.

The second demand which is dependent on the common good is that when appropriation of created things brings about a situation in which this common heritage given to humanity through creation is threatened, the common good demands the expropriation of certain goods from the individuals responsible for their misuse in order to make the principle of the common good operational.[49]

The demands of the common good are constantly changing as time goes on, yet they are determined in its basic sense by the eternal law. When certain individual practices impede the general prosperity of the people, such as someone transferring a considerable part of his or her financial income outside the country purely for personal advantage, or if the possession of certain estates create extensive misuse of land, these practices could be curtailed by the state and the lands expropriated in favor of the common good.[50]

c. *Octogesima Adveniens*

This encyclical by Paul VI commemorated the eightieth anniversary of *Rerum Novarum* in 1971. It was addressed directly to the Catholic faithful in order to urge them to incorporate more seriously a sense of Christian responsibility into all phases of their lives. There is a new theme introduced by this encyclical which the pope called "urbanization." The pope recognized the fact that individuals in modern society are facing a new kind of loneliness that comes from the anonymity, poverty, indifference, waste, and over consumption which is often found

---

[48]HEBBLETHWAITE P., *Paul VI: The First Modern Pope*, pp. 483-84.

[49]*Populorum Progressio*, ns. 22-24 in O'BRIEN D.J., SHANNON T.A., *Catholic Social Thought: The Documentary Heritage*, p. 245.

[50]Ibid., n. 24, p. 245.

178 Health Care and the Common Good

in city life. When this takes place, as in the large "megalopolis" which group together millions of persons, very large areas of the population can become unable to satisfy primary needs. These primary needs are things that all human beings share in common as needs, but find harder and harder to provide for all. Human beings begin to lose sight of this common good and become the slaves of the objects that they themselves have made.[51]

Paul VI recognized that this phenomenon of urbanization was irreversible and challenged humanity to "master its growth, regulate its organization, and successfully accomplish its animation for the good of all."[52]

d. The Synod Document "Justice in the World"

With the idea of implementing the Second Vatican Council, Paul VI started a regular synod of the world bishops to deal with different topics that would be addressed by the pope in future writings.

The Synod of Bishops in 1971 produced the document *Justice in the World*. Right from the beginning of this document, the bishops of the world recognized that the crisis in a sense of universal solidarity among all peoples was being combated by a new understanding that the resources which support human life on earth are precious and limited. These resources must be saved and preserved as part of a unique patrimony which belongs to all humanity.[53] The basis for this realization is the recognition that human beings have common needs secured by common goods which can be endangered through human irresponsibility and sinfulness. All the members of the Church, and of society as well, have the right and duty to promote the common good before all.[54]

---

[51]*Octogesima Adveniens*, nos. 8-9 in O'BRIEN D.J., SHANNON T.A., *Catholic Social Thought: The Documentary Heritage*, pp. 267-68.

[52]Ibid., n. 10 in D.J. O'BRIEN D.J., SHANNON T.A., *Catholic Social Thought: The Documentary Heritage*, p. 268.

[53]*Justice in the World*, Chapter 1 in O'BRIEN D.J., SHANNON T.A., *Catholic Social Thought: The Documentary Heritage*, p. 289.

[54]Ibid., p. 294.

4. The Social Teaching of Pope John Paul II

Being the first non-Italian pope in more than 400 years, John Paul II was immediately the center of attention of the world when elected in 1978. Through his frequent trips all over the globe, he has been able to take the Church's message personally, following the tradition of traveling begun by Paul VI. His encyclicals on social doctrine are probably the richest in content and the most personal of his writings.

a. Laborem Exercens

This encyclical was published in 1981 commemorating the ninetieth anniversary of *Rerum Novarum*. It developed the theme of a philosophy and theology of work in the contemporary world.

The encyclical begins by recalling that only human beings are capable of work. It is work that occupies the existence of men and women in this world, thus "work bears a particular mark of man and of humanity." The pope describes this mark as the one "of a person operating within a community of persons."[55] This mark constitutes the very nature of a human being. Work is something that is familiar to every man and woman, no matter what shape and form that work takes. Work is a good thing for all people, and in spite of the toil (the pope believes that maybe because of the toil) that comes with it, work is still a benefit for all people. This is so not only in it being a worthy thing, but also in the sense that it corresponds to something in the dignity of human beings and increases it. Even some virtues cannot be understood without a reference to work.[56]

It is clear that in the mind of John Paul II there is an acknowledgment of certain universal goods, and work is one of those realities that is part of a common heritage, given by God in His creating act, and part of the common good which every human is entitled to.

---

[55] *Laborem Exercens*, Introduction in O'BRIEN D.J., SHANNON T.A., *Catholic Social Thought: The Documentary Heritage*, p. 352.

[56] Ibid., n. 9, pp. 363-4. When the pope speaks about virtue he mentions specifically the virtue of industriousness: "Without this consideration it is impossible to understand the meaning of the virtue of industriousness, and more particularly it is impossible to understand why industriousness should be a virtue: For virtue, as a moral habit, is something whereby man becomes good as man."

b. *Sollicitudo Rei Socialis*

This encyclical was issued in 1987 to commemorate the twentieth anniversary of Paul VI's *Populorum Progressio*. The topic of "solidarity" is a central one for the pope. Authentic human development is seen as the solution for the problems created by both East and West. Solidarity itself is one of the fruits of interdependence.

The right of economic initiative is tied to the common good in the encyclical. The pope says:

> It should be noted that in today's world, among other rights, *the right of economic initiative* is often suppressed. Yet it is a right which is important not only for the individual but also for the common good. Experience shows us that the denial of this right, or its limitation in the name of an alleged "equality" of everyone in society, diminishes, or in practice absolutely destroys the spirit of initiative, that is to say *the creative subjectivity of the citizen.* As a consequence, there arises, not so much a true equality as a "leveling down." In the place of creative initiative there appears passivity, dependence and submission to the bureaucratic apparatus which, as the only "ordering" and "decision-making" body—if not also the "owner"—of the entire totality of goods and the means of production, puts everyone in a position of almost absolute dependence. . .[57]

It is important to notice that when the pope speaks about economic initiative he treats it as a common drive and a characteristic of every human person. Being part of the common good is what makes the protection of this right important in light of systems that take away such right. Economic initiative can be curtailed by totalitarian systems but also by a system in which not everyone is capable of being in a position to exercise such initiative. When this happens, our common heritage and dignity demands that the appropriate corrections be made so that everybody in the system can exercise economic initiative and become actively engaged in procuring his or her future.

The appeal of the pope goes beyond the frontiers of faith. He expresses the hope that even men and women without an explicit faith would realize that the obstacles to integral development are not only economic in nature but "rest on more profound attitudes which human beings can make into absolute values." Those who are responsible, in one way or another, of providing and securing a more human life for their

---

[57]*Sollicitudo Rei Socialis,* n. 15 in O'BRIEN D.J., SHANNON T.A., *Catholic Social Thought: The Documentary Heritage,* p. 403.

The Common Good 181

fellow human beings, should become aware of the "urgent need to *change the spiritual attitudes* which define each individual's relationship with self, with neighbor, with even the remotest human communities, and with nature itself; and all of this in view of higher values such as the *common good*."[58]

c. Centesimus Annus

John Paul II wrote this encyclical to celebrate the centenary of *Rerum Novarum*. He offers a review of the main principles of Catholic social teaching by using the key teachings of Leo XIII's encyclical. One of the main objectives of *Centesimus Annus* is to restore harmony between the various social groups.

With the end of the Cold War and the downfall of the communist regimes of Central and Eastern Europe, the pope takes the opportunity to deal with the errors of socialism in order to caution the world and prevent such mistakes from happening again. Socialism considers the individual person simply as an element, a molecule within the social organism. The good of the individual person is totally subordinated to the way the socioeconomic mechanism functions. There is no reference to the free choice and responsibility that every human being has in choosing good or evil. In the words of the pope:

> Man is thus reduced to a series of social relationships, and the concept of the person as the autonomous subject of moral decision disappears, the very subject whose decisions build the social order. (...) A person who is deprived of something he can call his own and of the possibility of earning a living through his own initiative, comes to depend on the social machine and on those who control it. This makes it much more difficult for him to recognize his dignity as a person, and hinders progress toward the building up of an authentic human community.[59]

In other words, it is the human person that must control the social machine and not the other way around. There is an intrinsic goodness, in the sense of well-being, that must be sought and secured for every human being and it must start by respecting the very nature of the human person.

---

[58]*Sollicitudo Rei Socialis*, n. 38 in O'BRIEN D.J., SHANNON T.A., *Catholic Social Thought: The Documentary Heritage*, p. 421.

[59]*Centesimus Annus*, n. 13 in O'BRIEN D.J., SHANNON T.A., *Catholic Social Thought: The Documentary Heritage*, pp. 448-9.

The pope then adds that the Christian vision of the person offers a contrast to the socialist understanding from which follows a correct picture of society. "The social nature of man is not completely fulfilled in the state, but is realized in various intermediary groups, beginning with the family and including economic, social, political and cultural groups which stem from human nature itself and have their own autonomy, always with a view to the common good."[60]

Finally, in the encyclical the pope acknowledges that all human activity takes place within a particular culture. In order to form this culture there is a need for the involvement of the whole human person. By this he means that men and women must be allowed to exercise creativity, intelligence, and their knowledge of the world and of peoples and thus display their capacities for self-control, personal sacrifice, solidarity, and readiness to promote the common good.[61] This is the principal service that the Church must offer to the world: To promote those aspects of human behavior that favor true culture as opposed to other models in which the individual is lost in the crowd.[62]

5. The National Conference of Catholic Bishops of the United States

The National Conference of Catholic Bishops (NCCB) of the United States began getting involved in social issues since the year 1919 with their program for social reconstruction. They later offered guidance to the country in critical times like during the great depression in 1929 or the civil rights struggles of the 1960's. Yet never before had the bishops been involved in such an intense and open fashion as they have been since the 1970's beginning with a pastoral letter on the problems of war, which was the result of a broad consultative process that culminated with *The Challenge of Peace*, published in 1983. This pastoral letter was drafted by a committee headed by the late and then Bishop Joseph Bernardin. While this committee was completing the work on this letter, another committee was established with Archbishop Rembert Weakland of Milwaukee as chairman. This new committee began drafting a pastoral

---

[60]*Centesimus Annus*, n. 13 in O'BRIEN D.J., SHANNON T.A., *Catholic Social Thought: The Documentary Heritage*, p. 449.

[61]Ibid., n. 51, p. 477.

[62]Ibid., p. 478.

letter on the American economy which sought to follow Paul VI's directives to apply Catholic social teaching to the problems in the United States. Both of these letters marked a significant development in Catholicism in America by incorporating justice and peace into every aspect of the life of the Church. We will concentrate for the purposes of this section on the topic of the common good in the letter on the economy.

The pastoral letter on the U.S. economy was entitled *Economic Justice for All,* and was published in 1986. The bishops stated their reasons for writing as "to share our teaching, to raise questions, to challenge one another to live our faith in the world."[63] They speak in the document as moral leaders and as Americans trying to draw from the social teaching of the Catholic Church and from traditional American values. One of the achievements of this document is to have restored to a prominent place the classic Catholic concept of the common good.

The document itself was written in a very unique way. There were a series of drafts that were published for the sake of criticism and then the whole draft was re-examined in order to incorporate parts of the critique. It is agreed that the most significant changes took place between the first and the second drafts. The notion of the common good was not at the center of the first draft. On the second draft, the theme of the common good was not either at the center of the argument—concern for the care of the poor was—but clearly the common good was given a position of prominence. In the first draft the text used vaguely the definition of the Second Vatican Council which stated that the common good is "the sum of those conditions of social life which allow social groups and their individual members relatively thorough and ready access to their own fulfillment." This text of the council repeated almost literally the definition of *Mater et Magistra* already quoted above which said that "the common good embraces the sum total of those conditions of social living, whereby men are enabled more fully and more readily to achieve their own perfection." In the second draft it was much clearer that the common thread of these definitions was their emphasis upon the fulfillment of the person.[64]

---

[63]*Economic Justice for All,* n. 4 in O'BRIEN D.J., SHANNON T.A., *Catholic Social Thought: The Documentary Heritage,* p. 572.

[64]M. Novak in his book *Free Persons and the Common Good,* p. 157, mentions that Hollenbach suggests that the purpose of the bishops when defining the common good is to incorporate part of the "liberal" tradition spoused by

From the very beginning of the document, there is an admission

writers such as Rawls, Dworkin, Gutmann, Galston, and Ackerman, and part of the "communitarian" tradition of writers like Sandel, MacIntyre, Walzer, and others. "Hollenbach summarizes the four commitments of each tradition as follows:

Liberal Commitments:
1- The fundamental norm of social morality is the right of every person to equal concern and respect.
2- The basic political, economical, and social structure of society should be organized in a way that will insure that society is a fair system of cooperation between free and equal persons.
3- Under conditions of pluralism, free and equal persons hold different and sometimes conflicting philosophical, moral, and religious convictions about the full human good; therefore, any effort to implement a comprehensive vision of the good society through law or state power is excluded, since that would violate the rights of some persons to equal concern and respect. This perspective is summarized by affirming that the right is prior to the good.
4- Because persons cannot be said to deserve the circumstances of their birth, such as special talents or economic advantages, the tendency of these circumstances to lead to disproportionate outcomes must be counteracted by appropriate societal intervention, although not to the exclusion of all inequality of economic resources or political power.

Communitarian Commitments:
1- The human person is essentially a social being. A person's communal roles, commitments, and social bonds are constitutive of selfhood.
2- The determination of how persons ought to live depends on a prior determination of what kinds of social relationship and communal participation are to be valued as good in themselves. Therefore the good is prior to the right. In fact the very notion of "rights" as it functions in liberalism, denies the constitutive role of community in forming the self.
3- Human beings do not know the good spontaneously, and they cannot learn it either by deeper and deeper introspection or by philosophical analysis of selfhood apart from the ends the self ought to pursue. Therefore, if we are to know how persons should live and how communities should be organized we must be schooled in virtue. That is, we must serve as apprentices in a community with a tradition that has taught it virtue.
4- How society as a whole ought to be organized will depend on a vision of the integral good of the whole community, that is, the common good. But because of the deep pluralism of modern social life, we lack a civic community with the traditions and virtues that are needed to teach us what the common good is. Therefore, for the time being, we must concentrate on learning these virtues in communities that are smaller than humanity as a whole or than the nation, that is, in local and intentional groups that do share a vision of the human good.

of the strength, productivity, and creativity of the American economy, yet at the same time there is an acknowledgment of those in the country who have been left behind through the progress generated by the economy.[65] An economic system is judged by the way it allows all people to participate in it.

Right from its initial pages, the pastoral letter sets as one of its basic moral principles that human dignity can be realized and protected only in community. The person is not only sacred but social. The precept of loving our neighbors has certainly an individual dimension but it requires as well a social commitment to the common good.[66] This common good is what is achieved, for example, when family life thrives in our society, and spouses can contribute to it through their work at home, in the community, and in their jobs, and when children develop a sense of their own dignity and their responsibility to help others.[67]

In the words of the bishops, there is a need to complete the American experiment by providing justice for all people. In order to do this there needs to be new forms of cooperation and partnership coming from those whose work is the source of prosperity and growth in the country. There needs to be a renewed commitment by all citizens to the common good and a new sense of participation in the commonwealth considering not only rights but obligations as well.[68] There is a clear call to strengthen the virtues that bring about this change of mentality, as well as the development of the institutional arrangements needed to support these virtues.

The pastoral letter reminds the reader that the founders of the country took care of fostering structures of participation, mutual accountability, and widely distributed power to make sure that all people had their rights and freedoms respected. There is a need today to take similar steps to expand economic participation, increase the sharing of economic power, and make decisions dealing with the economy more

---

[65] *Economic Justice for All*, n. 9 in O'BRIEN D.J., SHANNON T.A., *Catholic Social Thought: The Documentary Heritage*, p. 573.

[66] Ibid., n. 14, p. 574.

[67] Ibid., n. 18, p. 582.

[68] Ibid., n. 296, p. 646.

accountable to the principle of the common good.[69]

C. THE PRESENT DAY DEBATE ON THE COMMON GOOD

One of the most significant ethical debates in society today is the one on the meaning of the common good. This pre-modern theme has gained great notoriety in recent years and has shown profound disagreements especially between the individualist / contractarian and the communitarian / common good traditions. Other traditions have also tried to incorporate the theme of the common good into their ethical formulations. Michael Novak, for example, who is well known for defending democratic capitalism, argues that "individuals rather than larger social institutions such as the government are in the best position to judge what will make for success and prosperity." To him, the best way to achieve the common good of society is if each member exercises his or her reasoning ability and intelligence to the maximum in whatever economic activities he or she is involved in.[70] It is through the free market that human potential is maximized.

In Novak's mind, individual human beings cannot know what is good for society as a whole, but instead what is good for him or her. The notion of a total common good is too complicated for any one person to identify. His argument, which is not individualistic in its anthropological presuppositions, tends to endorse the modern arguments based on the writings of Locke and Adam Smith which free the individual from past social bonds.[71]

For other writers, such as Joseph Bower, who is a senior associate dean of the Harvard Business School, the notion of the common good corresponds to something much more complicated than what Novak's argument presupposes. The modern corporation is nothing like what Adam Smith had in mind when he wrote *Wealth of Nations* in 1776. Corporations today are tied to the rest of society in very complicated ways which exert tremendous influence upon the rest of society. The

---

[69]*Economic Justice for All*, n. 297 in O'BRIEN D.J., SHANNON T.A., *Catholic Social Thought: The Documentary Heritage*, p. 646.

[70]HOLLENBACH D., *"The Common Good Revisited,"* Theological Studies 50: 72, 1989.

[71]Ibid.

interdependent communities around the great corporations are greatly affected by the way the latter makes decisions. Large corporations today who want to be successful must remain connected to the more comprehensive goals of society as a whole and secure the well-being of the interdependent communities already mentioned. Some notion of the common good must be part of managerial planning.[72]

The difficulties expressed above have been traced back to the changes that have occurred in the American life since the nineteenth century. Back then, economic and social relationships were visible and, in spite of all their imperfections, interpreted as being part of a larger common life. Today we see a society which is more integrated and interrelated economically, technically, and functionally, yet the individual person has a very difficult time understanding himself or herself and his or her activities as related in morally meaningful ways with those activities of other Americans.[73]

This lack of connection to others has reshaped the individualism that lies at the core of the American culture. There is an American tendency to regard anything that could violate the right to think for oneself, make one's own judgments and decisions, and live one's life as one sees fit, as completely un-American. This understanding, helped by the lack of social connection experienced by individuals in the present day society, has helped in transforming the concept of individualism into a kind of ontological perception where the individual is prior to society. Society comes into existence by the voluntary contract of individuals seeking their own advantage. This kind of conception of the individual, totally withdrawn from the larger whole, is not capable of sustaining a true notion of individuality which is to be nurtured both in the public and private life.

This notion of individuality was not the one conceived by the founding fathers in the revolutionary generation of the late 1700's. They insisted that the government of the new republic to be born could only survive if animated by the virtues and a true concern for the public good. In *The Federalist Papers,* number 45, James Madison warned that the "public good, the real welfare of the great body of the people, is the supreme object to be pursued; and no form of government whatever has

---

[72]HOLLENBACH D., *"The Common Good Revisited,"* Theological Studies 50: 72-73, 1989.

[73]BELLAH R., et al., *Habits of the Heart,* p. 50.

any other value than as it may be fitted for the attainment of this object."[74]

The founders of the country did not expect the common good to come about without some help. It would become a reality as the citizens were instructed in public virtue.[75] The understanding in this was that the people, when trained in public virtue, would choose officials and representatives who would place the public good above their own good.

Michael Sandel claims that there are two main concerns that lie at the center of democracy's discontent today. The first one is the fear that, individually or collectively, we are losing control of the forces governing our lives. The second concern is that in every sphere of modern society—meaning family, neighborhood, and nation—there is an erosion of the whole notion of community. Our liberty in a democracy depends on the very sharing in self government. Politics is one way in which this is accomplished. Yet, according to republican political theory, sharing in self-government also means having fellow citizens deliberate about the common good in order to shape a destiny of the political community. In order to do this well, there is a need to know public affairs in the sense of having a concern for the whole. There needs to be a moral bond that manifests that the fate of the community is at stake.[76] Politics cannot be neutral towards the values spoused by the citizens of the republic. The conception that government should be neutral in regards to the common

---

[74] MADISON J., HAMILTON A., JAY J., *The Federalist Papers.* (Edited by KRAMNICK I.), p. 293.

[75] In *Habits of the Heart* there is an interesting discussion which mentions that the founding fathers such as Madison, Hamilton, Jefferson, Adams, and others knew that the aristocratic republics had been more enduring than democracies. They were students of the philosophy of Montesquieu who had defined a republic as a self regulating political society whose mainspring was the identification of one's own good with the common good, calling this identity civic virtue. In the mind of Montesquieu, the virtuous citizen understood that his personal welfare depended on the general welfare. For this character to be formed there was a need of an understanding that personal welfare and general welfare are coincidental. "For a specialized ruling group, an aristocracy, this conjunction of private and public identity is, other things being equal, more likely than it is in a democracy whose citizens spend most of their time in private affairs, taking part in government only part-time." [*Habits of the Heart*, p. 254].

[76] SANDEL M.J., *Democracy's Discontent: America in Search of a Public Philosophy*, pp. 3, 5.

good is a very recent idea. Political theory in the past held strongly that the very purpose of politics was to cultivate human virtues and promote them among the citizens.

There is also a cultural criticism related to the theme of the meaning of the common good which enters into this present day debate. This criticism deals with the question of whether it is possible under contemporary cultural and historical conditions to identify the common good. The book *Habits of the Heart* by Bellah and his co-authors has the goal of reviving the strong commitment to the common good in the American culture, while trying to retain a commitment to modern freedoms and rights that have come to be treasured as part of the American experience. The authors claim that the values and commitments of the founders and framers of the American experiment have been "nearly swamped by the rising tide of individualism associated with traditional styles of entrepreneurship and more recent therapeutic models of self-realization."[77] If people are cut loose from any connections to the larger common good, the society in which they live easily dissolves into anarchy or an authoritarian tyranny. The alternatives are either Hobbes' state of nature in which life is "solitary, poor, nasty, brutish, and short," or else the government of Hobbes' Leviathan.[78] Allowing society to foster a connection to the common good is acknowledged by the authors of *Habits of the Heart* as being a complex and delicate enterprise.[79] For them "modern individualism seems to be producing a way of life that is neither individually nor socially viable, yet a return to traditional forms would be to return to intolerable discrimination and oppression." The question for them is "whether the older civic and biblical traditions have the capacity to reformulate themselves while simultaneously remaining faithful to their

---

[77]HOLLENBACH D., *"The Common Good Revisited,"* Theological Studies 50: 74, 1989.

[78]Ibid., pp. 74-5.

[79]The authors of *Habits of the Heart* have been criticized by writers such as John Wilson and Barbara Hargrove because of what is perceived by them as a lack of sensitivity and inclusiveness of all the traditions that have shaped the American culture. As examples of these traditions, the authors quote the Native American, black, feminist and populist movements contributions. See review of *Habits of the Heart* in *Religious Studies Review* 14: 304-316, 1988.

own deepest insights."[80] For Bellah and other thinkers from the communitarian tradition such as Sandel and MacIntyre, this reformulation is indispensable in today's society.

Other writers emphasize another point of view. For example, the issue of the common good has also been raised in relation to the way that a government is called to treat all citizens as equal. Ronald Dworkin argues that there are two fundamental ways of answering this question. On the one hand equal treatment to citizens could be provided by making political decisions independent of any notion of the good life. This would be necessary since the moment that one conception of the good life is chosen, many others may be left aside since different groups of people have different notions of what the good life is all about. This is the position strongly advocated by Dworkin. On the other hand, equal treatment cannot be totally independent of a notion of the good life or the human good since the very meaning of treating all citizens equally presupposes a certain way that the truly wise person would like to be treated. A good government should foster and recognize what the human good and the good life are all about.[81]

It is obvious that the very idea of the common good is a problem for liberals like Dworkin and Rawls, among others, and for communitarians like MacIntyre and Sandel. For the liberals, any attempt to secure a vision of the common good in the pluralistic context in which we live, could only foster tyranny and oppression. For those who come from a more communitarian tradition, it is precisely the recovery of a notion of the common good which is urgently needed in today's society, and this is completely dependent on individuals being part of a community with a shared tradition through which they can be educated in virtue. There have been two prevailing attitudes in relationship to the possibility of establishing such a common notion of the common good. For those like Rawls, for example, who share a liberal philosophy, the only way for a common notion of the common good to be reached would be by the exercise of the virtues of tolerance and readiness to meet other people half-way through reasonableness and a sense of fairness. The pattern of justice, which Rawls claims to be derived from a procedural ethic, must always be seen in relationship to the overall effect, and would be

---

[80] BELLAH R., et al., *Habits of the Heart*, p. 144.

[81] DWORKIN R., *A Matter of Principle*, p. 191.

acceptable if it benefits the least well off. Others like MacIntyre, who come from a communitarian tradition, would not agree with such a conception of a kind of "average virtue," and would disagree with the possibility of sustaining society with such a weak notion of the common good. The tendency for those who think like MacIntyre has been to either abandon or weaken the importance they attribute to a common notion of the human good.[82] In MacIntyre's view, the ideas and social institutions that have developed after the Enlightenment have done away with the possibility of having a universal and rational notion of the foundation of morality. For him, moral language in today's world is only used to express disagreement. We have lost any kind of coherent moral vision and the institutions needed to secure the possibility of such a vision.[83] This moral breakdown becomes most dangerous in the inability to agree on the meaning of justice in American society, which is the central virtue of political life. The inequality that is engendered through this incapacity of generating a notion of the common good which makes justice impossible translates into a kind of domination of certain elements in society and a radical deprivation of basic needs.[84]

---

[82]HOLLENBACH D., *"The Common Good Revisited,"* Theological Studies 50: 77-78, 1989.

[83]MACINTYRE A., *After Virtue*, pp. 6, 104-5.

[84]WALZER M., *"The Concept of Civil Society,"* in WALZER M. (ed.), *Toward a Global Civil Society*, p. 19.

SIX

DISTRIBUTIVE JUSTICE

The whole notion of justice is of great relevance to any discussion that deals with ethical questions. It is one of the cardinal virtues in the teaching of the Church, and thus, it is often invoked. At the same time, justice is the subject of many disputes and arguments because of the difficulties encountered when trying to define this virtue. We have already seen in chapter four, how the different philosophies can appeal to an specific notion or definition of what justice should be, by adapting their definitions of justice to the principles spoused by them. Unless the virtue of justice is seen as satisfying general objective norms, then the particular expressions of this virtue may become mere servants of the popular philosophical tendencies of the time.[85] With that in mind, it is important to trace the origins of the notion of justice before expanding on the teaching of the Church concerning this virtue and its particular applications.

A. A HISTORICAL SURVEY OF THE NOTION OF JUSTICE

There is a definition of justice which has had a predominant place in all of the discussions about this topic since the Middle Ages and reaching all the way to our modern period. This is the definition attributed to Ulpian, a Roman jurist of the third century. His understanding of justice is expressed in the first sentence of Justinian's *Institutes,* written in the sixth century. It says: *"Justitia est constans et perpetua voluntas ius suum cuique tribuens,"* which means "justice is the constant and perpetual will of giving to each his own right." There is another statement attributed to Ulpian as well which may help in clarifying this notion. It says: *"Iuris præcepta sunt hæc: honeste vivere, alterum non lædere, suum cuique tribuere,"* which means "the precepts of rights [as in right conduct] are these: to live honestly, to harm no one, to give to each his own." This last phrase can be called the precept of justice or the element of justice in right

---

[85]CALVEZ J-Y, PERRIN J., *The Church and Social Justice,* p. 139.

action. Notice that in this second quote there is no mention of *"ius,"* or "right." Justice is mentioned simply as giving to each one "his own." This notion of "his own" means what is due to a person in the strict sense as it arises from the very nature of the individual as person. What is rendered to the individual in justice is as much as is his due. If less is given to him, then justice is not perfectly achieved; if more is given to him then some other virtue such as charity or liberality is in operation.[86]

This raises the question whether justice can be defined without a reference to rights. It is important to clarify, though, that the notion of "right" or *ius* can be ambiguous. It may mean "what is right" as in the second quote by Ulpian, or it can mean what is "a person's right," as in what is owed to the person. The first notion is usually called objective right, while the second one is referred to by most continental authors as subjective right. This does not mean that the latter is dependent on subjective opinions, but it means that it is seen in relation to the subject who receives what is owed to him.

Both statements come from the teachings of the Stoics. In Plato's *Republic* it can be found the probable background for Ulpian's definition of justice when he cites the saying of Simonides, the poet: "to give what is owed to each is just." Ironically, Plato himself rejected this definition, but offered one of his own which said that justice is "the having and doing of one's own and what belongs to oneself."[87] Plato believed that the state existed for the sake of the wants of human beings. Individual persons are not independent of one another, but in need of the aid and co-operation of other people in order to produce the necessities of life.[88]

Ulpian's definition of justice and his emphasis on a constant and perpetual will, also has some characteristics that are similar to the ideas of Aristotle concerning virtue in general. The Philosopher's notion of virtue is that of a trained disposition which is developed through practice. In Aristotle's work *Rhetoric,* there seems to be a basis for Ulpian's definition when it says: "Justice is that virtue on account of which everyone has his

---

[86]GAYDOS F.A., *Distributive Justice and Public Education in the United States,* p. 44.

[87]BLOOM A., *The Republic of Plato,* [434 A], p. 112.

[88]COPLESTON F., *A History of Philosophy,* Vol. 1, Part 1, pp. 249-251.

own in conformity with the law."⁸⁹ In Aristotle's *Nicomachean Ethics,* he distinguishes between universal justice and particular justice.⁹⁰ The first one is the practice of the virtue in general toward someone else, and the second one is concerned with the practice of justice in the distribution of honor, wealth, and other community assets. The opposite of particular justice is what he calls "pleonexia" which means grasping more than one's share. In Ulpian's definition it is not clear which one, if any, of these kinds of justice he has in mind.

St. Thomas Aquinas discusses in detail the distinctions made by Aristotle in the II-II of the Summa Theologiae, especially in questions 57-79. He approves of Ulpian's definition in question 58, and accepts that it is basically the same as Aristotle's, who describes justice in his *Nicomachean Ethics* as the habit according to which a person is said to be active by choosing that which is right.⁹¹ The originality of the Thomistic thought in regards to justice is found in his explanation of the distinction between general and particular justice. General justice is also called legal justice and is interpreted as the objective norm of social relationships. Particular justice, on the other hand, is the subjective expression of this norm. It is important to understand that in the Thomistic conception of these particular kinds of justice, there could be no meaning attributed to them unless they be embodied within the general objective norm of social relationships.⁹² Actually, this is the central theme of St. Thomas in his *Summa Theologiae,* which is in full conformity with his theory of society and the common good. Thomas defines justice as "the habit whereby a man renders to each one his due by a constant and perpetual will."⁹³

In the analysis of Thomas Aquinas it is important to distinguish between two aspects of justice which correspond to two different dimensions of one man's relationship with another. That "other" may be

---

⁸⁹*Rhetoric,* I, 9,7 in MCKEON R., *The Basic Works of Aristotle,* p. 1354.

⁹⁰*Nic. Ethics* V, in MCKEON R., *The Basic Works of Aristotle,* pp. 1002-1022.

⁹¹Ibid., V,5, 1134a1, p. 1012.

⁹²CALVEZ J-Y, PERRIN J., *The Church and Social Justice,* p. 139.

⁹³ST. THOMAS AQUINAS, *Summa Theologiae,* II-II, q.58, a. 1. Cfr. CALVEZ J-Y., PERRIN J., *The Church and Social Justice,* p. 140.

considered as an individual, but also ought to be considered as a social being. Particular justice refers specifically to the relationship between human beings as individuals. General justice applies to the relationships between each and all to the social whole. In the Thomistic understanding, the good of the part ought to be subordinated to that of the whole. St. Thomas Aquinas, in reference to this, states: "As the part and the whole are in a certain sense identical, so that which belongs to the whole in a sense belongs to the part."[94] In this way, particular justice itself is subordinated to justice. These different aspects of general and particular justice are bound together in an indissoluble way since relationships with others considered as individuals, are not to be separated from considering the place of each individual in society as a whole. In the same way, the existence of society cannot be separated from the varied inter-relationships of individuals which constitute it. When Thomas adds the qualification "general" to justice, it is an indication of the subordination of the acts of particular justice to the general well-being of the people to which the virtue of justice directs. General justice is directed toward different particular dealings, that when realized in a righteous way, promote the righteousness of the whole as well. The very acts of particular justice are righteous depending on their conformity to the well-being of the whole. When this theory is well understood, it will not be difficult to realize that it is precisely through the varied ways that particular justice is manifested that general justice can become a reality.[95] According to Thomas,

---

[94] ST. THOMAS AQUINAS, *Summa Theologiae,* II-II, q. 61, art. 1, ad 2m.

[95] These thoughts are relevant since recently some authors have questioned the convenience of dividing the virtue of justice in the traditional way, namely general and particular, with the latter one being divided into commutative and distributive. Failing to understand the Thomistic connection between particular and general justice, these authors believe that the traditional division separates general justice from distributive justice, placing the two in different and basically opposed categories. They believe this since they see general justice as trying to achieve the common good while distributive justice refers to the particular good. They disagree with placing together commutative and distributive justice under the same category of particular justice, since it seems to them that distributive justice should be better connected with general justice. To them both general and distributive justice refer to the social organism, or presuppose the *factum sociale.* These authors fail to see that even commutative justice presupposes the social state, and have proposed other categories such as dividing justice into organic and inorganic, and placing under the organic category both the

particular justice is divided into commutative justice and distributive justice.[96] The first one is the justice that relates to the transactions between equivalent moral agents, whether they are from individual to individual or group to group. The second one regulates the relations of a community with its members. It demands that benefits and burdens be distributed in the community according to proportional equality. Distributive justice will be the main focus of the discussion in the remainder of this part.

1. The Common Good and Distributive Justice

Principles of distributive justice presuppose that human beings are in society together and collaborating with each other. There is no need for distributive justice in the state of nature. The principles of distributive justice differ from those of justice among independent agents because of this social reality. What makes for such a difference? It is crucial to realize that distributive justice is not some kind of inferior type of justice whereby a person is given his moral due, or *quasi* due. There is a definite obligation on the part of the human community and a definite right on the part of the individual to promote a just distribution of the goods of society. In other words, this is not just a moral obligation as would exist for example in cases where gratitude is owed.[97] This obligation of the community and right of individuals have their bases on what is required in order to bring about the common good. The concept of distributive justice was further developed by John of St. Thomas (1589-1644)[98] Since

---

general or legal justice and distributive justice while placing commutative justice under the inorganic category. (Cfr. BERNA A., et al, *Curso de Doctrina Social Católica*, pp. 198-199).

[96]ST. THOMAS AQUINAS, *Summa Theologiae*, II-II, q. 61, a. 1.

[97]FAIDHERBE A.J., *La Justice Distributive*, pp. 39-47.

[98]John of St. Thomas attempted to determine the exact foundation of this obligation of the community when he wrote: "... distributive justice has a right and an obligation founded not in something given or received by some person, but in the very notion of the common good."JOHN OF ST. THOMAS, *Curs. Theol.*, Vol. III, Q. 21, disp. 6, a. 4, p. 547. (Cfr. FAIDHERBE A.J., *La Justice Distributive*, pp. 39-47.)

distributive justice is ordained towards another, it is necessary that the obligation existing in the point of departure *(terminus a quo)* have as a correlative a right in the point of arrival *(terminus ad quem)*. When considering commutative justice the right is founded in the person subject of this active right. When considering distributive justice, it is based on the law of the common good. This right is also a strict one, but different from that right which resides in the point of arrival *(terminus ad quem)* of commutative justice. The right in a case of commutative justice is a real right or a *dominium*. In the case of distributive justice, the member of the community is the subject of a personal right.[99]

The individual then does not have a *jus in re* to the goods of the community as he would have to his own property, but rather a personal right *(jus ad rem)*. In order to determine in what measure the individual person has a right to the goods of the community or in what measure the community has an obligation to the individual person, it is important to remember that according to the definition of distributive justice covered earlier, the goods and burdens must be allotted according to the merits, fitness, and necessity of the individuals who make up the community. There would be an injustice committed by society if goods and burdens were allocated on a perfectly numerical basis. Those who have a greater part in society by contributing more than the others, merit a greater reward from society, while those who are in greater need are deserving of more help from the custodian of the common goods. As was mentioned before, Aristotle and later Aquinas called this measure in distributive justice a "geometric proportionality" which involves a proportion between goods and persons.[100] The Aristotelian notions of distributive justice are related to some notion of the good since he held a social view of humanity that said that an essential constitutive condition of seeking the human good was

---

[99]John of St. Thomas clarified the right in the case of distributive justice when he wrote: ". . . distributive justice, in itself and intrinsically *(per se et ab intrinseco)* regards only that which is rendered to a particular person by reason of a debt of dignity and according to a proportionality, not by reason of a right of property *(jus in re)* which he has, but rather by reason of a right to property *(jus ad rem)*." JOHN OF ST. THOMAS, *Curs. Theol.*, Vol. III, p. 551. (Cfr. FAIDHERBE A.J., *La Justice Distributive*, pp. 39-47.)

[100]See for ARISTOTLE *Nic. Ethics* V, 3, 1131, 1132 in MCKEON R., *The Basic Works of Aristotle*, pp. 1006- 1009, and ST. THOMAS AQUINAS, *Summa Theologiae*, II-II, q. 61, a.2.

bound up with being in society. Through a just distribution of the goods of society, the common good is realized.

Outside of society, human beings could find themselves defending not so much a concept of distributive justice, but one of independent possession. Entering society would be only for the sake of protecting these rights. But once human beings are seen as social animals, then a certain kind of structure of society would be an essential condition of human potentiality. This would define the subject to whom distributive justice is due.[101] In praising justice as the first virtue of political life, Aristotle suggested that a community which lacks an agreement as to a conception of justice, also lacks what is needed to establish a political community.[102]

B. MAGISTERIAL DOCUMENTS AND DISTRIBUTIVE JUSTICE

For many years the Church has developed a Christian understanding of justice and the teaching on distributive justice that gives substance to such understanding. In order to study the Church's teaching on distributive justice it is necessary to study this topic as it has evolved in the major documents of the magisterium of the Catholic Church.

In the previous section on the common good we gave a brief introduction to the most important social documents of the Church, which allows now to discuss the documents directly as to how they describe distributive justice.

1. The Classic Texts

a. *Rerum Novarum*
With respect to distributive justice the encyclical recognizes some very important realities. There is an understanding that human beings are always in need. What is more, those human needs never die out. There is a constant recurrence of those needs, and even when we may be satisfied for one day, there is an on-going process which makes fresh supplies for tomorrow a necessity.[103] Nature must provide for man a stable

---

[101] TAYLOR C., *Philosophy and the Human Sciences*, p. 295.

[102] MACINTYRE A., *After Virtue*, p. 244.

[103] *Rerum Novarum* n. 7 in CARLEN C., *The Papal Encyclicals*, p. 243.

source from which he might look to draw continual supplies. Because of this, human beings have the right of providing for the basic needs of their bodies even prior to a consideration of the role of the state. The rulers of the state have the foremost duty to make sure that the laws and institutions that relate to the administration of a commonwealth, should be instrumental in bringing about the public well-being and the prosperity of all peoples. The state should consider the interests of the people as equal. To neglect one portion of the population in order to favor another would be irrational, thus the administration must provide for the welfare and the comfort of all the classes so as not to violate the law of justice that requires that each human being shall have his or her due.[104]

One interesting element of the encyclical is how Leo XIII deals with the whole notion of ownership and labor. He never acknowledges this in the encyclical itself, but his thinking on this subject seems to be influenced by St. Thomas Aquinas. The Theologian does dedicate the whole question 66 of the II-II of the *Summa* to human dominion over things and the issue of the right to property. He asks in article one whether it is natural for human beings to have external things. His answer is affirmative based on the reasonableness of human nature. Yet it is not until article two that he begins to speak of private property when he asks if human beings can possess something legitimately as their own. For Aquinas the dominion that can be considered natural to human beings as rational creatures is equivalent to the basic dominion that could be realized in social forms. By this, their personal participation in the use and reasonable disposition of goods, would be guaranteed. In article two Aquinas speaks of private property while feeling strongly the weight of a Christian tradition that leans to the holding of goods in common. He answers in regard to private property that human beings should hold these external things as though they were held in common, placing them at the disposition of others. The pope in *Rerum Novarum* states that by working on a part of nature, we can award ourselves such a part as private property. This is so since our work leaves an imprint on it. Leo XIII's notion is similar to the one held by John Locke, who said that by mixing one's labor with a good of nature human beings can claim property as their own, as long as it remained within the limits of what can be reasonably put to

---

[104]*Rerum Novarum* n.337 in CARLEN C., *The Papal Encyclicals*, p. 249.

use.[105]

Rerum Novarum most importantly, though, brings the language of justice to the social debate by promoting just wages for workers, and their right to free association. It also clearly points out that among the grave duties of government leaders in order to do their best for the people, the most important one is to act with strict justice—namely distributive justice—without making any class distinction.[106]

b. Quadragesimo Anno

Forty years after *Rerum Novarum,* Pius XI dealt again with the issue of private property in the encyclical that bore the name commemorating the fortieth anniversary of Leo XIII's encyclical. In *Quadragesimo Anno* the social function of private property is clearly stressed. The teaching begun by *Rerum Novarum* is now brought to new depths and evolves into much greater challenges.

The encyclical begins by affirming that the right of property has to be distinguished from its use. It acknowledges the fact that commutative justice requires a sacred respect for the division of possessions which prohibits the invasion of others' rights by exceeding the limits of one's own property, yet, at the same time it states that the duty of owners to use their property in a right way does not come under commutative justice but under other virtues and obligations.[107]

There is a call issued by the pope to encourage those who, while trying to preserve harmony between themselves and the Church, seek to define the nature of these obligations and how to limit the right of property or its use by analyzing in which way they are circumscribed to the necessities of social life.[108]

The way goods are distributed is of crucial importance to the pope since not every distribution among human beings attains in a satisfactory way the ends intended by God. The growing riches resulting

---

[105]See *Rerum Novarum,* n. 8 in O'BRIEN D.J., SHANNON T.A., *Catholic Social Thought: The Documentary Heritage,* p. 17.

[106]Ibid.

[107]*Quadragesimo Anno,* n. 47 in CARLEN C., *The Papal Encyclicals,* p. 422.

[108]Ibid., n. 48, p. 422.

from the economic-social developments in the world, must be distributed among individual persons and classes in a way that the common advantage of all will be secured.[109] One class is forbidden to exclude another class from a share in what is produced. In the words of the encyclical: "each one, therefore, must receive his due share, and the distribution of created goods must be brought into conformity with the demands of the common good or social justice. For every sincere observer is conscious that, on account of the vast difference between the few who hold excessive wealth and the many who live in destitution, the distribution of wealth today is gravely defective."[110]

Quadragesimo Anno acknowledges a crucial issue having to do with the principle of subsidiarity. This principle states that it is gravely wrong to take from individuals what they can accomplish on their own in order to give it to the community, since there is no need to assign to a greater or higher association what a lesser or subordinate one can do. The encyclical describes this principle as a weighty one. Nonetheless, it makes clear at the same time that history abundantly proves that many things which were done by smaller associations could only be accomplished now by larger ones.[111] This is an implication drawn from the principle of subsidiarity which clearly applies to many issues in the world today. In other words, the principle of subsidiarity is not meant only to prevent the larger association from taking over what the smaller can accomplish in a better way, but it is also meant in essence to obligate the higher or greater association to take care of what the smaller or lesser association cannot do. The encyclical implies that it is as wrong to take from the individuals or lesser associations what they can accomplish on their own, as it is to leave the individuals or lesser associations on their own to accomplish what only the higher association can effectively accomplish. The role of the state, for example, is to deal with the things that it alone can do effectively such as directing, watching, urging, and restraining according to requirements and needs.

---

[109]*Quadragesimo Anno*, n. 57 in CARLEN C., *The Papal Encyclicals*, p. 424.

[110]*Quadragesimo Anno*, n. 60 in CALVEZ J-Y, PERRIN J., *The Church and Social Justice*, p. 149.

[111]Ibid., n. 79 in CARLEN C., *The Papal Encyclicals*, p. 428.

The economic life of the state cannot be left to the forces of free competition. This can be beneficial if kept within certain limits, but it clearly cannot be the sole director of economic life. It results in an evil individualistic spirit that fails to see the requirements of the social life. A situation should not be created in which private ownership has a kind of sovereignty over society which is contrary to all other rights. Such sovereignty, the encyclical reminds us, belongs not to the owners, but to the public authority.[112] This exaggerated competition promotes greed, usury, speculation, fraud, and the accumulation of wealth in the hands of a few. This creates the possibility of monopolies that hold and control money through despotic economic domination. The result is a fierce battle among industrialists to have control of the state to the point that government becomes a slave tied down to human passion and greed while business owners delegate management to non-owning directors who commit injustices and fraud beneath the obscurity of the common name of the corporate firm.[113]

The encyclical ends this section with a very strong note: "For certain kinds of property (...) ought to be reserved to the state since they carry with them a dominating power so great that cannot without danger to the general welfare be entrusted to private individuals."[114]

Those involved in producing goods are not forbidden to increase their fortunes in a lawful way, since it is fair that those who render a service to the community should be made richer according to their position. The encyclical defends this, provided that this is sought with "due respect for the laws of God and without impairing the rights of others and that they be employed in accordance with faith and right reason."[115]

---

[112]*Quadragesimo Anno*, n. 114 in CARLEN C., *The Papal Encyclicals*, p. 433.

[113]Ibid., n. 107, p. 431.

[114]Ibid., n. 114, p. 433.

[115]Ibid., n. 136, p. 437.

2. The Transition in Catholic Social Thought

a. Mater et Magistra

The encyclical sees many of the problems of the day as a result of the growing complexity of modern society and from the progress made in science, technology, and communications. It confronts the evolution of the "organization man"—the individual whose life is dominated by the company for which he works—but reminds us that all these developments have come about through the efforts of men who are free and autonomous by nature.[116] As society becomes richer and more complex, according to the Pope, the duties of the states must increase accordingly, as it carries out its power of co-ordination and regulation as demanded by the good of all.

The state must monitor social production. It should be present to promote in a suitable manner the production of a sufficient supply of material goods.[117] It is not enough to assert the right to own private property and the means of production as an inherent part of human nature. There must be an insistence on the fact that these rights must be extensive in practice and not just in theory to all classes of citizens.[118] That is why, besides production, the state's major responsibility is to establish a just and equitable distribution of goods in society. John XXIII summarizes this teaching when he says: "The economic prosperity of a nation is not so much its total assets in terms of wealth and property, as the equitable division and distribution of this wealth. This it is which guarantees the personal development of the members of society, which is the true goal of a nation's economy."[119] Human beings are by nature social beings, thus the cause and the end of every social institution.[120] *Mater et Magistra* also emphasizes that this equitable distribution should be kept in mind to show

---

[116]*Mater et Magistra*, n. 63 in The Staff of the Pope Speaks Magazine [Commentaries by CRONIN J.F., et al.] *The Encyclicals and Other Messages of John XXIII*, p. 266.

[117]Ibid., n. 20, p. 255.

[118]Ibid., n. 113, p. 278.

[119]Ibid., n. 74, p. 269.

[120]Ibid., n. 219, p. 305.

social solidarity not only within a particular country but between nations as well. Countries and governments should seek the economic good of all peoples on a world-wide scale, while developed countries must provide nonopportunistic emergency and infrastructural help to underdeveloped ones.[121] John XXIII also encouraged through the encyclical a heightened sense of local, national, and international interdependence among individuals and social groups. There is an emphasis on human interrelationships and a decrease in the importance given to individualism. In what is believed by many to be a key passage of the encyclical, the Pope observed approvingly: "Certainly one of the principal characteristics which seems to be typical of our age is an increase in social relationships, in those mutual ties, that is, which grow daily more numerous and which have led to the introduction of many and varied forms of associations in the lives and activities of citizens . . ."[122]

b. Pacem in Terris

Pacem in Terris beautifully traced Catholic teaching on peace but also on human rights. The pope presented to humanity in a clear, simple, and eloquent way the foundations of society. Even when we fail to live up to such ideals because of weakness or selfishness, we are still capable of acknowledging the truth and what should be the ideal of any society.

Society is a rich combination of interrelated associations, with the civil state as its highest organ. The civil authority is a result of human nature, thus of God who created this nature. By participation in civil society, human beings, both as individuals and members of lesser organizations, contribute to the general welfare of all. Through civil society they harmonize their own interests with the needs of others in

---

[121]*Mater et Magistra*, n. 25 in The Staff of the Pope Speaks Magazine [Commentaries by CRONIN J.F., et al.] *The Encyclicals and Other Messages of John XXIII*, pp. 258-259. For other references in the same encyclical see *Mater et Magistra* ns. 80, 158, 161 which deal with emergency aid, no. 163 which deals with infrastructural aid, and ns. 170, 171, 173 which deal with the importance of nonopportunistic aid.

[122]Ibid., p. 265. The wording of this passage has been controversial because of the translations of the Latin phrase *"socialium rationum incrementa."* For a discussion of the translation problems see KIRWIN J.R., *"Christianizing the New Society: A New Translation of Mater et Magistra,"* in Catholic Social Guild, *The Social Thought of John XXIII*, England: Samuel Walker Press, 1964, pp. 90-93.

society.

Pacem in Terris gives for the first time a list of things that the Church considers to be rights of every man and woman. These are: the right to bodily integrity and to the means necessary for the proper development of life, namely food, clothing, shelter, medical care, rest, and the necessary social services.[123]

Human beings must be capable of engaging in economic activities that are suited to their degree of responsibility. Workers are entitled to a wage determined in accordance with the principles of justice. What a worker receives must be sufficient to allow him and his family a standard of living that is consistent with human dignity.[124]

Rights give rise to corresponding duties in others. According to the encyclical, it is useless to admit that there is a right to a necessity of life unless everything possible is attempted to supply a person with the means sufficient to obtain such necessity. Society must not only be well ordered, but must provide all people with abundant resources.[125] In the modern world it is clearly seen that political, economic, or cultural inequities among the citizens tend to be greater when public authorities fail to take appropriate actions concerning these areas of social life. When this happens, human rights and duties are rendered completely ineffective. The civil authorities must strive to promote and foster the good of all and not to favor any particular citizen or category of citizens among the people. There is a possibility that in accordance with the principles of justice and equity, the state and those in power may pay more attention to the weaker members of civil society due to the fact that usually these are at a disadvantage when defending their rights and securing their legitimate interests.[126]

---

[123] *Pacem in Terris*, n. 11 in The Staff of the Pope Speaks Magazine [Commentaries by CRONIN J.F., et al.] *The Encyclicals and Other Messages of John XXIII*, p. 329.

[124] Ibid., n. 20, p. 332.

[125] Ibid., ns. 30-32, pp. 334-335.

[126] Ibid., n. 56, p. 342.

3. The Second Vatican Council and Post-Conciliar Teaching

a. *Gaudium et Spes*

Gaudium et Spes begins its analysis of the social question by dealing with the inequalities found in the world today. On the level of race and social class there are tensions between the affluent and the underdeveloped nations. In the midst of all the conflicts, there stands the human person as the one affected by, as well as the one creating the conflicts.

The social nature of human beings signals to the fact that there is an interdependence between personal or individual improvement and the betterment of society. Life in society is not something extrinsic to man, but part of his very essence. This is his only way to achieve his destiny.[127] All human beings have been created in the image of God, thus while there are rightful differences between people, their equal dignity as persons requires that society provides for fair and more humane conditions. The economic and social disparities in the world among the different classes of people of the one human race is a constant source of scandal which speaks against social justice and equity.[128] Human beings must be seen as the source, the focus and the end of all social and economic life.[129] With the increased efficiency in the methods of production and distribution of goods, the economy has become an instrument that can better meet the needs of human beings in society. Yet many times, it is precisely the progress mentioned above that becomes the main reason for the enormous differences between rich and poor, at times even holding the underprivileged in contempt. While there are people in the world lacking the essential necessities for a dignified human life, there are others who squander their wealth.

The Constitution *Gaudium et Spes* made a strong call to all human beings to make every effort to put an end to the "immense economic inequalities which exist in the world and increase from day to

---

[127]*Gaudium et Spes*, n. 25 in FLANNERY A., *Vatican Council II: The Conciliar and Post-Conciliar Documents*, p.926.

[128]Ibid., n. 29, p.930.

[129]Ibid., n. 63, p.968.

day, linked with social and individual discrimination."[130]

Human goods have been destined by God to be shared fairly by all. It does not matter what the structures of property are in the different countries and among the different peoples of the world, human beings must always keep in sight the universal destination of human goods. These are not exclusive to one person but common to others as well in the sense that they benefit everyone. Every human being has a right to possess a sufficient amount of goods that contribute to his livelihood and that of his family. When someone is in extreme need, he has the right to supply for such need out of the riches or surplus of others.[131]

b. Populorum Progressio

The aspirations of human beings are summarized in *Populorum Progressio* as freedom from misery, the assurance of finding subsistence, health, and fixed employment, a share of responsibility without oppression, and better education.[132]

When discussing the purpose of created things, the pope used St. Ambrose to describe what takes place when someone gives to another person in need. This is not strictly a gift from one person to another, but it is handing over to the poor person what is his, since what has been given in common for the use of all people cannot become an exclusive personal property. In other words, the right to private property is not to become an absolute or unconditioned right. No one can keep for his exclusive use what he does not need while others do not have what is considered a necessity.[133] If there is ever a conflict between acquired private rights and primary community exigencies, the public authorities have the responsibility of searching for a solution with the help of individuals and social groups.

Industrialization in modern society has introduced a system that considers profit as the "key motive for economic progress, competition as

---

[130]*Gaudium et Spes* n. 66 in FLANNERY A., *Vatican Council II: The Conciliar and Post-Conciliar Documents*, p.971.

[131]Ibid., n. 69, p.975.

[132]*Populorum Progressio*, n. 6 in O'BRIEN D.J., SHANNON T.A., *Catholic Social Thought: The Documentary Heritage*, p. 241.

[133]Ibid., n. 23, p. 245.

the supreme law of economics, and private ownership of the means of production as an absolute right that has no limits and carries no corresponding social obligation."[134] It is not sufficient to increase wealth for it to be distributed equitably or to promote technology in order to make the world a more humane place, unless a parallel development, which promotes man as the one whom economics and technology must serve, occurs. And the only way for man to be truly man is by mastering his own acts and being the judge of their worth according to the nature that was given to him by his Creator.[135] A dialogue must begin based on man and not on commodities or technology that will bring benefits of self-betterment and spiritual growth to the human family.[136]

c. Octogesima Adveniens

In *Octogesima Adveniens* the pope emphasized justice as a personal responsibility of all Christians. While there is tremendous growth that has been achieved in society through scientific and technological progress, there are two aspirations that have made themselves felt in the reality of the modern world: the aspiration for equality, and the aspiration for participation. These express human dignity and freedom.[137] The Gospel teaches clearly about the preferential respect due to the poor in society, and how the more fortunate are called to renounce some of their rights in order to place their goods at the service of the needs of others who are less fortunate.

Human progress, seen in the western societies as a never-ending, breathless pursuit, has become for many a kind of ideology. Yet, the encyclical talks about a crisis that has developed regarding the meaning of such an indefinite pursuit that seems to elude the one who thinks that it can be enjoyed in peace. Merely quantitative economic growth has not offered the long-lasting solutions that could satisfy humanity. Mere economic growth does not by itself address "the quality and truth of human relations

---

[134]*Populorum Progressio,* n.26 in O'BRIEN D.J., SHANNON T.A., *Catholic Social Thought: The Documentary Heritage,* p. 246.

[135]Ibid., n. 34, p. 248.

[136]Ibid., n. 73, p. 257.

[137]*Octogesima Adveniens,* n. 22 in O'BRIEN D.J., SHANNON T.A., *Catholic Social Thought: The Documentary Heritage,* p. 273.

and the degree of participation and of responsibility," which according to Paul VI "are no less significant and important for the future of society than the quantity and variety of the goods produced and consumed."[138] Genuine progress is to be found in the development of a moral consciousness which will direct human beings to exercise a greater solidarity and openness to others and to God.

There needs to be in the world today a new attitude of greater justice in sharing goods which will enable every country to promote its own development with no threat of economic domination from outside. Many nations through the ambition that leads them to unrestricted competition to attain technological, economic, and military supremacy are led away from setting up structures based on greater justice that would correct the inequalities that result from a system that creates a climate of distrust and constant struggle.[139]

d. The Synod document "Justice in the World"

The 1971 synod dealt with the topics of the priesthood and justice in the world. The latter topic became the focus of attention in the Church, and resulted in a strong, positive statement which challenged the people to a more active and vigilant attitude in regards to the problems of justice and peace in the world. Structural change in society was one of the main challenges of the document that came out as a result of the synod.

Justice in the World affirmed that the strong drive that exists toward global unity, the unequal distribution of wealth in which one third of the human race holds three fourths of all the income, the insufficiency of merely economic progress, and the new awareness of the material limits of the biosphere, have given rise to the fact that there is a need to develop new ways of understanding human dignity.[140]

---

[138]*Octogesima Adveniens*, n. 41 in O'BRIEN D.J., SHANNON T.A., *Catholic Social Thought: The Documentary Heritage*, p. 280.

[139]Ibid., n. 45, p. 282.

[140]*Justice in the World*, in D.J. O'BRIEN D.J., SHANNON T.A., *Catholic Social Thought: The Documentary Heritage*, p. 290.

Injustice is mentioned by this document as a grave sin.[141] In the Old Testament, God is recognized as the liberator of the oppressed through the observance of the duties of justice. In the New Testament, Christ brings together in an inseparable fashion the relationship between man and God and the relationship of human beings among themselves. The concentration of power consisting in the total domination and control of the economic realities, research, investments, and other necessities, should be balanced in a progressive way through institutional arrangements that would strengthen the power and opportunities of developing nations as they are provided full and equal participation in organizations that promote development.[142] The efforts to promote the transfer of a precise percentage of the annual financial income of the well to do countries in order to assist the developing ones, must be fostered, while at the same time move in the direction of paying fairer prices for raw materials and the opening of the markets of developed nations to the developing ones.[143]

4. The Social Teaching of Pope John Paul II

a. Laborem Exercens

The main interest of this encyclical in connection to the topic of distributive justice has to do with the way the pope deals with the distinctions between labor and capital and the priority of the first over the second one, arguing against the evaluation of labor only in accordance with its economic purpose.

When analyzing the problems having to do with the present day situation and human work, the pope makes clear that the conflicts that have evolved have been created by man. Labor must always be placed before capital. It must be always considered the primary efficient cause in the process of production while capital must remain an instrumental cause. This also applies to the different phases of the production of any good, in which the first and most important phase is the relationship of man with the riches offered by nature. What comes from man through the

---

[141]*Justice in the World*, in D.J. O'BRIEN D.J., SHANNON T.A., *Catholic Social Thought: The Documentary Heritage*, p. 293.

[142]Ibid., p. 299.

[143]Ibid., p. 298.

process of economic production and technology, presupposes the riches and resources of the world which man did not create.[144] Man continually comes across these gifts of nature that are meant to be used by him correctly in the productive process. The concept of capital includes natural resources which are available to man but it also includes the innumerable means by which human beings appropriate natural resources transforming them in accordance with their needs. All these means are part of the historical heritage of the whole of humanity and not just one person.[145] Human beings are then to be considered as the subject of work and independent of the work they do, while capital is simply a collection of things. Human beings must have the primacy over the production process. There needs to be no enmity between capital and labor.[146]

The Holy Father traces the conflict between capital and labor to what he calls the error of "economism." This error consists in considering human labor only according to its economic purpose and is also mentioned as an error of practical materialism since it places the material over the spiritual and the personal.[147] The pope reasserts the right to private property, but reminds his readers that the Christian tradition has never upheld this right as absolute or untouchable. Actually the tradition has recognized the right to private property within the broader context of a right common to all in relationship to the goods of creation. John Paul II expressing essential agreement with earlier encyclicals, rejects, on the one hand, Marxist "collectivism" with its tendency to restrict personal liberties, and, on the other hand, liberal "capitalism" with its tendency to protect freedom at the cost of economic equity. He concludes in the Thomistic tradition by saying that "the right to private property is subordinated to the right to common use; to the fact that goods are meant for everyone."[148] The socialization of certain means of production cannot be excluded in consideration of human work and common access to the

---

[144]*Laborem Exercens*, n. 12 in O'BRIEN D.J., SHANNON T.A., *Catholic Social Thought: The Documentary Heritage*, p. 367.

[145]Ibid., p. 368.

[146]Ibid., n. 13, pp. 368-69.

[147]Ibid., p. 368.

[148]Ibid., n. 14, p. 371.

goods meant for human beings. Because of this, "rigid" capitalism, which defends an exclusive right to private ownership, remains unacceptable.[149] Furthermore, the pope clearly expresses that, for certain well-founded reasons, exceptions can be made to the principle of private ownership.[150]

b. *Sollicitudo Rei Socialis*

There is a persistent and widening gap between what is known as the developed North and the developing South. Yet the encyclical points out that this geographical terminology should not obscure the fact that the frontiers of wealth and poverty are found within the countries themselves, regardless of whether they belong to the North or the South. The encyclical, though, makes it clear that the search for equality among individuals cannot come by the suppression of the right of economic initiative. The creative subjectivity of every citizen must be preserved since what is being sought is not to diminish or to "level down" the individuals who compose society, but a true equality in which their spirit of initiative is respected and fostered.[151] There is a better understanding today that the mere accumulation of things, even when they benefit a majority of the population, is not sufficient for the realization of human happiness. Actually the experience today is that even the greatest technological breakthroughs, if not guided by a moral understanding, can come back to oppress humanity.[152]

John Paul II remembers the distinction made by Paul VI in *Populorum Progressio* between "being" and "having," and the dangers in a mere multiplication of things instead of examining how those developments enrich the value of "being." Then he adds: "One of the greatest injustices in the contemporary world consists precisely in this: that the ones who possess much are relatively *few* and those who possess almost nothing are *many*. It is the injustice of the poor distribution of the

---

[149]*Laborem Exercens*, n. 14 in O'BRIEN D.J., SHANNON T.A., *Catholic Social Thought: The Documentary Heritage*, p. 372.

[150]Ibid., n. 15, p. 373.

[151]*Sollicitudo Rei Socialis*, n. 15 in O'BRIEN D.J., SHANNON T.A., *Catholic Social Thought: The Documentary Heritage*, p. 403.

[152]Ibid., n. 28, p. 412.

goods and services originally intended for all."[153] The picture that arises from this is one where the ones who possess much are hindered by a cult to "having" and do not really succeed in "being," while the many who have nothing cannot fulfill their basic human vocation because of being deprived of essential goods. The problem is not simply in the "having" since in itself there is nothing wrong with that. The problem arises when "having" is realized without any regard for equality or an ordered hierarchy which subordinates goods and their availability to "being" and the true vocation of human beings.[154] Development is not limited to its economic dimension. The moment this happens, it ends up turning against the very people it is meant to benefit.

Individuals and peoples of the world must be able to enjoy a fundamental equality which is based on a right of all to share in the process of full development. Solidarity and freedom are the two conditions or frameworks through which development can be claimed to be genuine, and to sacrifice one of the two would discredit the whole process.[155]

The framework of solidarity within society is valid when the members of each society recognize one another as persons. Those who have a greater share of the goods in a society because they have more influence, should have a responsibility for the weaker and less influential members of society and be ready to share with them what they possess. The basis for this solidarity is that the goods of creation are meant for all. What human industry produces through processing raw materials through human work must serve all peoples equally.[156] The right to private property is valid and necessary, but it does not annul the above mentioned principle. The pope even says that private property is under a "social mortgage," which means that it is intrinsically endowed with a social function.[157]

---

[153] *Sollicitudo Rei Socialis*, n. 28 in O'BRIEN D.J., SHANNON T.A., *Catholic Social Thought: The Documentary Heritage*, p. 412-13.

[154] Ibid., n. 15, p. 413.

[155] Ibid., n. 33, p. 418.

[156] Ibid., n. 39, p. 422.

[157] Ibid., n. 42, p. 426.

c. Centesimus Annus

From the very beginning of the encyclical the pope makes it clear that human beings cannot be understood on the basis of economics alone, neither on the basis of class membership. When re-reading the teaching of *Rerum Novarum* which relates to economic goods and private property, the pope concludes that the same questions that Leo XIII raised in his time can be raised today in what concerns the origin of material goods that sustain human life, satisfy human needs, and are objects of human rights.[158] God gave the earth and its goods to all human beings.

The free market is distinguished in the encyclical as the most efficient instrument for utilizing resources and responding to human needs effectively at the level of both, individual nations and international relations. Yet, the pope is quick to add that this would be true only for those goods which are considered "solvent," meaning endowed with purchasing power, and "marketable," meaning capable of obtaining a satisfactory price.[159] There are many human needs which will not fulfill these two requirements, and thus have no place in the market. Fundamental human needs must not be allowed to go unsatisfied, and those who have such needs should not be allowed to perish.

John Paul speaks in the encyclical of what he calls "the human environment." He contrasts this with the need to take care of the natural environment by saying that human beings in many instances have failed to show concern for human realities that are more important than the ones of nature. These are realities such as the family, child bearing, and culture. He then adds that it is the duty of the state to "provide for the defense and preservation of common goods such as the natural and human environments, which cannot be safeguarded simply by market forces."[160] Just like at the time of what he calls primitive capitalism, the state had the duty of defending the basic rights of laborers, with the new forms of capitalism now, not only the state, but all of society has the duty of defending the collective goods which have become the essential elements for the pursuit of personal goals by each individual member of society. Here is where the limits of the market are clearly seen, since there are

---

[158]*Centesimus Annus*, n. 31 in O'BRIEN D.J., SHANNON T.A., *Catholic Social Thought: The Documentary Heritage*, p. 461.

[159]Ibid., n. 34, p. 464.

[160]Ibid., n. 40, p. 469.

many goods which cannot be satisfied by market mechanisms. The pope is very clear that "there are goods which by their very nature cannot and must not be bought or sold (. . .) goods which by their nature are not and cannot be mere commodities."[161]

5. The National Conference of Catholic Bishops of the United States

The U.S. economic system emphasizes freedom, nevertheless, it also recognizes that there needs to be a limit to market forces when it comes to fundamental human rights. Some goods are not to be bought or sold, especially when doing so causes harm to vulnerable members of society.

For the bishops distributive justice requires that the allocation of resources, by which they include income, wealth, and power, in society, are to be evaluated in light of how they affect persons whose basic material needs are unmet. Quoting the Second Vatican Council, they remind the reader that everyone has a right to a share of goods which would be sufficient not only to oneself, but also for one's family. There is a recognition that minimum material resources are an absolute necessity for dignified human living. Only an absolute scarcity of resources would prevent from this being the case, and such a situation is clearly not the case in the United States.[162] Basic justice calls for the establishment of a basic level of material well-being for all people. There are particular obligations on society and upon people with greater resources. This should call into question a situation in which there are extreme inequalities in regards to income and consumption when many lack those basic necessities. This does not mean that an arithmetical equality of income and wealth is necessary, but it means that inequalities that threaten the solidarity of the human community must be avoided.[163] These differences we see today, plus the concentration of privileges for some classes in society, are the result of institutional relationships which distribute power and wealth inequitably. These patterns must be critically analyzed if the

---

[161]*Centesimus Annus*, n. 40 in O'BRIEN D.J., SHANNON T.A., *Catholic Social Thought: The Documentary Heritage*, p. 469.

[162]*Economic Justice for All*, n. 70 in O'BRIEN D.J., SHANNON T.A., *Catholic Social Thought: The Documentary Heritage*, p. 595.

[163]Ibid., n. 74, p. 596.

demands of basic justice are to be met.¹⁶⁴

The fundamental rights of a person are the prerequisites for a dignified life in community. These rights are given to human beings by God and grounded in the nature of the human person. These rights are not created by society, which has the duty and obligation to secure and protect them.¹⁶⁵

The bishops point out the existing economic inequalities in the nation. Twenty-eight percent of the total net wealth is held by two percent of the families in the country. The wealthiest ten percent of the families hold fifty-seven percent of the net wealth. In 1984 the bottom twenty percent of American families received 4.7% of the total income. If the bottom forty percent is considered, they only received 15.7% of the nation's wealth. In contrast to this, the top twenty percent received 42.9% of the total income.¹⁶⁶ These numbers suggest the high degree of inequality that exists in America and the uneven distribution of power in society. When evaluating this unequal distribution, there should be some priorities to be considered, like for example the meeting of the basic needs of the poor and the importance of increasing the level of participation by all peoples in society.

The United States shows pride in both, its competitive sense of initiative and its spirit of teamwork. Throughout the years it has become more and more clear, that competition alone will not yield the needed results. There are too many negative consequences when competition is left unrestricted. Good citizenship means recognizing, not only rights, but also obligations. The virtues that lead people toward justice must be strengthened if society is truly going to move beyond mere competition and seek for the good of all.¹⁶⁷

In what concerns government intervention, the bishops point out that the principle of subsidiarity calls for government involvement when smaller or intermediate groups are unable or unwilling to do the things needed to promote justice. Government should ensure that basic justice

---

[164] *Economic Justice for All*, n. 76 in O'BRIEN D.J., SHANNON T.A., *Catholic Social Thought: The Documentary Heritage*, p. 596.

[165] Ibid., n. 79, p. 597.

[166] Ibid., ns. 183-184, p. 620.

[167] Ibid., n. 296, p. 646.

is protected in society while at the same time protecting the rights and freedoms of all agents involved. In other words, this does not need to be a one-sided centralization by the public authorities. A just and rational coordination among individuals, free groups, and local work centers and complexes must be secured.[168]

C. THE PRESENT DAY DEBATE ON DISTRIBUTIVE JUSTICE

Some widely published authors in biomedical ethics, consider that distributive justice is the core or key issue for biomedical ethics today.[169] There are some, as for example Tom Beauchamp and Ruth Faden, that when discussing the topic of whether there is a right to health care due to the fact of scarce health resources, believe that limiting themselves simply to the study of "rights" fails to appreciate a more fundamental concern. They believe that if there is a right to health care it can only be because there already exists an obligation to allocate such resources for assistance. Norman Daniels, for example, believes that the only way to justify a right to health care is if it is derived from an acceptable general theory of distributive justice.[170] The major issues about rights to health care are related to the justification of social expenditures and not primarily to a notion of a natural, inalienable, or pre-existing right.[171] In other words, for these authors, the right to health care does not

---

[168]*Economic Justice for All*, n. 314 in O'BRIEN D.J., SHANNON T.A., *Catholic Social Thought: The Documentary Heritage*, p. 651.

[169]Among these authors we can mention Joseph Fletcher in *Ethics and Health Care Delivery: Computers and Distributive Justice* in VEATCH R.M. and BRANSON R, (eds), *Ethics and Health Policy*, Cambridge: Ballinger Publishing Co., 1976, pp. 99-109. Also Paul Ramsey, who considers the task of rationally ordering medical priorities and overall social priorities as "the most incorrigible social and ethical question." See RAMSEY P., *The Patient as Person*, New Haven: Yale University Press, 1970.

[170]DANIELS N., *"Rights to Health Care and Distributive Justice: Programmatic Worries,"* Journal of Medicine and Philosophy 4(2):174, June 1979.

[171]MCCULLOUGH L.B., *Justice and Health Care: Historical Perspectives and Precedents*, in SHELP E.E.,(ed.), *Justice and Health Care*, Dordrecht, Holland: D. Reidel Publishing Co., 1981, Vol. 8.

stand independently from a notion of justice, but emerges from it.

For writers like Michael Walzer, certain goods that we produce or provide in common, require a justified distribution especially when justified by the very nature of the good provided. In modern western democracies, where universal citizen self-rule has become central, the exercise of essentially political power, which is based on the ownership of property, has been rendered illegitimate.[172]

At the same time a second kind of argument, while recognizing that certain goods provided have a social perspective as they are realized in a common structure, states that certain people contribute more to the common good than others and thus deserve more since we are more in debt to them.

In order to solve the difficulties brought about by this apparent contradiction posed by the two arguments, a third one has been suggested which says that although the contribution to society by different individuals may vary in value, as members of a community who sustain in unison certain kinds of relations in regards to civility, mutual respect, etc., their mutual indebtedness is totally reciprocal in nature. If not fully reciprocal, at least close enough so that any kind of judgment would be impossible.[173] Once this principle is accepted, then we can take a look at the situation today in the world and accept it in one of two ways: It can be held that because of a common good or a common life in our society, we must accept certain principles of just distribution which take into account the real balance of this mutual indebtedness in relation to this good. In other words, we owe each other much more equal distribution than what we might agree upon based solely on an economic criteria due to the fact that we are involved in a society of mutual respect and common deliberations. The other way would be to acknowledge that a certain kind of society, namely one of mutual respect and common deliberations, represents the kind of society that would help to maximize human potentiality, but most societies have not yet reached this point in their common life.[174]

There is also an argument that states that the demands of distributive justice will differ according to the society and the moment in

---

[172]TAYLOR C., *Philosophy and the Human Sciences,* pp. 296-7.

[173]Ibid., p. 298.

[174]Ibid., pp. 298-9.

history for a particular country.[175] Sometimes these variations may lead outside the range of distributive justice altogether. Sandel has shown how certain associations, for example the family, are of such nature that demanding distribution by entitlement may be of a destructive nature. Distributive justice, in a sense, could be said to be excluded from these associations for their own good.[176]

An understanding of distributive justice in no way implies that there is a cessation in the belief that there are certain inalienable rights. The mistake of writers like Nozick is to try to make an asocial, atomist conception of society the sufficient basis for distributive justice in society. In today's world there has been a consistent putting aside of all views that embodied a differential order which had been formerly justified on unbridgeable differences of status. Today there is no longer a way to justify one group of people receiving perpetual systematic treatment that would make them have a different lot than another group. Actually, with the advancements of modern technologies and the modern industrial economy, even inequalities between different regions are no longer easily justifiable or beyond remedy. There is an obvious resistance to this equalization. As Charles Taylor reminds us: "When have the comparatively better off liked distribution?" Nevertheless, he himself acknowledges that this resistance is taking place in a certain climate brought about by the intent by western industrial societies to break up the old local communities and bring about a kind of "privatization" of life in which the picture of the good life is the individual alone.[177]

This privatization has the effect of making people see society as a set of necessary instruments and not the place where one can develop to the fullest human potential. There is a tension that is created where the less favored in society have a sense of grievance against the ones who can cope with a highly independent society in which arrangements can be made at will. At the same time, since the measures of redistribution seem to be in favor of the less endowed and the less hard-working people, and

---

[175] This is one of the most crucial points in MICHAEL WALZER'S *Spheres of Justice*, New York: Basic Books, 1983.

[176] For a discussion of this see Chapter 1 of SANDEL M.J., *Liberalism and the Limits of Justice*. Cambridge, London, New York, New Rochelle, Melbourne, Sydney: Cambridge University Press, 1984 (3rd edition).

[177] TAYLOR C., *Philosophy and the Human Sciences*, p. 304.

Distributive Justice 221

this violates the principle in a "privatized" society that one should receive according to his or her contribution, it brings about a sense of grievance by the affluent as well. The real question underneath these problems is: What principles of distribution animate the truly good society? The basic error of an atomist, privatized conception of life is that it fails to take into account the degree to which an individual is only possible within a certain kind of society. Like Walzer has said: "The primary good that we distribute to one another is membership in some human community. And what we do with regard to membership, structures all our other distributive choices."[178] To be left out of this community places an individual in a condition of infinite danger. Without the development of certain institutional practices, law, the bases of equal respect, cultural development, and the habits of common deliberation and association, there would be no conception of the individual in the modern meaning of the term.[179] The underlying idea behind the privatized notion of the individual is that all those things exist for the purpose of protection, and the self understanding of the individual is something given. Over time this notion would tend to atrophy because the conditions that should sustain it would be consistently suppressed. The meaning or sense of the goals achieved by an individual must be nourished by a free exchange with others and held responsible for the direction of public affairs. It is not enough to sustain the practices and institutions which defend liberty but also those which maintain the *sense* of liberty.[180] To the extend that humanity sees itself as formed by the collective history of past institutions and practices, an obligation will arise to maintain them so that the good we have received can be passed on to other generations. If public institutions, in the Lockean conception, are only meant to protect individual liberties, all kinds of inequalities could exist. If on the other hand, these institutions are meant to nourish the sense of liberty through common deliberations, disproportionate inequalities would be unacceptable.[181] Each society will have to deal with the practical ways of putting into effect distributive justice according to what is appropriate, given its history, economy, and

---

[178] WALZER M., *Spheres of Justice*, p. 31.

[179] TAYLOR C., *Philosophy and the Human Sciences*, p. 309.

[180] Ibid., p. 310.

[181] Ibid.

the degree of social integration at a particular time.

As MacIntyre has pointed out, the moral breakdown signified by the individualistic tendencies in today's society, manifests itself most dangerously in our inability to achieve agreement about the meaning of the central virtue of political life, namely justice. He goes as far as to describe our situation as that of a new "dark ages."[182]

Distributive justice deals with the relationship of the whole to the parts. It may be defined as the virtue which obligates society through its representatives to distribute its goods among its members according to their merits, fitness, or necessity, while distributing its burdens according to their ability to bear them.[183] When society has amassed a certain amount of wealth from its citizens, it must decide how and in which way to return these resources to the people. Crucial to the conception of a just society is that risks and harms, as well as benefits, be distributed fairly among its citizens. Yet, this distribution must correspond to a proportional equality of the goods to be distributed to the person. Distributive justice must consider the subject and not just the goods or burdens in themselves. Society would be unjust to distribute its goods and burdens on a perfectly numerical basis. There is a subjective element present in distributive justice that is not part of commutative justice. This latter one involves a quantitative or arithmetical equality based on the goods themselves, while distributive justice depends on a proportional equality which includes the relationship to the person. He who is in greater need in the society is deserving of more help from the custodian of the goods meant for the whole of society. If this was not the case, then distributive justice would basically be satisfied with a kind of egalitarian justice that would not take the subject's needs into account. It would only consider the equality of distribution without any consideration of personal needs and communal benefits. This measure in distributive justice was called by Aristotle and St. Thomas Aquinas a "geometric proportionality"

---

[182]MACINTYRE A., *After Virtue*, pp. 6, 104-5, Cfr. HOLLENBACH D.,*"Justice as Participation: Public Moral Discourse and the U.S. Economy,"* in REYNOLDS C.H., NORMAN R.V. (eds.), *Community in America: The Challenge of "Habits of the Heart,"* pp. 218-19.

[183]MERKELBACH B.H., *Summa Theologica Moralis*, II, N. 611.

which involved a proportion between goods and persons.[184]

A theory which included the notion of distributive justice would give more importance to the societal aspect of human existence and avoid the individualism that comes from adopting simply a notion of equalitarian justice. This theory would never admit that individual rights are in conflict with the requirements of just distribution. Justice includes proportional equality as much as arithmetical equality.

Distributive justice recognizes and acknowledges that a just distribution must consider the goods to be distributed as well as the cost of such distribution. These two factors must be seen as related, and, in many situations, when the cost of distribution makes a just distribution impossible, the first goal of a theory of justice must be to examine the structures that are responsible for the unjust distribution and correct them. Even when conceptually, distribution and costs can be considered separately, it would be a mistake to consider them as totally unrelated, or as if costs could be the only factor to blame for the impossibility of a just distribution of goods in society. This should be especially the case when we are talking about goods that are to be considered basic for every human being, such as health care.

The notion of distributive justice refers principally to political society and much less to economic relations. There exists in political society a necessary authority over persons as well as over the functions that such persons have to perform. Economic relations are not directed solely by concerns for distributive justice, which takes persons into account without dealing directly with the goods exchanged; yet this does not apply when the political society exercises distributive justice in legitimate interventions of economic relations because of their connection to the common good. When there is an action that must be taken by political society because it is needed to defend the good of all, then the application of distributive justice to such situation is not only called for but morally required.[185]

The concept of distributive justice makes specific the claim that all persons have to share in goods which are essentially public or social. Among these goods there could be mentioned: the fertility of the earth, the

---

[184]See for ARISTOTLE *Nic. Ethics* V, 3, 1131, 1132 in MCKEON R., *The Basic Works of Aristotle,* pp. 1006- 1009, and ST. THOMAS AQUINAS, *Summa Theologiae*, II-II, q. 61, a.2.

[185]CALVEZ J-Y, PERRIN J., *The Church and Social Justice,* p. 160.

productivity of the economy that comes as a result of industrialization, and the security brought about by systems of health care and social insurance. These are considered by the tradition embraced in Catholic social teaching as the products of the social system as a whole. They cannot be the exclusive property of any one individual or class of individuals, since all members of society are at least indirectly involved in the production of such goods just by being members of society. By the mere membership in the human community a bond is created among human beings which is sufficient to ground at least a minimum claim to everything necessary to foster human dignity regardless of how much each person cooperates directly with society, or even if they are incapable of cooperating due to age or incapacitation. Distributive justice is the norm that clearly states this obligation of society and which specifies the requirements of mutuality and interdependence in those relations that determine the opportunity of every person to share or participate in essentially public goods. There is an equal right of all to share in the goods and opportunities that are needed in order to claim genuine participation in the human community. According to distributive justice, society has a strict duty to guarantee these rights to everyone.[186] What matters is the fair, equitable distribution in society which should be determined by justified norms which structure the terms of social cooperation. The scope of distributive justice are the policies that bring about diverse benefits and burdens such as property, resources, taxation, privileges, and opportunities. Public and private institutions should be involved in providing and securing this, especially the government and the health care system.[187]

In considering distributive justice as applied to health care, one thing that must be studied is the principle of need, which says that the distribution based on needs is just. When it can be said that someone has a fundamental need for something is equivalent to saying that a person will be harmed or affected in a fundamental way if such a need is not met.[188] Some have claimed that since ill health many times can be attributed to

---

[186]HOLLENBACH D., *Justice, Peace, and Human Rights: American Catholic Social Ethics in a Pluralistic Context*, pp. 26-27.

[187]BEAUCHAMP T.L., CHILDRESS J.F., *Principles of Biomedical Ethics*, p. 327.

[188]Ibid., pp. 329-330.

life-style, a merit conception of justice should be used since individuals must be responsible for the actions that directly affect their health. Yet, using this merit principle instead of need would be to subvert medical commitment to care irrespective of the cause of the need. Ill health is unevenly distributed, and we have only moderate control over it.[189]

Certainly there are problems to be faced when trying to develop a theory of justice. Even though it is meant to correct the utilitarian principle of providing the greatest good for the greatest number, still the modifications that such a theory would promote are in no way easy to implement. Some authors have pointed out the fact that such a theory would have to accept the establishment of a floor or accepted minimum, an allowance for differences in individual needs, the acknowledgment of the problems that come about from the distribution of indivisible and scarce goods, how to decide on a mode of distribution, and how to carry out the distribution itself.[190] Yet none of these obstacles are sufficient to make one desist in the attempt of developing a coherent theory of justice following the principles of just distribution concerning health care.

---

[189] CHURCHILL L., HAUERWAS S., SMITH H., *"Medical Care for the Poor: Finite Resources, Infinite Need,"* Health Progress 66(10):34, December 1985.

[190] For a discussion on these issues see Nicholas RESCHER'S book *Distributive Justice,* New York: Bobbs-Merril, 1966, or J.H. BRYANT'S article entitled *"Principles of Justice as a Basis for Conceptualizing a Health Care System,"* International Journal of Health Services 7(4):707-739, 1977.

SEVEN

TOWARDS A CATHOLIC THEORY OF JUSTICE

A theory of justice based on the notion of the common good and implemented by applying principles of distributive justice will be the theme of this chapter. A notion based on those principles, instead of rights, will be suggested as the best way to respond to the wall of individualism present in today's American society, especially in what concerns facilitating access to health care. It is imperative today that any account of what health care is meant to be, should arise within an account of just health care. The goal must be to achieve the social conditions that will allow people to reach their potential more fully and more easily. Decisions cannot be made only on the basis of what is good for "me," but on the basis of what is good for "us" as a community. Since this theory of justice will be applied specifically to the problems related to access to health care in the next chapter, it is important to first come up with the basic principles of this theory.

There are three specific ways that the Catholic Christian tradition, using the principle of the common good as an organizational or structural context and distributive justice as an implementing tool, can contribute to the development of a theory of justice. The first one is by moving beyond the current polarization of "statist" versus "market-dominated" solutions and focusing on the social nature of the human person which is the basis of civil society becoming the seedbed of true human freedom realized in community. Personal participation by human beings promotes social empowerment.

The second contribution has to do with a human understanding of the social elements in society. There is a civil conversation that can take place yielding a shared understanding of the social good or the common good. This can be true even through shared religious understanding. This is not solely related to personal preferences by individuals but ideas subject to the reasonable assessment of a community where genuine discourse is taking place.

The third contribution is by the promotion of a believe in the self-transcendence of the person, which all historical world religions have affirmed throughout the centuries, as essential not only to the achievement of freedom, but of genuine community. It is through this believe that human beings can go beyond their own personal desires and recognize the obligation of a just distribution according to human needs.

If we were to summarize these three elements and their significance, it has been expressed in this way:

> The first is an appeal to the dignity of the individual made in the image of God. The second is an understanding of the common good, which in contrast to secular liberal theory, sets forth an organic vision of society with duties incumbent upon institutions according to the purposes of society as established by God. The third theme, which follows (...) as an extension of the traditional emphasis upon the common good, is the regulative ideal of what is called social justice.[191]

A. A SOCIAL UNDERSTANDING OF THE PERSON

The first principle of a Catholic theory of justice is that human beings must be considered as social by nature. When it is claimed that individuals are social by nature is not merely a factual claim. There is also a moral relevance since individuals are by necessity embedded in a social network that provides goods for the benefit of each and all together. Therefore those basic commitments which we bring to any moral inquiry are such that they include obligations to society and to persons in society. This view of the social nature of humankind is best seen when contrasted with the concept of a private society in which the social or collective, is only valued as it advances personal gain. It is here that it can be clearly recognized that not every private good becomes necessarily a social good. For example, a person may enjoy the private good of financial stability, but if the activities involved in securing financial stability create a monopoly over the dominant resource of the region upon which millions of people depend for a livelihood, then it is questionable whether the private good of financial stability of some citizens is beneficial to the

---

[191] LUSTIG A.B., *"The Common Good in a Secular Society: The Relevance of the Roman Catholic Notion to the Healthcare Allocation Debate,"* Journal of Medicine and Philosophy 18(6): 572, Dec. 1993.

social good. Thus, the social good cannot always be the sum total of private goods.

There is a common nature of human goods that helps to uncover an expanded notion of the individual or what has been termed a "person." Human beings have a capacity to engage in moral activity that shows regard for others. This shared capacity for regard for others, generates a moral community in which others and they and their needs are to be respected. There is a difference between individualism, which denotes regard for self; and personalism, which denotes regard for others.[192] Even when in and of itself, personalism does not connate with regard for others, at the same time it is the whole understanding of the human person which is at stake. The consideration of the social dimension is part of personalism. Personhood, as understood within an ethical framework of personalism, bespeaks a notion of human goods that links them to persons in community, not to isolated individuals.

An individual is simply a member of a species; a person means an individual with a capacity for insight and choice, or in other words, for inquiry and freedom. From these derive the principles related to liberty and responsibility that are the bases for human dignity.[193] This was the dynamic idea of the writers of the U.S. Declaration of Independence when they spoke of the person as having certain inalienable rights given by their Creator.[194] The institutions created by human beings had to answer to this common human reality and protect this dignity found in every person. This had to be a social task since "a self-enclosed individualism would falsify the capacities of the human person."[195]

The human community is given immediately with the person. There is no such thing as a "private citizen," as much as we use that term. Both community and person are derived from, and are subject to, a moral order which is not at the disposition of any one individual. Due to this moral order, the individual person has needs which he or she cannot fulfil by him/herself and therefore needs to be a member of society. But as a person he/she has inherent dignity which constitutes him/her a member of

---

[192]MARITAIN J., *The Person and the Common Good*, pp. 31-46.

[193]NOVAK M., *Free Persons and the Common Good*, p. 35.

[194]Ibid., p. 36.

[195]Ibid., pp. 35-6.

the moral order that sustains the community as a moral entity: Dignity, because there are certain perfections that are inherent in every person due to his or her openness to the communications of inquiry and choice which require a life of relations or in relation with other persons. Needs, because the human person by himself or herself has certain indigence and limitations that demand the integration into a larger body of social communications without which the attainment of a full life and achievement would be impossible.[196] It is as a social being in society that the person receives the conditions of existence and development needed. These include not only material things, such as food, shelter or clothing, but the need of his or her fellows in acting according to reason and virtue. A human person is a political or social animal, precisely because he is a reasonable animal, whose reason, in order to develop, needs the teaching and cooperation of other human beings, thus discovering society and accomplishing human dignity. Reason requires the development that occurs through character training, education, and cooperative alliances with other human beings. In this sense the social becomes not only indispensable to accomplishing human dignity, but inseparable from human dignity.

Thus a Catholic theory of justice cannot consider the human person in any other way but as social by nature. By definition a human person relies on a certain sociability without which he or she could not exist as a member of the human community. Without this notion, the value of life itself would be constantly threatened. This is so not only in the sense that without the social protection given by the community, actual lives would be threatened, but also in the sense that the value and respect of human life would be undermined. Both situations would endanger human life. Any good or system which addresses the human person in true fashion, cannot exclude this inherently social notion of the person or place any other reality ahead of the human person socially understood since this would be contrary to a full and balanced notion of what a human being is. The absence of the correct notion of person could lead to the actual lack of social protection that could result in physical death, the undermining of a general respect for human life, and immoral acts against the norms requiring the protection of personal life.

---

[196]MARITAIN J., *Scholasticism and Politics*, p. 68.

B. A HUMANE UNDERSTANDING OF SOCIETY: THE COMMON GOOD

It is not only important for a theory of justice to develop a correct understanding of the person as a social being, but also to develop an understanding of society which includes due respect for the human dimension of that society. That is what is claimed by the concept of the common good. Society is more than an aggregate of individual persons. In other words, society and the state are not voluntary associations which individuals decide to join in, according to their own purposes. As we have seen, part of being human is being part of "the social." This is the way human beings *are,* and therefore, it can be claimed that social protection is required. This is what makes a human society different from any other animal "society." In the animal kingdom, it could be said that there is a good to be achieved according to the different species and the instincts that make them productive creatures, yet this good cannot be called "common." For example, among the bees, there is a good, namely, the good functioning of the hive, but not a common good, that is, a good received and communicated. The human person, because of its very perfections as person, has an inner urge to communicate knowledge and love which requires for him or her to relate to other persons. The common good must include "the sum or sociological integration of all the civic conscience, political virtues and sense of right and liberty, of all the activity, material prosperity and spiritual riches, of unconsciously operative hereditary wisdom, of moral rectitude, justice, friendship, happiness, virtue and heroism in the individual lives of its members, since all these things are, in a certain measure, communicable.[197]

In the human society there is not only a responsibility not to harm the public interest, but also the moral obligation to remedy social evils and overcome the problems that create a threat to human survival no matter who has caused them. There are rights that pertain to the individual, but the realization of the need to support a common good provides a useful counterbalance to the excessive claims of rights language and focuses on the obligations that we have as a society.[198] There is a need for a social

---

[197] MARITAIN J., *The Person and the Common Good,* pp. 41-43.

[198] For a good discussion about the missing language of responsibility and sociality in political discourse in the U.S. and the abuse of "rights" language see GLENDON M.A., *Rights Talk: The Impoverishment of Political Discourse,* New

coherence based on the very nature of human beings.

When the framework of the "common good" is used, it is equivalent to claiming that there can be a general consistency in the formal definitions of what enhances human life through the social arrangement adopted by a particular country. This general consistency, by definition, could not be achieved by individuals acting in an autonomous fashion, but through their interrelationship. This was precisely part of the American experiment which is reflected in the Constitution. The truths expressed in the U.S. Constitution are the product of human reason reflecting on the human experience and arriving at "human truths" of the kind that every person is bound to hold. The set of conditions which enable a member of a community to attain reasonable objectives, can be reached because there is an understanding of what constitutes the human good. As one author has put it:

> It is not so much an agreement on something that is at issue as it is an acknowledgment of who we are. The appropriate language is not one of choice but of knowledge and responsibility, of recognizing and owning up to who we are.[199]

The philosophical difficulty in achieving this notion lies in the liberal conception of citizens as freely choosing, independent selves, without any ties to the people before them in time and as the potential subjects of their concern and giving. This vision is very limited and cannot account for obligations we recognize as very important, such as loyalty and solidarity. As Michael Sandel says: "By insisting that we are bound only by ends and roles we choose for ourselves, it denies that we can ever be claimed by ends we have not chosen—ends given by nature or God, for example, or by our identities as members of families, peoples, cultures, or traditions."[200]

The greatest difficulty with the notion of the common good in a pluralistic society is that it could be argued that a society of free persons depends upon practical cooperation, but this can hardly be equated with

---

York: The Free Press, 1991, especially chapters four, five, and six.

[199] See PINKARD T., *Democratic Liberalism and Social Union*, pp. 44-48.

[200] SANDEL M.J., *Democracy's Discontent: America in Search of a Public Philosophy*, p. 322.

common purposes. Since in today's free societies individuals can have different aims, them having a common end does not seem to be realistic. The only way to achieve a common end is by showing that free individual persons do have common purposes.

In order to show this a group of authors have tried to develop points of agreement that could offer some basis for the possibility of such common purposes. There are five main points they have expressed:

1. Any good of higher order is greater than any good of lower order.

2. Within a given order, there is absolute primacy of the common good over any private good.

3. When a person is an absolute person (i.e. God), there is an absolute coincidence of common and personal good.

4. To the degree that a created person is a person there is a tendency toward a coincidence of personal good and common good.

5. There is no restriction on the primacy of the common good in its order; when this primacy disappears (3 and 4), this is not because the primacy then belongs to a private good, but that the problem of primacy disappears.[201]

Point four is the crucial one since it is when the human person acts with reflection and choice that the personal good and the common good tend to coincide. This notion evolves into a characterization of persons united in shared pursuits which, if taken seriously, would mean that the arguments based on the individual claims of a person cannot interfere with the claims of justice. What is owed to one must be calculated considering the claims of others. These common pursuits are not easy to separate into the private and public spheres. These pursuits are meant to protect the community in relation to its safety, the integrity of its basic institutions and practices, and the preservation of its core values. The goal being to accomplish the good life, human flourishing, and moral development. At the least, these core values must be recognized as values by any reasonable person, and must be best realized by the corporate effort of a political society. The promotion of political equality and the prevention of the exploitation of the weak by the strong must be part of

---

[201] This is the work of philosopher Ives R. Simon together with De Koninck and Maritain as quoted in NOVAK M., *Free Persons and the Common Good*, p. 32.

these core values. To accomplish this, human persons need institutions suitable to the task.

The common good of any society consists in treating every person as an end and never as mere means. It is important that the people of a society pursuing the common good live the virtues necessary to accomplish it, but virtue is not enough to cope with the structural problems inherent in republican societies. Self interest, factions and individualism must be stopped with institutions structured to cope with such diseases.

In practice, the term "common good" points to two facets of human nature. The first one, which was mentioned above, is that human beings are social and political animals who are in need of one another. The second one is that human beings are historical animals constantly striving for outcomes not yet achieved. The concept of the common good must be open to change, to invention, creativity and free choices. This is why it is not necessary to conceive of the common good as a collection of goods that everyone should have but more of an organizational context which will allow for all to share in the basic human needs and the goods that cover those needs. It is not enough to claim that the private pursuit of wealth results in the best outcomes for all of society since this would be to view the common good as a merely accidental consequence of other actions. By definition the concept of the common good obligates the citizens to confront the social whole in order to see where are there exclusion of citizens, unmet needs, or potentially future problems. The public cannot be missing from the discussion of these major issues in society. The common good of a civil society is equivalent to the measure of the communion of persons that is achievable in history.

Today a correct notion of the common good is crucial in not allowing the citizen to be swallowed up into the notion of "the economic man." Since economics seems to be the main model today, we are constantly being tempted to place our destinies in the hands of managers and experts. As Robert Bellah has expressed it: "What has failed at every level—from the society of nations to the national society to the local community to the family—is integration: we have failed to remember our community as members of the same body."[202] The extreme fragmentation of the modern world is the greatest threat to our true personhood and to a conception of a common good for all. Or in the words of Michael Sandel: "The public philosophy by which we live cannot secure the liberty it

---

[202]BELLAH R., *Habits of the Heart*, p. 285.

promises, because it cannot inspire the sense of community and civic engagement that liberty requires."[203]

Thus, a Catholic theory of justice would embrace the notion that it is possible to reach a definition of common human goods since they respond to the reality of what a human person is. There are certain levels, depending on whether they are considered a higher or a lesser good, in which there are no questions about the universality of the value of such good. This will depend on how close the good is in connection to the person and whether it allows the person to fulfill his or her potential. Some goods will be difficult to separate from the very notion of person, while other goods could enhance human life while remaining non-essential in fulfilling the human potential. Persons composing the human society, can determine which goods are in what category by observing the effects of marginalization experienced by the persons lacking the goods. Each society could agree on factors that would constitute evidence of this marginalization. An example could be participation in the political life of a democracy and the exercise of voting rights in free elections.

C. A JUST DISTRIBUTION ACCORDING TO HUMAN NEEDS

We have seen how the person is a social being and how the common good is based on a universal understanding of what is properly part of human nature. These goods recognized as common, must flow back to the persons who make up society. Once the social dimension of the human person is understood, and how this notion of the person helps in arriving at the possibility of holding a conception of the good life, then every effort must be made to facilitate this common good to all in society. In the words of a contemporary author:

> [T]he common good by its very essence, directs itself to the persons as persons and directs the persons as individuals to itself. It directs itself to persons in a two-fold way: first, in so far as the persons are engaged in the social order, the common good by its essence must flow back over or redistribute itself to them; second, in so far as the persons transcend the social order and are directly ordained to the transcendent Whole, the common good by its essence must favor their progress toward the absolute

---

[203] SANDEL M.J., *Democracy's Discontent: America in Search of a Public Philosophy*, p. 6.

goods which transcend political society.[204]

This is what a concept of distributive justice will do. Before distributive justice can be made functional in our society, there has to be a common understanding of the person and the common good, and also a realization that the individual is never absolute. Each human person self-transcends his or her immediate reality. This opens him or her to providing for the common good through the implementation of practices that help all to partake of the goods in society. When this is acknowledged, the relevant and crucial question for social ethics is no longer one of absolute rights of human beings, but whether in an affluent democratic republic with an abundance of resources, it is allowable to let basic human needs go unfulfilled. When seen in this way, providing for those basic human needs has more the quality of an obligation than a strict legal right in the Lockean sense. There is certainly a human right to own private property, but the use of private property is not absolute but governed by the communal destination of the goods of creation to serve the needs of all.

When dealing with basic human needs, there is an element of equality in the guarantees necessary for a person not to feel threatened by the lack of such needs, and for the knowledge and peace of mind necessary to know that when such needs occur, there is already a set mechanism in society to address them. One way of evaluating how successfully society is addressing this issue is by measuring the effects that the lack of basic needs has on the persons who are primarily affected. If these persons' needs are not addressed by society, then it is impossible to claim these people as part of the human community. As the U.S. Bishops said in their economic pastoral *Economic Justice for All:* "The ultimate injustice is for a person or a group to be treated actively or abandoned passively as if they were nonmembers of the human race."[205] The only exception to this would be when there is an absolute scarcity of resources to provide for those basic needs. There are particular historical circumstances that must be taken into account since the specific actions that must be taken cannot be removed from historical traditions, social relations, and roles of the individual persons. But even in such cases, a discriminate or partial

---

[204]MARITAIN J., *The Person and the Common Good,* p. 66.

[205]*Economic Justice for All,* n. 77 in O'BRIEN D.J., SHANNON T.A., *Catholic Social Thought: The Documentary Heritage,* pp. 596-7.

approach to allocate goods that are part of the basic human needs, would be difficult to justify. The allocation would still have to be reasonable in human standards and higher goods considered first.

Since the real world is characterized by people who many times fail to see their self-transcendence and rely on a limited perception of the person thus implementing selfish solutions, it is necessary to have the social structures needed to implement the programs that would facilitate distribution of essential goods. There has never been a political community in the world that did not provide, or try to provide, or claim to provide for the needs of its members as those needs were understood by them.

Thus a Catholic theory of justice would include the principles of distributive justice that strive to allocate basic human goods in ways that would take into account the universal need of such goods. Lesser human goods will have to make way for higher human goods when a just distribution of goods is at stake. This just distribution will recognize primarily that when certain common goods are critical for the full realization of the person, these goods must be distributed in a proportional fashion, according to the needs of those in a particular society. When dealing with basic human needs there is no other principle or value that should take precedence over justice in their distribution. An unjust distribution of resources can never be justified, but this is especially so when all the ethical alternatives to solve the problem have not been tried.

UNIT FOUR

REFORMING ACCESS TO HEALTH CARE

There is a need to reform the health care delivery system of the United States. The first unit of this work showed that there are major problems that need to be addressed in order to facilitate access to health services to all the people in the country. The inequalities that are manifested on a daily basis are not the result of a lack of concern on the part of Americans to offer equitable and efficient health care to everyone. In fact, there are probably as many heroic stories about medicine providing the needed attention to a particular tragic case as there are stories of people lacking the basic appropriate health care that would help them maximize their human potential. The problem with health care in the United States is a systemic one and not one merely based on a lack of concern coming from the citizens of the country to offer to all the best health care available.

It was very evident in the first chapter, that Americans have traditionally throughout their history considered health care as a critically important good. This notion has grown throughout the years, especially as people have seen the marvels that medical science has accomplished. It can be said that today there is an expectation by the people that, in case of need, the most sophisticated medical technologies will be made available to them, while all the other considerations will be of secondary importance.

It is important to remember that in many ways this attitude found in most of the population today is a direct result of the enormous progress that health care has made particularly in the second half of this century. As we get closer to the third millennium, it may be worthwhile to remember that in many cases the successes of the current health care system in the United States have been the end result of facing up to the problems.

This final section is meant to show how the principles of the common good and distributive justice, as discussed previously, are relevant to health care reform in the United States of America. This will be done in three main chapters. The first will name the main problems affecting access to health care today and the important concrete proposals that have been made to bring about some reform in the system with a discussion of each one of them. Chapter nine will show how the principles of the common good and distributive justice can provide a theological, moral basis that could be seen as common ground regarding health care, and how to apply these two principles to the American context. The tenth, and final chapter, will present a four-fold proposal for reform based on the two principles already-mentioned.

EIGHT

THE PROBLEMS AND THE PROPOSALS FOR REFORM

A. MAIN PROBLEMS AFFECTING ACCESS TO HEALTH CARE

There are different categories of problems that affect health care delivery in the United States today. Some of the ones that are constantly mentioned have to do with the high cost of health care, the inefficiencies found in the system, and the economic pressures of health care on the economy as a whole. But the most fundamental problem today in what concerns health care ethics has to do with the lack of access to health care experienced by large segments of the population. After all, health care is about patients, and enabling them to receive care. Throughout the years there have been more and more variables that have come into play in determining who gets access to the system and who does not. As was shown in chapter one, more and more Americans are beginning to realize that health care has become one of the great burdens in their lives. Whether it is that they feel trapped in their present job due to the fear of not qualifying for health insurance because of a pre-existing medical condition; whether there is hesitation in seeking health care because of the fear of draining financial resources needed for other needs such as food and rent; whether there is fear of losing their job; or whether it is the concern that providing for the health care of their employees will affect the survival possibilities of a new small business, the issues related to health care are usually at the top of the list of critical concerns in the minds of most American citizens today. Obviously, these concerns typically tend to increase when an unexpected need for health care arises within a family or for an individual due to illness or accident, which are not unusual occurrences.

1. The Uninsured

The most critical issue affecting access to health care in the country is the problem with the uninsured. Their number continues to increase every year, and, as was shown in chapter two, the breakdown of their statistics corresponds to the age distribution of the population in the whole country. In other words, it is a myth to think that only young, healthy, employed people who choose to be without insurance are part of this group. The number of the uninsured most often given, borders around the forty million mark.[1] Actually, the U.S. Bureau of the Census has estimated that during a typical year more than sixty-three million Americans are without health care insurance for at least one month.[2] This means that one quarter of the population of the country on any given month of the year lacks health care insurance. If we subtract the people over sixty-five years of age, who are covered by Medicare, from the total population, the result is more dramatic since any given month a third—one out of every three persons—of the American population lacks health insurance.

2. Poverty

In chapter one it was also shown how the differences in the socio-economic status of the people is the primary cause of unequal health care. Illness in our society cannot be seen as simply a chance occurrence over which we have no control. Today more than ever our society is coming to realize that there is a connection between illness and poverty. When society does not take steps to break the cycle of illness and poverty, the tendency is to see this connection become more explicit and evident in time.

There is a connection between low income and lack of access to health care. This connection holds even when employment or unemployment factors are considered, and also when the age factor is taken into account. In other words, among those who are employed, there is a correlation between the amount of income and the accessibility to

---

[1] In a recent article the number is said to be 41 million. See DICKERSON J.F., *Dr. Clinton Scrubs Up,* Time, December 8, 1997, p. 48.

[2] FRIEDMAN E., *The Uninsured: From Dilemma to Crisis,* Journal of the American Medical Association 265: 2491, 1991.

health care. Even with Medicare, elderly who have greater incomes tend to have better access to care than those with lower incomes. This problem is exacerbated when the insurance which is supposed to protect the poor—Medicaid—does not grow at the same rate as poverty, or is applied in very different ways according to individual states.

3. Cultural and Racial Factors

Another two factors affecting access to health care in the country are culture and race. As shown in chapter one, even if universal coverage would be granted immediately to the entire population, there would still be plenty of possibilities and opportunities for discrimination based on cultural and racial factors due to the structures that are presently in place to provide health care. The difficulties in accessing health care on equal terms that was seen when the patient was African-American, member of another minority group, a rural area resident as compared to an urban one, requiring a certain kind of treatment like coronary angioplasty or organ transplantation, undergoing delayed discharges due to racial prejudices, facing discrimination due to gender, or receiving inadequate pre-natal care in poverty stricken areas, were not coincidental. These statistics reveal a systematic pattern of unequal treatment that affects large segments of the U.S. population.

4. Market Mentality

Another critical problem affecting access to health care in the country is related to the market mentality that plagues health care delivery. When health care becomes a commodity with, not only a profit to be made, but also a potential for developing capital, it is clear that there is no great interest in treating those who cannot pay for services. The problems faced by the people who need health care do not correspond to other needs that would allow for a market to function fairly. This does not mean that there are certain inherent benefits of the principles that guide a market-conscious system. There are many occasions in which intelligent and informed choices by those receiving health care, not only help in recognizing the dignity and autonomy of the individual patient, but also can function as restraints on unnecessary spending. At the same time, most cases that require intervention from the medical field are not the kind that would make it irrelevant whether care is provided or not, and where the alternatives are so far apart in financial terms as to make decisions dependent mainly on the financial considerations. Even if this was the case, health care is so intimate to the person that no one should be forced to choose a less effective method or medical technique solely on the basis of money. In the first chapter it was shown how socio-economic differences among citizens has become the primary cause of lack of access to care. Ill health and poverty are connected, and the lack of financial resources has an impact on the kind and the timing of health care sought. This should not be the case since it could be said that health care is unlike any other human need in that, when it is offered, it is to be presumed by the patient that the remedy applied is the most effective one possible for a person, in the specific circumstances and medical needs.

It was shown in chapter one how the laws of supply and demand do not apply to health care. Once the market forces are allowed to control health care delivery what happens is that the basic rules of the market do not work as with other commodities, only causing an abundance of providers trying to satisfy the demand and giving them the opportunity to raise the prices of health care many times in order to pay for the investments of time and money they themselves have made. The disproportionate amount of specialists in the United States attests to the fact that many physicians are drawn to their specialties due to the financial liabilities that they acquired in the process of their education. This vicious circle of specialization in order to increase revenue has affected access to primary care enormously.

Also, due to the fact that the market mentality has taken such a central role in the provision of health care in the country, the importance attributed to preventive care has decreased overall. There may be some indications today that there is a renewed emphasis being placed on preventive care, but until access is improved, campaigns to motivate people to improve their health habits and to make use of the health care available, will not be as successful as they could be. The emphasis on illness prevention must be accompanied by ways in which people can have access to the system without the fear of not being able to carry through a health maintenance program. A system that emphasizes a market mentality will tend to be a reactive system rather than a proactive one. Future savings due to preventive medicine cannot be measured in actual financial terms, thus impossible to make such savings a factual information that could be shown in actual numbers. They would only be part of speculations that could not be proven with certainty, even when studies with control groups clearly have shown the effectiveness of good preventive medicine. One clear example of this was mentioned in chapter one in relation to effective prenatal care.

B. PROPOSALS FOR HEALTH CARE REFORM

There have been several proposals suggested for change in the health care system of the United States. All of them deal mainly with some significant element or elements of the system, according to what is considered in need of change, and have a common goal in mind: to improve access to health care especially among the people who have been left out by the present system. Some of these proposals will be discussed below, beginning with the less disruptive to the system, leading up to the ones calling for more radical changes. Taking a look at these proposals will provide a good idea of the structural reforms being suggested, and later in this unit it will be shown how the principles of the common good and distributive justice must be utilized to establish certain policy positions that could bring about true reform. As has been said by a distinguished Catholic author in social ethics: "Failure to move beyond the framework will leave a Church with a solid structural vision at the margins of the public debate."[3]

The proposals will be divided into five different categories: 1) The ones limited to reforms in the tax system in order to improve access to the private health system, 2) the ones that propose universal access while retaining the present system of Medicare-Medicaid-Private Insurance, 3) the ones that want universal access increasing public coverage while keeping private insurance and employment based insurance, 4) proposals for a unified national financing with administration by private insurers, and 5) proposals for a single payer national health insurance.

1. Tax Reforms

One of the most important ways in which the government of the United States helps to facilitate access to health care is through the tax system. This means that through tax policies that allow certain practices by businesses or individuals, the government ends up offering help for accessing health care. It should come as no surprise then, that a series of proposals for health care reform singles out the tax system as the single

---

[3]HEHIR J.B., *"Policy Arguments in a Public Church: Catholic Social Ethics and Bioethics,"* Journal of Medicine and Philosophy 17(3):362, June 1992.

most influential way that such reform can take place.

a. The Heritage Foundation Proposal

One example of such a proposal is the one made by the Heritage Foundation. This organization based in Washington D.C. has proposed that significant tax credits should be made available to people so as to help them with their expenses on health care. In order to understand this proposal, it is necessary to explain it in more detail.[4]

The tax-exclusion of employer-based plans for health insurance has certainly eased the anxiety of many families, but it has also been the cause for many people remaining uninsured and for the escalation of health care costs. The reasons for this have to do mainly with three kinds of problems. The first one is related to the existing inequity in tax assistance. Under the current system, highly paid executives may be able to receive tax subsidies worth more than 40% of medical costs, when tax relief is considered. Meanwhile, employees in the lower income brackets, even when in the same company, may be below the tax threshold and receive no tax break at all. The second problem has to do with job mobility disincentives, which means that families with severe health problems may find moving to a better job impossible without the risk of losing their health insurance, since insurance is employer-based. The insurability of such a family would have to be reassessed by another insurance company and subject to refusal due to pre-existing conditions. The third one is the inflationary pressure that results when the employee has no incentive to lower costs of health care since the employer is the one who covers medical costs. Physicians and hospitals are also affected by this since they know that their role is to provide the perceived value of the service since the patient will have no incentive to challenge the price charged to the insurer and ultimately the employer. It might be argued that greater central regulation is required to solve such problems, there are those, however, who maintain that on the contrary a better solution is developing a system based on active consumer driven market. This is the kind of system proposed by the Heritage Foundation. They have proposed that if the tax treatment of health care is reformed by changing the structure of tax relief, then two major goals would be achieved: First, an increase in the provision of health care to the uninsured and less help to

---

[4]The information explaining this proposal is taken from the article by BUTLER S.M., entitled *"A Tax Reform Strategy to Deal with the Uninsured,"* Journal of the American Medical Association 265 (1991), pp. 2541-2544.

those who do not need large tax subsidies, and secondly, the provision of greater incentives for consumers to challenge the costs offered by providers of health care since that way they would maximize the value of the services for their money.

There are two main steps in the proposal of the Heritage Foundation: 1) Replace the tax exclusions with refundable tax credits for health expenses, and 2) establish a health care social contract. The first step will phase out the current system over several years in order to bring the health insurance cost into the employee's tax forms. Any change of health plans or reductions in coverage by the company would require a cash value of the reduced benefits that would be manifested in the employee's paycheck. The tax credit given to a family, for example, would correspond to the ratio resulting from the family's total annual health spending as compared to its income. The higher this ratio, the higher the percentage credit. The credit would be designed in a way that net costs of health care will not exceed a certain percentage of family income.

The second step of a social contract will entail that each head of household will be required to enroll all family members in a health plan containing a certain basic package of services. Health plans will offer a series of premiums, based on different out-of-pocket costs, and the consumers will have to choose a plan meeting at least 10% of the requirements. Even when lower income families may face higher premiums, this will be offset by the larger tax credit available to them.

This proposal considers its greatest values to be: 1) the guarantee of basic health coverage to all Americans, 2) the fact that governmental help to offset health care costs will be based on actual medical expenses in proportion to employee's income which will make every employee eligible for exactly the same tax structure, 3) the strong incentive for employees to seek the best value for their money and thus reduce spiraling health care costs, 4) the drastic reduction of expensive administrative regulations by insurers and employers, 5) it would end the employment mobility problem, 6) it will result in a lower cost to the government, 7) it will reduce Medicaid and welfare costs and 8) it would reduce pressure for medically unnecessary state mandates on insurers.

b. President Bush's Proposal

In his January 28, 1992 State of the Union address, President George Bush gave another example of the importance of this kind of solution when he showed his own support for tax credits and proposed the following:

> My plan provides insurance security for all Americans while preserving and increasing the idea of choice. We make basic health insurance affordable for all low-income people not now covered. We do it by providing a health insurance tax credit of up to $3,750 for each low income family. The middle class gets help too. And by reforming the health insurance market, my plan assures that Americans will have access to basic health insurance even if they change jobs or develop serious health problems.[5]

In a follow up message by the President, he gave more details about the plan, which made the full amount of tax credit available only to those earning less than $7,000 a year. This was not good for the many families who, even though making more than $7,000 a year, are lacking in health insurance. Since health insurance for families can be very costly, the $3,750 figure does not solve the problem in many instances. Because of this, many authors have questioned such tax credit proposals, and criticized the President's proposal as having been done quickly and without much thought.[6]

Overall it must be acknowledged that health care reform based on tax-credit proposals would allow some people to improve their financial possibilities of purchasing health insurance. At the same time, it is unlikely that this type of approach would truly favor the great majority of those who find themselves without insurance today. This approach does not seem to address directly the flaws and inefficiencies that are inherent in the system and will only end up making more money available to be invested into an already inefficient system. At the same time, tax-credit proposals rely principally on a free market approach to solve health care problems in the nation. As we will see later, there are growing concerns that when it has to do with health care, the market approach is precisely the cause of many of today's problems. There is no question that the free market is valuable for the economy in general—a fact which the

---

[5]*The New York Times,* January 29, 1992, pp. A-16 and A-17.

[6]KEANE P.S., *Health Care Reform: A Catholic View,* p. 39.

The Problems and the Proposals for Reform   **249**

Church has recognized in official magisterial documents[7]—yet it seems clear today that it is not the best way by itself to solve some of our more pressing social problems.

2. Universal Access Retaining Present Mixed System

The proposals under this category have several things in common. First of all they want to use revenues from taxes to assure health insurance to the poor. Secondly, they promote the idea of all working people being insured through their jobs. Thirdly, they want to be able to achieve the first two goals while retaining the present mixed system of private insurance, Medicare, and Medicaid. Obviously these goals can be accomplished in a variety of ways, thus there are differences among the proposals.

a. Basic Health Care for All Americans Act

In 1987 Senator Edward Kennedy of Massachussetts and Representative Henry Waxman of California proposed the Basic Health Care for All Americans Act.[8] This bill developed into a series of proposals having to do with health care which required employers to insure all full time workers. The employers would pay 80% of the cost while employees payed the remaining 20%. It also had a provision to expand the Medicaid program in order to cover all of the poor and uninsured.

Concerning medical services that would be covered, the idea of the proposal was to offer a basic program of benefits and to limit the out-of-pocket expense per family per year to $3,000. Together with all this there would be a development of guidelines for medical practice and cost management strategies.[9] This bill was originally conceived as what is

---

[7]One important recent reference to this fact can be found in the encyclical by John Paul II, *Centesimus Annus,* n.42 in O'BRIEN D.J., SHANNON, T.A., Catholic Social Thought: The Documentary Heritage, p. 471.

[8]As was mentioned in chapter one, Senator Kennedy's proposals go back to the late 1960's. This Act proposed in 1987 has roots that go all the way to those early proposals by the Senator.

[9]Law Library of Louisiana Depository, Supreme Court Building, 301 Loyola Ave. Senate Bills, 101st. Congress, 1st Session, Microfiche 00108.

called a "play only" bill, meaning that every employer would be required to insure all full time employees. Later a new concept was introduced which labeled the bill "play or pay," meaning that employers could choose to be taxed for the employees they did not insure for health care.

b. Health Access America

The American Medical Association has proposed another plan that would fit under this category. It is called Health Access America. The aims of this plan are to require employers to provide insurance for full time employees, put Medicare on a sounder fiscal basis by requiring higher premiums, and have employers and employees contribute to the plan during their working years and not until after retirement. There are six fundamental principles that were presented by the plan[10]:

    1- Improvements to the American health care system should preserve the strengths of our current system.

    2- Affordable coverage for appropriate health care should be available to all Americans, regardless of income.

    3- Particular efforts are needed to assure continued access by the elderly to affordable health care services.

    4- Health care services should be delivered with high quality at appropriate costs.

    5- Patients should be free to determine from whom and the manner in which health care benefits are delivered.

    6- All physicians should be committed to the highest ethical standards in the delivery of care to patients.

The plan called for the federal and state governments to ensure access to medical care to all those with incomes below the poverty level. Medicaid eligibility must reflect the economic realities of each state, and this can be achieved by adjusting the federal poverty level to the state cost-of-living modifier. Medicaid must be able to provide for the medically

---

[10] TODD J.S., SEEKINS S.V., KRICHBAUM J.A., HARVEY L.K., *"Health Access America—Strengthening the US Health Care System,"* Journal of the American Medical Association 265: 2504, (1991).

necessary physician and hospital services, and should not differ greatly across state lines.[11]

In regards to the proposal of having employers provide health insurance for all full time employees and their families, tax incentives are to be provided and also risk pools developed, that would help small businesses to afford such coverage. Risk pools would help insure that no American would be unable to obtain health insurance at a reasonable price due to a health condition. There should be a slow phase-in of the program to allow all businesses to adapt to the transition.[12]

Health Access America called also for Medicare reform. An actuarially sound, pre-funded program is a necessity if assurance of access to quality care is to be given to senior citizens. This reform would entail individual and employer tax contributions to Medicare during their working years. These older citizens would retain freedom to choose a system of health care provision, and would be entitled to a voucher, if wanted, that would enable them to purchase health care in the private sector without having to pay a program tax.[13]

Finally, Health Access America proposes an expansion of long-term care financing through an increase in private sector coverage. This would be encouraged by tax incentives and an asset protection program. This would mean that persons who purchase long-term-care insurance would be able to protect assets they designate, up to the monetary value of the benefits, from being included in any eligibility determination for Medicaid coverage for such care.[14]

c. Consumer Choice Health Plan

Another plan that promotes universal coverage while retaining the present mixed system has been suggested by Alain Enthoven, who is a Stanford economist, and Richard Kronick. In a two part article in the New England Journal of Medicine they proposed the Consumer Choice

---

[11]Ibid.TODD J.S., SEEKINS S.V., KRICHBAUM J.A., HARVEY L.K., *"Health Access America—Strengthening the US Health Care System,"* Journal of the American Medical Association 265: 2504, (1991).

[12]Ibid.

[13]Ibid., p. 2505.

[14]Ibid.

Health Plan. This proposal is designated with two main goals in mind:

> To provide financial protection from health care expenses for all, either through enrollment in comprehensive health care financing and delivery plans or, for the irreducible minimum of people, through public providers of last resort, [and] to promote the development of economical financing and delivery arrangements, by requiring consumers to be conscious of costs in choosing among health care organizations.[15]

The Consumer Choice Health Plan comes out from an understanding that the American people are not completely sold to the idea of universal health care. This, according to the authors, bring fears of socialized medicine and total dependence of the health care delivery system on the government. These American cultural preferences have been considered by the authors before suggesting their proposal.

The goal is to have everyone not covered by an existing public program, be capable of buying affordable subsidized coverage through his or her employer or through "public sponsors." These sponsors would be created by the states through legislation powerfully influenced by incentives from the federal government. These sponsors would serve as brokers, selecting the coverage that is to be offered, contracting with health plans, managing the enrollment process, collecting premiums from those served, paying premiums to health plans, and administering the subsidies available.[16]

Medicare, Medicaid, and private insurance would remain intact under this plan. Employers would be required to cover full time employees and taxed 8% on the first $22,500 of the wages and salaries for any worker they are not required to cover. In addition, employers will offer those employees working at least 25 hours per week, a choice of qualified plans, and contribute at least 80% of the average cost of basic coverage including dependents.

A similar tax would apply to those who are self-employed, retired, or uninsured but capable of paying. The revenues from this will go to the public sponsors who will provide coverage to those not covered by Medicare, Medicaid, or other employer-based programs. Those people

---

[15]ENTHOVEN A., KRONICK R., *"A Consumer-Choice Health Plan for the 1990's,"* New England Journal of Medicine 320(1): 31, (1989).

[16]Ibid.

with incomes below 150% of the poverty line would be completely covered, and the deductibles or out-of-pocket expense for anyone could not be more than 100% of his or her insurance premium.

One of the main ideas of the plan is to offer incentives to consumers by making them—employers and employees—pay enough of the cost of health care that they would be motivated to seek for the plans that offer the best mixture of efficiency and quality care. Employers would be motivated to do this due to the fact that they would pay 80% of the costs. Employees' incentive will be related to the loss of some tax deductibility that is now part of their health benefits.[17] The other idea is to promote managed competition among providers of health care that will evolve into widespread private reform of the system.

Criticisms of proposals like this one have mainly emphasized the doubt as to how effective social changes can be without some level of governmental intervention, and at the same time whether individuals and private enterprises have the sufficient knowledge of medicine necessary to effectuate such efficient consumer controls in what relates to health care delivery.[18]

d. National Leadership Commission on Health Care

The last proposal that will be discussed under this section will be the one of the National Leadership Commission on Health Care. This Commission put out a document entitled *For the Health of a Nation* which was developed by a coalition of thirty-eight corporations, unions, and foundations.[19] The Commission worked under the assumption of agreement upon some fundamental principles: 1) there should be no financial barrier separating Americans in need of health care from access to care that is available; 2) providers of health care should be adequately compensated; 3) health policy should restore clinical freedom to the highest degree possible; 4) financial responsibility for the poor should be assumed by the government, individuals, and employers; 5) individuals

---

[17]ENTHOVEN A., KRONICK R., *"A Consumer-Choice Health Plan for the 1990's,"* New England Journal of Medicine 320(1): 36, (1989).

[18]KEANE P.S., *Health Care Reform: A Catholic View*, p. 42.

[19]Report of the National Leadership Commission on Health Care, *For the Health of a Nation*, Health Administration Press Perspectives: Ann Arbor, Michigan, 1989.

have a duty of securing adequate health care insurance for him or herself and for any dependents; 6) a basic package of health services to which all should have access is ultimately the responsibility of the federal government; and 7) the integrity of the doctor-patient relationship should be protected.[20]

There are many similarities of this proposal in relation to the ones previously discussed, including a $3,000 limit for out-of-pocket expenses and a call for preventive care especially in relationship to prenatal care and mental health care. There are some other recommendations that are unique to this proposal. For example, the National Leadership Commission proposes that each state should set up an uninsured access program which they call UNAC. This program would cover the poor and those in need of acute care through Medicaid.[21] This provision may help to foster the effectiveness of the Medicaid system by moving its administration totally to the states, but it would still leave three separate coverage systems.

Another thing proposed by the Commission is that employers and employees either contribute to pay for employee health insurance on a 75%-25% ratio, or else pay the equivalent tax to cover the cost of employees' insurance. The employers would be taxed 9.68% on the first $45,000 in wages per employee, while the employee would be taxed 2.04%.[22]

These four approaches presented above point toward a variety of reforms while keeping the present system with practically all its components. This reluctance to deal more directly with the system itself has generated the strongest criticism of these proposals and of the people who support them as the answers to American health care.

---

[20]National Leadership Commission, *For the Health of a Nation*, p. XXII.

[21]Ibid., pp. XXIII-XV.

[22]National Leadership Commission, *For the Health of a Nation*, pp. XXIII-XIV. There is a table given at the bottom of the page explaining the numbers. Notice that the tax is limited to the first $45,000, thus not fully progressive, but clearly the "play or pay" concept is enforced.

The Problems and the Proposals for Reform 255

3. Universal Coverage Increasing Public Coverage While Keeping Private Employment-Based Coverage

The three proposals that will be mentioned in this section still attempt to combine public programs with private health insurance offered mainly through employment. The difference of these plans from the ones mentioned in the previous section is that they call for more drastic changes in the government sponsored aspect of the plans.

a. MediPlan
The first proposal to be discussed is the program called MediPlan, which was introduced by Representative Pete Stark of California in 1990.[23] Under this proposal, employers could choose to provide private insurance or health maintenance organization coverage. Part C of the act, which deals with payments for benefits and financing, describes clearly that certain medical services such as those for mothers and children, will be considered as benefits that must be distributed as promptly and directly as possible. The coverage for nursing home is better, and there is a limit set on the costs that can be charged.[24] Americans that fall below the 200% of the poverty level would receive a full subsidy that would cover the full cost of health insurance. This would be administered by a new program which would eliminate the inequalities of the present Medicaid program and its differences from state to state. The MediPlan also includes a 4% tax on personal or corporate incomes of more than $16,000 a year. This tax will be necessary in order to pay the federal costs that would be incurred if the plan was enacted. To this sobering realism can be added the fact that the plan does little to simplify the already complex combination of private, employment-based insurance, and a federally managed health insurance program.

b. The Pepper Commission
Another plan that wants to reform the U.S. health care delivery while retaining the current system of private insurance is the one proposed by the U.S. Bipartisan Commission on Comprehensive Health Care. This commission was formed by the U.S. Congress in 1988, and in 1990 came

---

[23]Law Library of Louisiana Depository, Supreme Court Building, 301 Loyola Ave. House Bills, 101st. Congress, 2nd Session, Microfiche 00284.

[24]These costs are limited to $2,000 per individual and $3,000 per family.

up with its final report. The Commission was renamed the Pepper Commission in honor of its creator and first chairperson, Representative Claude Pepper (D-Fla). It was later chaired by Senator John D. Rockefeller IV of West Virginia.

The main proposal of this report was to build a consensus to make universal coverage for health care and long-term care a reality. The two tasks faced by the commission were to reform the nation's existing system for assuring health care, and to create a system that would assure long-term assistance to the people.[25]

The Commission's major findings have to do with the fact that job-based coverage is under siege. This is especially true for workers in small businesses. Even in large companies, employers are trying to cut benefits and shift health costs to employees. The answer is to build on and strengthen the current combination of job-based and public coverage. Patching the current safety net provided by Medicaid or giving poor people vouchers for health care cannot achieve the universal coverage desired. This would come at a very high price to tax-payers—something that the commission wanted to avoid. In summary, the Commission proposed the following measures as the elements that would make a new plan work: offering guaranteed coverage for workers through the workplace, bringing about private health insurance reforms and incentives to help small businesses fulfill this charge, subsidizing access to a public program in order to guarantee all employers access to affordable coverage, providing a good public plan for nonworkers or other employers who would prefer it, and securing quality and cost containment measures for the entire health care system.[26]

The Commission recommended that all workers should be entitled to receive health coverage through their jobs. In order to achieve this, special attention must be paid to small employers, meaning those with less than 100 workers.[27] In order to help small businesses the Commission

---

[25]ROCKEFELLER J.D., *"The Pepper Commission Report on Comprehensive Health Care,"* New England Journal of Medicine 323: 1005, Oct. 4, 1990.

[26]Ibid.

[27]Statistics show that those employers with less than 25 workers employ about half of those who are uninsured in the population, while those with less than 100 workers employ two-thirds of the total of uninsured people in the population.

proposed eliminating the long-list of state-mandated benefits and establishing a new federal minimal standard to ensure access to preventive, primary, and catastrophic care. Tax subsidies to small employers would also be offered. Predictable rates for insurance and prevention of discriminatory practices based on health status constitutes a third measure proposed by the Commission. Preexisting-condition exclusions would be eliminated, and everybody would be allowed to purchase insurance. The government must do its share in fulfilling its responsibility to provide coverage for health care. Thus a new federal program, which will not be welfare-based is recommended. This program would function as a safety net for the poor and unemployed, as well as an option for employers who may find this plan more affordable. National standards would be established for this program.[28]

The Pepper Commission clearly calls for a stop to unnecessary or inappropriate care. There should be private an public initiatives to promote the best value for each dollar spent in health care. The plan recommended to encourage employers to pursue the development of managed care in job-based coverage, but also to require those insurers offering managed care to large businesses to do likewise with small businesses.[29]

Overall, the Pepper Commission called for important reforms, but with its insistence of retaining a private and employer-based insurance while at the same time developing new federal programs to take care of the poor and the aged, it failed to address the systemic problems that will not be dealt with effectively. Even if health care would be assured to everyone through the proposals of this plan, it is still difficult to see how the inequalities of the present system will be corrected instead of shifted to a slightly higher level of health care assistance that would be still subject to high administrative costs and inefficiencies.

c. The President's Health Security Plan

The last proposal included in this section will be the 1993 Health

---

[28]ROCKEFELLER J.D., *"The Pepper Commission Report on Comprehensive Health Care,"* New England Journal of Medicine 323: 1006-1007, Oct. 4, 1990.

[29]ROCKEFELLER J.D., *"A Call for Action: The Pepper Commission's Blueprint for Health Care Reform,"* Journal of the American Medical Association 265: 2509, May 15, 1991.

Security Plan developed by the Clinton administration.[30] This proposal called for a new synthesis of market competition, new powers of government regulation, employment-based coverage, and the possibility of shifting in and out of Medicare by joining government regulated health alliances. Medicaid would be faded out, with the exception of the possibility of using the program for undocumented persons who need emergency services.[31]

The Clinton Plan, as it popularly was known, came about after a remarkable process of policy development. The First Lady, Hillary Rodham Clinton, was put in charge of directing the working group. A management expert and long time friend of the first couple, Ira C. Magaziner, worked in secret with more than 500 experts. By September 1993 the main outlines of the draft were ready, and the President made choices from the different options presented in the document in order to present it to the nation during a prime time address to Congress.

The plan proposed a system that would draw on managed competition as developed by several market-oriented economist, among which Alain Enthoven was one of the most prominent. Most people would obtain their health insurance through a new system of "health alliances" run by the individual states, who would set standards for local health plans, following federal guidelines. Consumers would be offered a variety of plans, all having the same basic package of health benefits. Health plans, organized mainly by private insurers, would compete for customers on the basis of price and quality. In order to control spending in health care, the plan proposed that the federal government impose caps on the growth of health premiums in order to keep them in line with the general inflation rate. A new National Health Board would be established in order to oversee national spending and to set national standards.[32]

Under this proposal, every person would be required to have health insurance and to contribute to its cost. Employers would be required to contribute 80% of the cost of premiums for their workers and their families. Employees would be responsible for the other 20%. There were three basic kinds of plans envisioned by the proposal: 1) low cost-

---

[30]The White House Domestic Policy Council, *The President's Health Security Plan,* Times Books: New York, 1993.

[31]*The President's Health Security Act,* p. 229.

[32]Ibid., pp. 44ff.

sharing plans, meaning by this HMO's in which patients would pay $10 per office visit when using affiliated doctors and services, 2) high cost-sharing plans, which would allow the freedom to visit any doctor or facility on a fee-for-service basis, but would require individuals to pay the first $200 and families to pay the first $400 of cost and 20% of any subsequent bills with a maximum spending of $3,000 per year per family, and 3) Combination plans in which the patients would pay little to use affiliated doctors and more to use others.[33]

The Clinton Plan did not pass Congress approval. In fact, it could be said that the plan was defeated long before it was up for a vote. The reasons for this were many, but there was a high level of distrust for the plan which developed mainly from the efforts to keep the evolution of the plan secret. Obviously this was intended to prevent outside pressure from influencing the work of the committee, but it ended up backfiring and practically discrediting the proposal completely. There is no question that the ignorance of the majority of the population of matters related to health care was a factor, but at the same time the proposal tried to bring together too many different elements in an attempt to satisfy every camp. The health care system proposed by the Health Security Act lacked a certain coherence due to an exceedingly complex structure and a bureaucratic approach which gave the impression at times that the patient was left in the bottom of the system supporting the whole structure. Keeping the employer mandate also was considered as a weakness since it would extend the practice of holding the rest of the economy hostage to the health care system, as is currently the case.[34]

4. Unified National Financing With Administration By Private Insurers

The next three plans to be discussed move toward the notion of a single national plan for financing health care while retaining private insurers. In these plans the role of the states will be of great importance since each individual state in the country will be responsible for the administration of the system and the approval of private health coverage plans as well.

---

[33]*The President's Health Security Act,* Charts in pp. 38-43.

[34]ANGELL M., *"The Beginning of Health Care Reform: The Clinton Plan,"* New England Journal of Medicine 329(21): 1570, (1993).

260 Health Care and the Common Good

a. The Health Security Partnership

The first proposal to be considered is the Health Security Partnership which was developed by a multi-disciplinary technical committee of the Committee for National Health Insurance and proposed by Rashi Fein of the Harvard Medical School.[35] The aim of this plan is to address the problems of access to health care and medical costs simultaneously. Since the different parts of the health care sector are interrelated, there is a need for a comprehensive program. This would be achieved through a partnership between the federal government and the different states. Since there have been many changes in the way health care services have been distributed in the different states, it is more appropriate to have different parts of the country structure payments for health care differently in order to address their economic and demographic needs.[36] States must be capable of addressing their current health needs according to what works with their diverse populations. Each state is to become a sort of national experimental laboratory.[37] In this way, health care related decisions will be brought closer to the people they affect.

Due to the states' involvement, the proposal made clear that it would be very difficult to describe how *the* program would work. There would be likely as many programs as there are states. Nevertheless, it is possible to outline what a typical state approach would look like. The first step of the plan is a definition by the federal government as to what constitutes the core benefits that would apply to all the states. This would be designed to promote equity and eliminate competition among the states. Federal authorities would then proceed to certify that an individual state has 95% of its residents enrolled in a health insurance program, whether private or public, receiving those basic benefits. The mechanisms to ensure enrollment and to generate the necessary funds would be left to the

---

[35]FEIN R., *"The Health Security Partnership: A Federal-State Universal Insurance and Cost-Containment Program,"* Journal of the American Medical Association 265: 2555-2558, May 15, 1991.

[36]Ibid., p. 2556.

[37]Dr. Fein quotes here the work of Justice Louis Brandeis, who held this position of making states in the nation serve as experimental laboratories. Cfr. FEIN R., *"The Health Security Partnership: A Federal-State Universal Insurance and Cost-Containment Program,"* Journal of the American Medical Association 265: 2556, May 15, 1991.

state government. One of the main goals of the plan would be to provide financial protection to individuals who enroll and full payment to providers through insurance. This would encourage health care providers to treat everyone in the state in the same way.[38]

The Health Security Partnership proposal would also allow individual states to determine the appropriate role of private insurance companies. Probably insurance companies that develop managed care programs and capitated health care delivery systems would develop a competitive advantage over the others. Not all companies would survive, but eventually expenditures would be lowered and this would help the companies that survived work more efficiently.

The proposal did not require the elimination of deductibles or coinsurance. These cost-sharing decisions would be left to the states. At times cost sharing may be deemed by particular states as not helping in the cost-containment efforts and adding complexity and administrative costs to the system. States can decide whether cost-sharing is beneficial for them or not. Annual limits would be set, though, amounting to deductibles of $200 for the individual and $500 for a family. There would be also a total out-of-pocket expenditure per family of $2,500. Payments by patients who are below the poverty line would be eliminated as well as for prenatal and postnatal services to individuals or families with incomes below 150% of the poverty line.[39]

b. *Health USA Act*

Another example of a proposal which takes a unified approach to funding health care while leaving untouched the private insurance industry is the Health USA Act proposed by Senator Robert Kerrey of Nebraska.[40] There are three main goals in this proposal: universal access to health care, containment of health care costs, and a single payer financing which would be independent of employment. A National Health

---

[38]FEIN R., *"The Health Security Partnership: A Federal-State Universal Insurance and Cost-Containment Program,"* Journal of the American Medical Association 265: 2556, May 15, 1991.

[39]Ibid., p. 2557.

[40]Law Library of Louisiana Depository, Supreme Court Building, 301 Loyola Ave. Senate Bills, 102nd. Congress, 1st. Session, Microfiche 00259-00260.

Care Commission would be created in order to set guidelines for the states, as well as for establishing national standards for health care and quality and cost control standards.[41] State programs would have to meet the requirements established by the Commission. It would be guaranteed that every citizen would be insured, and the minimum benefits would include physician services, hospital care, medical tests, preventive care, prescription drugs, drugs and alcohol abuse treatment programs, hospice care, skilled nursing facilities services, and mental health services.[42] In order to finance this proposal there would be national and state health care budgets, using federal funds to provide for the states. Each state would have a single payer system that would eliminate an employment-based health insurance system. The goal is to have an administratively simpler plan and thus more cost effective. States would have a choice of administering their own programs or engaging a group of competing private insurers in administering their health program. Also, when people are geographically closer to facilities in a state different from the one they live in, they can access the closer services in the neighboring state and still qualify. This would help especially in facilitating access in rural areas of the country.[43] The money that goes now into Medicare and Medicaid would be applied to the new program. In addition there would be a 5% payroll tax, a 2% tax increase on non-wage income, a top tax bracket tax of 33%, a 10% increase in corporate income tax, taxes on alcohol and tobacco, and an increased tax in social security benefits. Individuals would pay an annual deductible and a 20% copayment with a limit of $2,000 per year for a family of three or more.[44]

This proposal claims as its strength the fact that it can save the U.S. billions of dollars in health care costs over the next five years. This has not been proven convincingly, especially since the proposal would leave the private insurance industry untouched. This industry, being one of the main sources of administrative waste in the present system, needs

---

[41]Law Library of Louisiana Depository, Supreme Court Building, 301 Loyola Ave. Senate Bills, 102nd. Congress, 1st. Session, Microfiche 00260, p. 8.

[42]Ibid., p.15.

[43]Ibid., pp. 76ff.

[44]Ibid., Microfiche 00260, p. 65.

The Problems and the Proposals for Reform 263

drastic changes if real cost reductions and improved efficiency are going to take place.

c. Catholic Health Association Proposal

The Catholic Health Association proposed a value-driven systemic reform plan that would provide universal access to health care while keeping, in order to assure quality, an informed consumer choice and a state chartering of private provider networks. The plan also proposes, in order to assure overall expenditure control, a national budgeting process and extensive use of managed competition. The proposal bearing the title *Setting Relationships Right,* was adopted by the CHA Board of Trustees on February 20, 1992 as a model for systemic reform that would be consistent with the values articulated by the document itself.[45]

The main aim of the plan is not to adopt a system that assimilates that of other countries, but to develop a system that would enhance the strengths of American health care while addressing its weaknesses as well. Certain values are emphasized in order to promote just health care, which include the notions of service, human dignity, the common good, caring for the poor, stewardship, and the role of government.[46]

The working proposal begins with the importance of delivery reform instead of focusing on financing issues. This would be the best way to begin the systemic reform of a fragmented and costly system like the one in the United States. The idea would be to promote a better integration among primary care, acute care, and long-term care.

Funding would be derived from multiple sources. Some of the systems for funding already in place would continue to function. For example, Medicare revenues would continue to be collected through the FICA payroll tax, and the federal and state Medicaid revenues would continue to be collected through the programs already established. Even though these two programs will no longer exist under the CHA's proposal, their flow of financial revenues would be kept.[47] A new agency would be

---

[45]Catholic Health Association of the U.S., *Setting Relationships Right: A Working Proposal for Systemic Healthcare Reform,* CHA Press: St. Louis, MO, 1992.

[46]CHA, *Setting Relationships Right*, pp. ix-xi.

[47]Ibid., p. 17.

created under the title of the National Health Board (NHB), which would gather the revenues into a trust fund. The NHB would administer the trust fund by establishing annual expenditure levels and determining a comprehensive health benefits package for all people. There would be a new entity at the state level as well, called the State Health Organization (SHO), which would receive the NHB dollars, charter local networks of providers, assure that there is competition among them, and give them funds on a risk-adjusted, capitated basis. The local networks of providers would be private entities called Integrated Delivery Networks (IDN's) who would then compete to provide health care on a continuum basis and bear the risk of capitated payment. These IDN's would be privately organized but publicly chartered by the SHO's. All providers would be forced to join one or several IDN's in order to receive funding. There would be an open season during the year for people to choose among IDN's, who in turn cannot refuse enrollment regardless of the health status of the person. Premium payments would be eliminated, while client cost sharing would be based on income. Persons below the poverty level would have no cost sharing, while those between 100% and 200% of poverty pay would contribute on an sliding scale. The annual cost sharing would be limited to $2,000 for individuals and $3,000 for families. Supplemental benefits would be allowed to be purchased outside the IDN network but without any tax benefit.[48]

The health care coverage would be determined by the NHB, tailored to the individual states by the SHO's, and delivered by the IDN's. The NHB would be an independent public agency, modeled on the Federal Reserve Board which would be responsible for overseeing the whole system. This would include managing the national trust fund, recommending health care expenditure levels to the Congress, allocating the funds to the state agencies, and determining the benefit packages for all individuals. The SHO's would determine the community needs and authorize the IDN's in each individual state. They would assure competition among the different networks and provide the payments. According to the size of the state, more than one SHO would be possible to take care of different regions. The SHO's would also determine the rules for competition in each state or region.

As was mentioned already, the major public financing sources such as Medicare and Medicaid would be maintained. Instead of

---

[48]CHA, *Setting Relationships Right*, pp. xi-xii.

The Problems and the Proposals for Reform   265

premiums, employers and employees would pay a new payroll tax that would be 6.9% on all employers and 1.7% on all employees. The balance of the program would then be financed through an excise tax on alcohol and tobacco plus an increase in the federal income tax. Even with these increases, the proposal suggests that because of being freed from high insurance premiums, the average household would end up saving money. Most importantly, the proposal envisions more savings in the future due to a more efficient and quality oriented system.[49]

The CHA plan offers many advantages that would systemically change present day health care delivery. Its emphasis on quality and how to provide it is very significant. It is an acknowledgment that poor quality and high costs in health care are related. More money for programs of health care does not necessarily translates into better care. Poor quality can be very costly. The flexibility and pluralism of the IDN's will be expected to contribute to the creativity and innovation in lowering health care costs while maintaining a standard of quality.[50] Some of the concerns, though, would have to do with the support of a type of bureaucracy that instead of devoting its efforts to cost shifting, as is presently the case, would dedicate its efforts to monitoring quality.

There is also the possibility of promoting a two-tired system of health care, in which the people would be capable of accessing better health care outside of the IDN system. If these differences would be considered substantial in certain situations, it could work for the demise of a system promoting the basic minimum for all. The whole notion of a basic minimum of health care is such a fluid notion, that such a definition would need to be revised constantly. Probably as well, the high startup costs and inherent risks involved in entering a competing field of IDN's where capital would be needed, would make it very difficult for some agencies to begin, and for the system to promote true competition at all financial levels.

5. Single Payer National Health Insurance

The last classification of proposals to be discussed are the ones that call for the end of the private health insurance industry as it exists today, and for the establishment of a national insurance system to be

---

[49]CHA, *Setting Relationships Right*, p. 33.

[50]CHA, *Setting Relationships Right*, p. 25.

administered by the different states. There are two proposals to be discussed in this section.

a. The Physicians for a National Health Program

The first one is the Physicians for a National Health Program proposal. This was the work of a writing committee of thirty physicians from the Cambridge Hospital-Harvard Medical School. This committee was chaired by doctors David Himmelstein and Steffie Woolhandler, and the proposal they came up with has been signed by more than 400 doctors from all over the United States and from all fields of the medical practice.[51]

This plan would call for the replacement of the current mixed system with a single national public insurance plan to cover all necessary medical services. Co-payments and deductibles will no longer be payed by the patients. The reason for this is that these usually end up threatening poor people's health and have little effect on health care costs.[52]

All hospitals would receive an annual sum of their prospective payments from a national health fund. This lump sum of money would be based on past performance and the changes projected in the services provided by each hospital. Individual states would be the ones determining the size of the payments which would in turn be distributed by regional health-planning boards composed of experts and community representatives.[53] Physicians would be paid by billing the national health program for the services rendered to a patient. The taxes to be levied would include the current sources for Medicare and Medicaid funding, taxes on employers, which will tend to vary in how they affect the different companies according to how much was the employee covered by previous private plans. A company that provided generous coverage to their

---

[51] See the introductory note in the article by HIMMELSTEIN and WOOLHANDLER entitled *"A National Health Program for the United States,"* New England Journal of Medicine 320(2): 102, 1989, January 12.

[52] HIMMELSTEIN D., WOOLHANDLER S., *"A National Health Program for the United States,"* New England Journal of Medicine 320(2): 103, 1989, January 12.

[53] Ibid., p. 104.

employees, would end up realizing huge savings with the new system.[54] In the long run, overall costs would be reduced, since health costs would rise less steeply due to better planning and greater efficiency.

The most crucial aspect of this proposal is the elimination of the private insurance industry. There are more than 1,500 private insurers in the United States with an administrative cost that accounts for 8% of the total cost of health care while Medicare has administration costs of less than 3%.[55] This kind of unitary program could afford to pay expanded care from the savings that would be realized in administration without having to add new costs to the health care budget. This would free physicians from the many administrative intrusions that are currently a major part of health care practice.[56]

This proposal would create a single insurer in each individual state that would be subject to national standards. The structure of the insurer could vary according to the state's preferences. This means that the insurer could be placed under a government agency or under a commission elected by the citizens.[57]

Everyone would be fully insured for all medically necessary services. The practice of sending itemized patient-specific hospital bills would cease. Practitioners who function on a fee-for-service basis would submit all their claims to the state. A fee schedule for physician services would be negotiated. The expenses related to billing would be minimal, while physicians would receive full payment for virtually all services and

---

[54]The Chrysler Corporation, for example, would reduce payments per employee annually from $5,300 to $1,600, a figure that was calculated by the total spending today on health by employers by the total number of full-time-equivalent, non-government employees. See HIMMELSTEIN D., WOOLHANDLER S., *"A National Health Program for the United States,"* New England Journal of Medicine 320(2): 106-7, 1989, January 12.

[55]HIMMELSTEIN D., WOOLHANDLER S., *"A National Health Program for the United States,"* New England Journal of Medicine 320(2): 103, 1989, January 12.

[56]GRUMBACH K., BODENHEIMER T., HIMMELSTEIN D., WOOLHANDLER S., *"Liberal Benefits, Conservative Spending: The Physicians for a National Health Program Proposal,"* Journal of the American Medical Association 265: 2549, May 15, 1991.

[57]Ibid..

an extra payment for any bill that is not paid within 30 days. Physicians could also choose to work on a salaried basis for hospitals or clinics with a global budget, or a health maintenance organization that would receive a capitated payment for all non-hospital services.[58]

b. The Universal Health Care Act

A second proposal for a national health insurance program is the Universal Health Care Act of 1991 which was introduced by Representative Marty Russo of Illinois.[59] This bill was jointly sponsored by twenty-five other members of Congress and endorsed by several labor unions and other organizations. The Russo bill offers the same structure as the proposal offered by the Physicians for a National Health Program. It does, however, offer more specific information on the administrative, financial, and cost related factors of a national health insurance program. At the national level the program would be administered by the Department of Health and Human Services.[60] The individual states could administer the program themselves or they could contract only one private firm to handle claim processing. Insurance premiums would be substituted by a 6% tax on employers. There would also be a 4% increase in corporate taxes, a top rate of 38% in the federal income tax of those earning over $200,000, a long term care premium increase for the elderly of $25 over the current Medicare Part B premium, and the consideration of 85% of Social Security benefits as taxable income.[61] Once again the Russo bill makes a strong case for the benefits that could be achieved through the simplification of the present health care system and the resulting reductions in administrative costs. The Russo bill asserts that hospitals' administrative and billing expenses constitute 18% of total costs, and that 45% of the income received by doctors can be spent on

---

[58]GRUMBACH K., BODENHEIMER T., HIMMELSTEIN D., WOOLHANDLER S., *"Liberal Benefits, Conservative Spending: The Physicians for a National Health Program Proposal,"* Journal of the American Medical Association 265: 2550, May 15, 1991.

[59]Law Library of Louisiana Depository, Supreme Court Building, 301 Loyola Ave. House Bills, 102nd. Congress, 1st. Session, Microfiche 00120.

[60]Ibid., pp. 20ff.

[61]Ibid., pp. 28ff.

costs related to billing.[62] If this proves to be true, the strategies presented by a single payer national health insurance proposal may prove to be the best equipped to deal with the systemic problems of the present system.

---

[62]KEANE P., *Health Care Reform: A Catholic View*, p. 49.

NINE

COMMON GOOD, DISTRIBUTIVE JUSTICE,
AND HEALTH CARE

There are many useful and helpful elements in the proposals mentioned above. All the different suggestions attempt to offer what is perceived as the best way to make health care delivery a more just, efficient, and economical reality. What is lacking in all of them is an adequate ethical component in that they do not articulate the principles on which they are based, nor indeed take sufficient cognisance of the ethical dimension. It is true that a couple of the proposals deal with the ethical foundations and the values involved in health care, but none of them deals with the nature of health care upon which such values are built.[63] By the nature of health care it is meant the intimate link that exists between the human person and medical care.

In unit three we presented the subjects of the common good and distributive justice as two notions that have been developed by Catholic theologians and Church teaching in order to help human beings give guidelines for cooperative social living, and at the same time facilitate proper distribution of basic human needs. Health care is part of the heritage of humanity, and it is certainly a basic human need. This means that health care today is the product of the commulative effort of millions of people throughout history, and that every human being, by simply belonging to the human race, has a claim upon medical care. The ethical implications then as to how to develop a system of health care, are great.

---

[63]The reference here is to the plan by the Clinton administration of 1993 and the Catholic Health Association proposal from 1992. Both have sections dedicated to the ethical dimensions and values related to health care, yet obviously the primacy of these values when placed against other values such as free enterprise and libertarian notions of human freedom, is precisely what is being questioned. Unless the deeper dimension of the nature of health care is addressed, there is a risk of never fully comprehending the obligations that are part of such nature.

The concepts of the common good and distributive justice could help us focus on the true nature of health care and on the person subject to health care, thus giving us a better understanding of the direction that it should take in the future. Granted that providing health care is an obligation, there is evidence that the fulfilment of this obligation will encounter much complexity. As it has been shown, this is not happening at this time in the United States. Adequate health care for all is the most important link in providing an organizational context in which all human beings can flourish, and the principles of the common good and distributive justice can provide the bases for the obligation of providing such a context.

As it has been shown already, health care has gone through great historical changes in the U.S. which have brought medical science to unparalleled levels of recognition. Historical circumstances, though, have been critical as well in facilitating a health care delivery system in which health care is considered as a commodity. Technology has made a commitment to health care. Society has learned to depend on health care. Yet a lack of understanding of the nature of health care has promoted and accepted a kind of system that is destined to collapse. No consumer good can bear the burden of having an unlimited demand, no desirable alternative, critical life-sustaining capability, escalating costs, and great economic potential, while at the same time pretend to be able to effectively satisfy the needs of the whole population. The lack of ethical foundations in the proposals for reform have contributed to a faulty analysis of the situation concerning health care in the country. The problem is that the issue has been dealt with a presumption that health care is to be considered merely as a commodity, without attendant ethical values, a kind of attempt at "value free" analysis. This will not do. Unless the true nature of health care is studied, and solutions which correspond to this nature are proposed, no reform proposal of universal health care will be effective. The reason for this is that unless health care is seen as a societal obligation, and not simply as one more good in the marketplace, there would always be the possibility of accepting and justifying less than universal health care as a solution. It was shown at the beginning of the text that this would be done at the expense of many people not receiving timely and necessary care.

1. Moral Basis for Health Care Reform

As was shown in the previous chapter, one of the great controversies in the pluralistic world of today is whether it is possible to have a common notion of the good life. This controversy is more closely connected to the specifics of certain proposals that have been suggested for health care reform. When dealing with health care in general, there are certain primary principles that all human beings can agree upon. As one contemporary author has said: ". . . it is true that there are great differences between civilizations where it is difficult to find a unique intellectual vision, however the fact that we can recognize them all as moral visions bespeaks the fact that there is a deeper unity even if we are incapable as yet of describing and analyzing it."[64] It is in this "deeper unity" that a notion of the common good must be found.

A call for reform in what concerns access to health care is clearly one of these moral visions that have a universal value. Certainly in the United States, judging by the amount of literature on the subject, access to health care is an important national concern. There are certain principles concerning health care that touch upon this deeper unity which is found in all peoples.

The notions of the common good and distributive justice provide the framework that enables us to reach certain basic agreeable principles concerning health care. These principles are to become the building blocks from which health care should be structured in the U.S. We will first discuss such principles which will in turn become the reference points to later help us consider how to apply them to the American context.

a. The nature of health care

Health care reform must be based primarily upon the nature of health care itself. Medicine is intrinsically a moral activity. This is so because everything that medicine does is related to making a decision for a particular person who is in need due to illness or distress. The focus of medicine is on making the right choice for a needy patient based on universal values and scientific knowledge. Choices based upon these values must be justifiable by following ethical standards of conduct. These ethical standards tend to have a universal dimension since health policy, regardless of country, race, or faith should be a fundamental concern of all human activity. Health care considered in this way, is a basic necessity of all human beings which originates independently of considerations of utility, property, professional prerogatives, or the willingness of society to finance the cost of the services required.

---

[64]KENNEDY T., *Doers of the Word*, p. 62.

Health care is unique among social goods. There are many other needs that people have in today's world such as housing, food, clothing, education, and recreation among others, yet, in all these, the needs are approximately equal. No human being needs more housing than another. In the case of health care the same is not true. Legitimate need for medical help varies tremendously. These needs develop many times when least expected. As persons we are all equally subject to pain, suffering, disability, and death. Ignoring health care needs arbitrarily is incompatible with the basic principles institutionalized in society.[65]

There are some things that can be considered more important than health, but not many. Some absolute rights such as life, liberty, freedom of expression, and justice may be some of them, for example. Yet, when a person is ill, it can be said that these absolute rights cannot be fully exercised. It is evident that in a society that professes to be democratic, affluent, and with abundantly available medical resources, the fundamental and universal human need for health care should not go unfulfilled.

b. Stewardship of resources

Another principle that can be generally accepted by all human beings has to do with the way medical resources are to be considered. We have a common stake to develop a health care system that meets our needs as they change throughout our lives. Since we all age and usually develop greater health needs with the passing of time, we must share fairly the benefits and burdens of a good health care system across generations. This common claim we have, results in the fact that considerable public dollars are spent on health care. These public dollars have for decades underwritten a significant share of the cost of medical education and important research from which we have all benefited, as well as provided needed medical services affecting the demand for certain treatments.[66] It is also public institutions that provide much of the environment and structure in which medical activity occurs. In summary, health care is not simply "private property." It "belongs" to all human beings and to society as a whole. This is so since health care is the result of the cooperation of

---

[65]VEATCH R., *"Just Social Institutions and the Right to Health Care,"* Journal of Medicine and Philosophy 4(2):172, June 1979.

[66]JECKER N.S., PEARLMAN R.A., *"An Ethical Framework for Rationing Health Care,"* Journal of Medicine and Philosophy 17(1): 85, February 1992.

generations of physicians, scientists, patients, as well as sources coming from other private and public concerns.[67]

As human beings we share as well in a general property right to natural resources. It can be said that we own, as members of society, natural resources such as viruses, molds, minerals and plants. Many basic health care resources are produced from these natural ones which we, as a society, own. One in four prescription drugs in the United States comes from natural resources.[68] This does not say that the people who invest the capital and labor needed to make products from natural resources have no additional share in those resources. But it does say that this is not an absolute share since we hold natural resources in common.

Another way of considering this same argument is by what can be called an argument from collective social protection. Threats to health are comparable to those presented by crime, fire, and a polluted environment. Freedom from assault, for a society that intends to guarantee it, means establishing a police force, with its necessary personnel, equipment, and facilities to operate. It also means the establishment of a judiciary system to try violators and enforce penalties. In other words, it means judges, lawyers, courts, and relevant legal support. There are many collective schemes already at work to protect health, which include programs for air and water sanitation among others. Consistency in this regard, demands that the essential health care assistance in response to the threats to health that come from illness and distress should likewise be a collective responsibility. These concepts should not remain abstract, but should be based on a true sense of community and of the recognition of our common vulnerability and finitude.

c. Universal access

Due to the nature and common claim that every human person has upon health care, there should be universal access to it. When this requirement is translated into the language of society and government it means that there should be a national plan that provides health care for the whole population. This is clearly not the case in the United States. The concept of a national health insurance has been consistently misunderstood

---

[67]BOUCHARD C.E., *"Healthcare Reform's Moral, Spiritual Issues. The Problems are not Just Political,"* Health Progress, p. 59, May-June 1996.

[68]JECKER N.S., PEARLMAN R.A., *"An Ethical Framework for Rationing Health Care,"* Journal of Medicine and Philosophy 17(1): 85, February 1992.

and villainized throughout the centuries in the history of the country. Its implementation would be the only certain way to assure that the poor, the needy, and the marginalized receive appropriate and timely health care. Health care should never be considered by any citizen as a burden that should be avoided because of its lack of affordability now or in the foreseen future.

The best way to ensure appropriate, timely, comprehensive, and continual care is to ensure access to primary care. This is one of the most noticeable differences between health care in the United States of America and in countries such as all the ones in Western Europe, Canada, Japan, Australia, and New Zealand. In all those countries, forty to fifty percent of all clinical physicians are general practitioners, while in the U.S. only fifteen percent are.[69] In all of them, there is an explicit commitment to universal access to primary care. It is interesting that even though the U.S. has a higher standard of living than those nations, all of them, without exception, have a longer life expectancy of their population and lower infant mortality rates. Primary care is a universal need which imposes a claim on society and the professions, especially the medical profession. Even when this claim is not considered absolute by some authors, it is nevertheless a very strong one in a kind of society like the one in the U.S.[70]

Any way one looks at it, the situation in the United States is one in which universal coverage is not a priority. Even when at times some studies point to the fact that in many instances the publicly insured are worst off than the privately insured and even the uninsured,[71] the main reason for this is that there is no clear commitment to universal care.

---

[69]DOUGHERTY C.J., *American Health Care: Realities, Rights, and Reforms*, pp. 13-14.

[70]PELLEGRINO E.D., THOMASMA D., *A Philosophical Basis of Medical Practice: Toward a Philosophy and Ethic of the Healing Professions*, p. 224.

[71]BASHSHUR R.L., HOMAN R.K., SMITH D.G., *"Beyond the Uninsured: Problems in Access to Care,"* Medical Care 32 (5): 418, 1994 May. The argument of these authors is that offering public health care to the whole population will not solve the problem since they attribute the problems of the current health care system in the U.S. to the lack of efficiency of the public health care. The authors fail to analyze the lack of coordination in the whole system which ends up maldistributing resources.

There are plenty of good conservative reasons to cover everyone: The great number of "baby boomers" are getting older, and there is a need for a healthier work force; there is a lot of money wasted through the misuse of trauma care when people are uninsured; the underwriting practices of insurance agencies compromise employer integrity in terms of protecting all workers; health care providers are taking too much of a hit; the system is irrational; the newly available foreign workers have access to care and will compete with the American work force. Regardless of all these good reasons, there is still great resistance to the idea of a universal health insurance in the country. This in spite of the general agreement among the people that health care needs can be objectively ascribable even when the person is not completely aware of them. Health impairments constitute deviations from an individual's normal structure and function which also reduces an individual's fair share of what some authors have called the "normal opportunity range."[72]

There are several objections to a national health insurance initiative. One of them is that it would involve spending more money on health care. It has been shown, though, that properly designed, universal health insurance would provide the best way to curb the expenditures on health care as has happened in the rest of the industrialized world.[73] The U.S. lacks the financial control that a comprehensive health insurance program would produce. It is interesting that in 1965 the U.S. spent about the same percentage of the Gross Domestic Product (GDP) on education (6.2%), health care (5.9%), and defense (7.5%). Since then, the military share will go closer to 5% by the end of the 1990's, education has increased over 7%, but the health care share had gone to over 14% by 1992 and the Congressional Budget Office estimates it to reach the 17.5% or 18% mark by the year 2000.[74] This huge change in the allocation of national resources is taking place with no public understanding or discussion of the future effects that such trend could have in the national economy. At times this growth has been blamed by the population on

---

[72]VAN DER WILT G.J., *"Cost-effectiveness Analysis of Health Care Services, and Concepts of Distributive Justice,"* Health Care Analysis 2(4):299, November 1994.

[73]STARR P., *The Logic of Health Care Reform: Why and How the President's Plan Will Work,* p. xxxvii.

[74]Ibid., p. 13.

factors based on incorrect hypotheses. For example it has been said that the escalation of health care costs is connected to defensive medicine and the fear of malpractice coming from physicians, yet malpractice insurance represents less than 1% of the overall costs. Actually, malpractice insurance premiums have remained constant as a share of costs.[75] Another group that have served as scapegoats to blame for the rise in health costs have been the elderly. Yet, aging has been only of secondary importance for cost expansion. According to one study, aging alone caused a very small 0.3% annual increase in the use of health services in the forty years between 1946 and 1986. It is true that with the improvement of life-support technology and the advanced care offered to the elderly today there has been an effect on the national costs of health care, yet, what really matters is not how many elderly people the country has, but how is the health care provided to them managed. The truth is that the U.S. system, as it is run today, brings about high costs for all Americans, especially the aged, who have become, not the cause, but the key focus of the problem.[76]

Another criticism is that national health insurance will limit free choice. This old argument is losing credibility today. The truth is that Americans are already losing freedom under the current system as has been already mentioned in conjunction to employer-based insurance, for example. For those without any insurance, "free choice" is a cruel way to describe their need of an emergency room for routine access to health care. Universal coverage could really enhance the real options that citizens have. National health insurance would provide access to a mainstream standard of coverage on the basis of citizenship rather than employment.

d. Comprehensive similar benefits

As mentioned before, health needs should be the primary bases for the health care that is to be provided. Any other factor should remain secondary according to circumstances. Due to the nature of health care, health needs provide the most legitimate measurement of the kind of assistance required. Every society should strive to abide by the principle of justice that if anyone has an opportunity to receive a service or good that satisfies a health need, then everyone "who shares the same type and

---

[75] STARR P., *The Logic of Health Care Reform: Why and How the President's Plan Will Work*, p. 20.

[76] Ibid., pp. 21-22.

degree of health need must be given an equally effective chance of receiving that service or good."[77] What this principle does is to remove health care from the possibility of determining distribution according to factors that are not intrinsically part of what it takes to promote good health. Obviously, there are circumstances that could limit such distribution. The most obvious one is the scarcity of resources or the technological capabilities of a particular nation. There are certain limits that even the great advances in medical science have not been able to surpass. Following this principle, every country would be morally obligated to offer the greatest amount of health care available in a way that would not discriminate on any other basis than health need as to who receives what kind of treatment.

Health needs in essence are the same, regardless of race, language, and socio-economic status. When these factors begin to affect the way health care is distributed, then the whole reason for providing care can deteriorate in the process, and health care would lose its "soul." This is precisely what Rawls tries to communicate through his ideas on the "veil of ignorance." The objection to Rawls, which was raised in chapter two, is precisely that this notion of certain basic similar needs is so much a part of the human reality that even without the veil of ignorance, reason would affirm the importance of providing for the uncertainties of life through just health care. The veil of ignorance is not as important as a veil *from* ignorance. This veil from ignorance will not keep us outside real life, but, on the contrary, will allow us to keep ideas that go against basic human intuition and common sense excluded from our decision-making. The highest quality of health care possible for all would be made available in this way, and there would be a constant challenge to evaluate whether this goal is being achieved and if all the possibilities to make of this provision a priority are being considered.

e. Integrity in the physician-patient relationship

By its very essence the medical act is an ethical act. This means that the relationship between physician and patient has certain ethical connotations which are very important in delineating the different roles that will be assumed by the two parties while there is a professional relationship. This covenant that is established between the doctor and his or her patient is based on the trust that develops from the very first

---

[77] RHODES R.P., *Health Care: Politics, Policy, and Distributive Justice: The Ironic Triumph*, p. 23.

interview. It is through this trust that both, doctor and patient, decide to collaborate with each other with the common objective of combating the condition which gave place to the initial interview.[78] There is a certain sanctity of this covenant that is in the best interest of both patient and physician. It could be said that this trust should be extended as well to any health care provider. During illness or need the patient is in a very vulnerable situation in which there should not be an unreasonable concern about the sincerity and the motivations of the health care provider.

It has been mentioned already in chapter two how the physician's role has been changing to one of what has been called "gatekeeper." Obviously there is a responsible role of a physician to be such a "gatekeeper" since he or she is called to practice rational medicine in which guidelines should be to provide just the right degree of economy of means in diagnosis while offering just those treatments that are demonstrably beneficial and effective. By doing this the physician fulfills the moral obligations of avoiding unnecessary risk to the patient from dubious treatment while conserving the financial resources of both the patient and society. The ethical dilemma of gatekeeping arises when economic incentives and disincentives modify the physician's duty to act on behalf of the patient. The physician should never become the agent of a hospital or system at the expense of the patient, and the patient should never become primarily a source of income. Physicians, nurses, and health care providers have an obligation not to abandon their patients simply to optimize resources. Every rational person would agree that when it comes to something as important as health, the covenant established between health care provider and patient must be safeguarded to its ultimate consequences unless we are willing to put up with a system in which human life is totally devalued in favor of economic incentives.

2. Application of Moral Basis to the American Context

How are then the principles discussed above applied in the context of American health care? There are several things that would need to take place in order to put into practice the principles that the notion of the common good highlighted.

a. Patient as the priority

---

[78]DE LAS HERAS J., *"La Relación Médico-Paciente,"* in Manual de Bioética General, (ed.) DR. AQUILINO POLAINO-LORENTE, Ediciones RIALP: Madrid, 1994, p. 271.

Health care is about patients and how to provide them with the medical assistance necessary to help them live up to their human potential. The patient and his or her needs should occupy the center-stage in any health care system. Most proposals for reform in the country emphasize dealing with financial incentives first and only then see how the system can be better designed to respond to the medical needs of individuals and families. A patient-centered system would reverse this trend. By focusing first on the financial arrangement of the system, there is a lack of consideration of the step that would address the fundamental flaws in the way health care is organized and delivered. Only if the patient's needs are considered the most important aspect of the new system, a procedurally fair system could be put in place. This would be a system in which there would never be a denial of care coming from a unilateral decision from a non-physician manager, but, on the contrary, such a decision would be always subject to review by a health care professional and the patient.[79]

The good of the patient should always be considered first. The structures upon which health care practices depend, must reflect this reality. This notion of the patient's good should be seen in a broader context that brings in the social dimension of the patient as well. One of the tendencies that has favored a more individualistic system of health care and the present emphasis in health care as a commodity, has been the consideration of the patient's autonomy as the most important value in medical care. This way of understanding autonomy has been developed without a recognition of how the principle of autonomy is connected with the good of the patient or the principle of beneficence. Autonomy and beneficence are not conflicting views. Respecting the patient's autonomy leads to the good, since people know their own interests better than other people. The problem may arise when respecting the autonomy of the patient may not realize the individual's medical or social good. In order to keep the patient as the center of health care, when assessing the total good, it is important that each level be understood and respected. Some authors have spoken about the need of "deabsolutizing autonomy." They have emphasized that "beneficence takes into account, but does not capitulate to autonomy."[80] In this way beneficence and autonomy are not

---

[79]GOSTIN L.O., *"Health Care Reform in the United States,"* Journal of Law, Medicine and Ethics 21(1):8, Spring 1993.

[80]PELLEGRINO E.D., THOMASMA D.C., *For the Patient's Good: The Restoration of Beneficence in Health Care,* p. 279.

removed from the conception of the social good or the common good.
In order to develop a patient centered system, there is a need to include the general population in the decision making processes that involve health care issues. One of the major problems in the country has to do with the ignorance of the general population when it comes to medical care.[81] The citizens of a society should have opportunities to have the different alternatives of health care provision explained to them, and they should be able to be part of boards and committees that deal with such problems. At the same time they should be engaged in some kind of voting and filling out satisfaction surveys. Forums that address the whole population and that strive to eradicate the ignorance related to health care should be encouraged and developed by the government and health care organizations. The bottom line always should be what is in the best interest of the patient.

b. A comprehensive approach to health care
Functional health, as described earlier in the text, is not enough for a comprehensive approach to health care. This is the kind of health that allows a basic functioning of the person without any consideration to his or her total well-being. It is certainly true that health is a very fragile reality and that, in many instances, becoming functionally healthy is as much as can be expected. Yet, this does not allow health care providers to limit their provision of health care to what is needed to reach a functional minimum. Feeling healthy is a holistic experience for the person, and providing all the treatments that promote good health must be considered as resources allow. Many times the demands of the taxpayers, health professionals, and health care financiers for the rights to follow and satisfy their own individual interests, have affected the development of a comprehensive health care system.

One of the crucial problems related to the provision of a comprehensive health care system has to do with what kinds of services are meant to be part of such a system. This issue, as well as who is responsible for making such decisions, has been one of the major controversies with no clear answer. Many times this has been used as an excuse for the impossibility of establishing some kind of unified system of

---

[81]For an excellent article on this lack of knowledge of the American population regarding issues of health care today see BLENDON R.J., et al, *"The Beliefs and Values Shaping Today's Health Reform Debate."* Health Affairs, [Spring] (1): 274-284, 1994.

health care. In some ways this argument is similar to the debate about whether it is possible to have a conception of the common good in a pluralistic society.

The notion of the common good that has been defined in this work is not a static one. The human appreciation of what constitutes the common good of society can change with time. A lack of consensus at any particular time should not be an obstacle for reaching some kind of definition as to what comprehensive health care should be. This lack of consensus should be expected due to the very nature of the common good. As long as there is a consensus on the social dimension of human beings, the importance of a human understanding of society where higher or lesser values can be distinguished, and the fact that human beings are the only creatures that can go beyond themselves in order to provide for the needs of others, there should be sufficient vocabulary available to sustain a "meaningful conversation" in our society. Health care matters are especially significant since these are services that are intimately connected to the person. It is true that the developments in the health care field have been astronomical in the last few decades, yet at the same time it is true that even in that comparatively short period of time, we as a society have enough information to determine the effects of the lack of health care provision. In other words, there are many treatments that should be clearly considered part of comprehensive health care simply because we know very well the marginalizing effects that the lack of such services can create for people in our communities. Surely there are many things that are being developed in health care as we speak, which are still in experimental and study phases. Nevertheless, this does not mean that the whole health care science is beyond our intuition and reason to decide as a society what should be included in comprehensive health care.

c. *The role of government*

There is a prevailing attitude today in the United States of mistrust toward the government. The reasons for this are mixed. It depends on who one asks and how that person has fared in society whether the answer will emphasize a lack of action from the part of government which is seen as increasingly protecting the interests of the upper classes, or criticism about too much action and control which has confiscated hard-earned income and redistributed it to the less productive members of society. The bottom line regardless of whether the criticism comes from the left or the right of the political spectrum is that the dissatisfaction and distrust of government comes as a result of the lack of capacity in today's

American culture to see government as part of a much greater reality. The different motivations for our collective distrust of the government make consensus on appropriate health care reform difficult. At the same time, in many instances government has become an individual entity with a life of its own and sometimes with very little connection to actual people and their needs. In order to implement the moral bases of health care reform the people and not only the government must understand that there is a legitimate role for the government to play when it comes to social issues in society. In a time when the emphasis is on rights and not on a societal response to the issues that affect people's lives, it is not difficult to see how the government can become more of an obstacle than a help.

When considering adequate health care to the members of a particular society, it is imperative that health care be recognized as part of the common good. If this is the case, then the first body responsible to offer this service must be society as a whole. The government, functioning as the entity which should voice the needs of the people, has an obligation to participate in this societal response. This does not mean that the government necessarily should have the sole responsibility or even the principal responsibility. The argument that should be developed to provide for the health care needs of the population should be systemic but not necessarily statist. In other words, health care provision does not necessarily need to be a state-sponsored program. Yet, the state should be obligated to work in whatever way necessary to make sure that every person in society can have his or her health needs taken care of. There are two important roles for the government in what relates to health care: 1) It must be the final guarantor that needed health care will be provided, and 2) it should be willing to collaborate with other agencies even when those agencies are the principal means through which health care is being offered. The health care professions have to be the primary agents of health care provision with a clear understanding of their duty to cover the health needs of their society. The role of the state in many instances will be determined by a correct understanding of the principle of subsidiarity, which, as mentioned before, does not only say to leave to the smaller organizations what can be accomplished at their level, but also that there may be certain things that can only be handled well at a governmental level. It is the duty of a society to analyze, understand, and critique the different alternatives that would be possible to follow in order to provide for the health needs of the community. The goal should be to plan how to provide for the health care needs of all, and, once that is the main consideration, then see how it could be done more effectively and efficiently without leaving huge sections of the population out. The state can regulate such procedures as directed by the will of a well informed population, but it does not need to necessarily operate the system. The ultimate and most important role of the state is to facilitate the common good, remembering that primarily this is not meant to be understood as maximizing the sum total of individual goods, but providing the appropriate structural framework for the common good of all to flourish in society.

d. Care over administration

The emphasis of health care should be on care rather than on administration. The over concentration in administrative matters has had a detrimental effect on health care provision in the country. Administration of health care is no longer a tool to facilitate the best and more effective health care available, but actually has become one of the major contributors to the problem. Excessive waste in administrative expenses in health care has come about as a consequence of the development of a system where care is not the main incentive but wealth. The United States pays more for health care than any other industrialized country in the world. Not only this, but the country also uses a higher proportion of health care expenditures for administrative expenditures than any other nation, which interferes with quality care and diverts resources from the delivery of effective services. This certainly puts a tremendous strain on the private economy leaving less resources for housing, education, and other needs. A renewed emphasis on care will allow stewardship concerns to surface in a way that the duplication, the waste, and other factors that make the system so expensive will be challenged.[82]

It is estimated that 22% of the health care dollars is spent on billing and other administrative tasks.[83] There is a normal increase in health care costs throughout the years in every country. This is a result of higher prices for health care goods, a greater volume of goods and services which can be explained by the utilization of goods, the increase in the complexity or intensity of the goods, general inflation, and the continued population growth and shift to an older population. These account for

---

[82]UNITED STATES CATHOLIC BISHOPS, *Resolution on Health Care Reform,* Origins 23(7): 99, July 1, 1993.

[83]ETZIONI A., *"Health Care Rationing: A Critical Evaluation,"* Health Affairs 10(2): 90, Summer 1991.

approximately 60% of the increase in costs. Nevertheless, there is a 40% growth in the cost that comes directly from administrative costs. In the realities of health care provision today, this constitutes an enormous amount of money since we are talking of health care expenditures of approximately 1 trillion dollars a year.[84]

Cost inflation will not be primarily the result of implementing a national health program. This is a misconception that has fueled the talk against any kind of national health insurance. The statistics say that our two closest linguistic and geographic neighbors, England and Canada, have successfully contained costs of health care while embracing systems in which, respectively, there is government ownership of the facilities, and in which the provincial and federal governments pay and regulate health care providers. In the United States the number of health care administrators increased by 171% between 1970 and 1982 while the number of doctors and health care personnel increased 48% and 57% respectively.[85]

Private insurers in the U.S. contribute significantly to the administrative waste. In 1983 the private health insurance companies in the U.S. received $110.5 billion in premiums while paying $100 billion in benefits. The $10.5 billion overhead paid for marketing, processing bills, office furniture and structures, and profits. If one would add the administrative cost of Medicare and Medicaid plus other administrative costs for that year, it comes out to $15.6 billion in order to administer health insurance in the country.[86] Yet, since private insurers see themselves as losing more from the implementation of effective cost controls which threaten their very existence, they invest mightily in political goodwill to fight any cost-containment effort. It is estimated that between 1980 and 1991 medical, pharmaceutical, and insurance companies contributed more than $60 million to candidates running for

---

[84]JOST T.S., TANENBAUM S.J., *"Selling Cost Containment,"* American Journal of Law and Medicine 19(1-2): 98, 1993.

[85]HIMMELSTEIN D.U., WOOLHANDLER S., *"Cost Without Benefit: Administrative Waste in U.S. Health Care,"* New England Journal of Medicine 314: 442, February 13, 1986.

[86]Ibid.

congress.[87]

A good portion of the administrative expense happens as a result of the current reimbursement system which requires that each of the more than 1.6 billion hospital admissions and visits to the doctor by patients each year be attributed to a particular person. By instituting a national health service much of that type of expense could be eliminated. In Canada, for example, hospitals have virtually no billing department and much less of the internal accounting structure that is necessary in the U.S. to attribute costs and charges to individual physicians and patients. Administration has become the master of medicine instead of its servant. Two contemporary physicians and authors have said that administration of health care has gone "from a handful of support personnel dedicated to facilitating patient care to a vast apparatus increasingly influential in medical decision making. Each new reform in the health care system deposits yet another layer of administrators who have the power to say 'no' but not 'yes'."[88]

A deeper understanding of the common good as related to health care matters should be helpful in tilting the balance once again to the side of care rather than administration. This is needed not only to curb the current trend of administrative waste, but also to restore health care to its true role in our society which is to provide for the health care needs of all.

e. Promote local responsibility

It was mentioned above how the present day distrust of government by the citizens should be addressed in a way that would underline the importance of understanding the state as an instrument of the people that should be at their service. At the same time it is important to recognize that this same present day tendency to distrust big government has had a positive effect in calling people to consider anew the importance of smaller, local organizations. As it was shown in the section where the different proposals for reform of health care were presented, the importance of the role of the individual fifty states in the country has received much attention recently. Part of this comes from the belief that

---

[87]JOST T.S., TANENBAUM S.J., *"Selling Cost Containment,"* American Journal of Law and Medicine 19(1-2): 104, 1993.

[88]HIMMELSTEIN D.U., WOOLHANDLER S., *"Cost Without Benefit: Administrative Waste in U.S. Health Care,"* New England Journal of Medicine 314: 445, February 13, 1986.

many of the country's problems can be solved in a more efficient way at a local level.

Related to health care this means that in order to address the needs based on the common good of a very heterogeneous population, as the one which exists in the United States, it would be important to reinstate community-based health planning mechanisms. Local health planning agencies could have a very important role in approving or disapproving of capital expenditures that would exceed a certain monetary limit. This kind of approach would help in creating a more leveled field among the different hospitals and other health care providers and thus diminishing the growing conflicts between hospitals and medical staffs while preventing the unnecessary duplication of health facilities and services. This would help in containing the growth of health care spending.[89]

This approach would also help in dealing with the limits that exist in health care resources by providing health care in a more informed, specialized way, addressing the specific issues related to the different geographical and cultural areas in the country. There is no need for a non-flexible uniformity in the system when clearly there are areas in the country that are doing better than others. The main goal of bringing health care back into a more localized level of organization would be precisely to emphasize the genuine role of health care which always should have patient care as the priority.

f. Terminology needs to change

Before policy engineering can change, verbal engineering has to change. One of the great obstacles concerning radically changing access to health care in the country has to do with the way most Americans understand health care today. There has been a clear development, guided mainly by what has been experienced as problems related to cost of medical care, to deal with health care as a market commodity. The patient has been more and more removed from any direct involvement with the financing of health care. With the development of intermediary organizations responsible for paying medical services, patients tend to lose perspective as to their connection to health care financing. Insurance agencies and health care providers have been brought into a situation in which their providing of health care to the population must be guided

---

[89]BERMAN H.J., KLEIN D., *"Pieces of the Puzzle: Steps Toward Affordable Health Care,"* Hospital and Health Services Administration 37(1): 10, Spring, 1992.

Common Good, Distributive Justice, and Health Care   289

primarily by whether such provision is financially beneficial to them. Those people who want some decent level of health care in time of medical need, must make arrangements to enter into a contract with one such company or agency at a time when they will not become a financial burden. In view of the cost of medical technology, the payments to such companies can be high, effectively leaving out from access to quality care those who cannot afford it.

Developments such as these have turned health care in the nation to something that by nature it is not. Receiving adequate health care has become almost "making the right move at the right time." In other words, health care has become at times a matter in which people have to take certain *risks investing* what they are capable of paying while determining what kind of coverage is sufficient. All this obviously without knowing what the future has in store for them, and many times finding out in not such a distant future, that their health care coverage was inadequate.

Nationally the talk is about reducing the *costs* of health care, making *competition* the center-piece of cost reduction, developing new *managing strategies* that would keep health care costs under control, rationing the distribution of health care *goods,* and motivating people to *buy* the most comprehensive (and expensive) type of insurance. Businesses offer people, whose physical condition qualifies them for the employer-based insurance, comprehensive health plans for which high premiums from their salaries are required.[90] Notice how the whole terminology connected to health care has become the one that corresponds to big business.

Health care terminology has to change from competition to collaboration, from management to social obligation, from health care goods to health care services. Continuing to use the business terminology that has plagued health care in the last three decades only promotes greater

---

[90]A recent newspaper article warns the population that after four years of near stability brought on by managed care, the premiums that most Americans pay for health insurance will rise significantly next year. This increase is predicted to be at least 5% which is more than twice as much as wages and inflation have been rising. This rise is motivated by insurance companies who want to recapture profits that they were losing after they froze or cut premiums in an intensely competitive market for their patients and their employers. Employers have been forced to negotiate with insurance companies, and some times premiums have gone up by more than 10%. See KILBORN P.T., *"Health Care Premiums to Surge,"* in *The Times Picayune,* Monday, October 20, 1997, p. A-7.

hesitation from the part of society to push for governmental responsibility, keeps more and more people in society from a sense of any kind of entitlement to health care, and promotes a mentality from the members of the community who have some kind of health insurance that someone else is paying for it. These three situations work against a greater social understanding of how access to health care is an issue that should involve the whole community in seeking for just and equitable ways of providing and contributing to the health needs of all.

Our society has been able to motivate people to use what has been called "politically correct" language by promoting a new consciousness that there are certain words and expressions that are derogatory toward certain groups of people in society. These efforts, mostly disregarded in the past, have been very successful in changing the way people speak and drawing certain limits as to what terminology will be acceptable in our society. The consequences of challenging what is acceptable by appealing to freedom of speech have been disastrous for some public figures.[91] Considering this in a pastoral way, this process has been successful in bringing about change in the language people use by making them more sensitive to social factors in today's society. This could be applicable to the health care world by educating the population and by socially encouraging the mass media to utilize the more socially minded terms which manifest in a better way what health care is all about.

3. Distributive Justice in Practice

It has been shown above how the notion of the common good as presented in chapter three of this work can be influential in highlighting several principles that society as a whole could subscribe to. It has also been shown that there are certain ways that such principles of the common good could be applied to health care provision in the United States. It was mentioned earlier that the implementation of the common good requires a way of expression; a way of making the common good a part of society. This implementation would take place with the help of an understanding of distributive justice as an expression of the self-transcendence of every

---

[91] We can only think of the many public television commentators and writers who have even lost their jobs and acceptance in professional circles by using words or ideas that are considered "politically incorrect" by our society. I am referring to utterances or articles regarding race or gender in which the authors used words or ideas that are unacceptable by society's standards.

human being, which makes it possible to look beyond personal needs and into the needs of all. Such an understanding of distributive justice would help in dealing with three of the most difficult obstacles in the country that prevent just health care from becoming a reality.

a. Health care is not simply a market commodity

Health care cannot be considered a market commodity. Nevertheless, there is a trend today to ignore this notion and to continue moving in the direction in which health care is stripped of its *raison d'etre*. We have seen throughout this work how this trend to continue dealing with health care as a commodity has been defended in many different ways. Historically it was shown how every time there was a possibility to change this approach, something happened that detracted from any concrete change taking place. A scapegoat to eliminate any kind of notion of social responsibility was always found. The particular historical realities which had the private sector better organized than the public one at the time when health care financing was being considered, prevented the establishment of a national approach to health care provision. In most decisions which had to do with how to provide health care to the population there was little consideration of the moral, ethical problems that had to be considered prior to a decision being reached. The heterogeneity of the population plus an exaggerated notion of personal rights at the expense of any conception of social responsibility developed into a social unresponsiveness to the needs of others. Even when it has been shown that health care does not behave like any other market commodity, still nothing has been done to change that basic approach. The defenses for keeping health care as it is, continue to be many, while at the same time more and more Americans see their lives affected by a lack of appropriate care. The "buck" continues to be passed on, as health care expenses for those who have any kind of insurance are assumed by businesses and private insurers who are more interested in keeping their expenses low and their profits high than in serving the public. People for the most part have lost perspective as to who ends up paying their health care needs, developing a "someone-else-is-paying" mentality , and have grown more and more detached from any understanding of the health care system. Many feel the lack of freedom that comes from having given up such an important part of their well-being to an impersonal company that does not care necessarily for the experiential health of its employees, while at the same time, many companies are beginning to wonder how did they ever get into insuring workers for their health needs.

The excuses today for treating health care as a market commodity continue to be many. Some claim that in order to continue having the best health care system in the world, there is a need to keep a level of competition in place. Without the financial incentives that come from being able to make money from health care investments, few health care agencies would continue to research and improve medical equipment. Any time there is talk about any kind of national insurance, private insurance companies scare the whole population by talking about how much their freedom of choice will be restricted, and end up paying millions of dollars in advertisement campaigns to communicate their opposition. This factor alone should be enough to alert the population that there is something suspicious in such tactics. The only reason an attack like that from insurance companies is successful is because, for the most part, only the most vulnerable and poor members of our society are affected in an extreme way by the lack of adequate health care. The numbers here are shifting, though, and every year more and more people are experiencing the inadequacies of health care provision in the country. There is less trust in the medical profession which has been sold to managed care in ways that threaten in a real way for the first time in American history the clinical autonomy it should enjoy. Even at the time when doctors took care of slaves in the southern plantations, there was no other way in which health care was provided to the rest of the population. In essence it can be said that the doctors who took care of the slaves for a fee were the ultimate way of providing health care in that society. That is not the case today when doctors who receive a capitation fee make important choices for companies that affect the lives of their patients through needed services that are not facilitated or allowed. For some patients the whole process of requesting what they believe are necessary and prudent treatments, has become an obstacle course and a constant battle with their physicians or health care providers. When the aim of those choices is to save money with at least a partial disregard of the patient, it cannot be said that those patients have received optimal health care.

      Besides all these factors which show why health care should not be considered a market commodity, there are other ways as well to answer some of the main objections, especially the ones related to the future of health care being curtailed unless free enterprise is left in place. It is clear that health care is here to stay. In other words, there is such a clear recognition in the world today and especially in the United States of the importance of effective and efficient health care that it is very unlikely that changes in the way it is offered and financed will have a major negative effect. There is an understanding today as never before of the direct connection between certain medical procedures and the restoration of health. The risks involved in many procedures that used to be considered highly risky and complicated are minimal today. This is so to the point that, regardless of the lack of financial means, preventing a person from receiving such benefits which are clearly effective and directly connected with assured healing or at least an improved quality of life would be immoral. This is so in procedures that are considered very expensive today. Most of the discriminatory practices outlined and documented in chapter one are not necessarily the result of a lack of concern for the needs of the people but the logical evolution of a system that is not structured to provide health care to all in an efficient, effective way. Obviously health care provision will always involve money transactions. Doctors and health personnel are entitled to a way of making a living from their services. What should have no place in the health care profession is to see hospitals, that at one point were operated by a single administrator, evolve into business empires with all kinds of layers of associates representing all kinds of pursuits. Many of these officials are excessively paid with even non-profit organizations having administrators that enjoy compensations of close to half a million dollars every year.[92] With the current statistics showing that many people lack appropriate basic health care it must be considered unethical the practice to build what some have described as "luxurious emporiums, with all rooms private, supplying such luxuries as color TV's, bedside telephone, valet parking, and other comforts which run up costs but have no bearing on the patient's treatment and recovery."[93]

While health care continues to be treated as a market commodity in the country, the practice of distributive justice coming from a notion of a societal obligation to provide for the health care needs of all, will be impossible. The very essence of the market mentality creates distinctions which may work very well with certain goods in society, but provision of health care is certainly not one of them.

---

[92]HOLLOWELL J.W., *"The Health Care Crisis—How We Got There,"* Virginia Medical Quarterly 120(4): 222, Fall 1993.

[93]Ibid., p. 223.

b. Rationing is not the solution

As has been mentioned before, the literature concerning health care reform today is enormous. The moment one types the words "health care reform" into a computer data bank, one has to be prepared to see thousands of references to books and articles on the topic. Invariably one of the topics that has received extraordinary attention within this literature has been health care rationing.

It has already been mentioned earlier what rationing stands for in the medical field, and specific plans, such as the Oregon Plan, which dealt with rationing of health care resources, were discussed in chapter two. In many circles rationing has been hailed as the only way to solve the health care crisis in the country. It has been described as a compelling reality. For many authors it is clear that not everyone can have complete access to the highest-quality health care available. This mentality, for the most part, has been behind the push to make physicians the gatekeepers and designated guardians of society's resources. Some authors have detected a certain hypocrisy in this understanding of rationing. For example, two prominent contemporary authors have this to say:

> We argue that the line of reasoning that leads to rationing and physician gatekeeping is morally unsound and factually suspect; that there are conditions under which rationing might be morally justifiable, which are not met by current plans; and that we ought to minimize, rather than enhance, physician self interest as a motive in medical and health care provision. We are well aware that this position resists the current popularity of justice and access discussions, which assume that rationing is a forgone conclusion and assign new roles to physicians.[94]

Other authors have questioned the honesty in thinking that only the health care budget is in need of rationing. They have argued in the following way:

> Why not rationalize the whole government budget and look for non-health items that could be curtailed with much less sacrifice of people's needs and preferences? The problem lies in our present political system. Congress is so dominated by special interests that allocations are driven more by who pays most for the enormous costs of re-election than by any other

---

[94]PELLEGRINO E.D., THOMASMA D.C., *For the Patient's Good: The Restoration of Beneficence in Health Care*, p. 173.

criteria.[95]

Rationing is certainly morally justifiable when its whole object is to deal with limited resources. Any system of health care would be foolish to offer an unlimited access to health care independently of the costs of that system. There are always limitations to be dealt with which are just part of a reality that cannot be ignored. Every country must strive to guarantee to its citizens the best health care possible according to the resources available. This is what can be morally required.

The problems with rationing when considering health care in the United States is that a system of rationing can be inherently evil if it is based on inequitable distribution of goods and services in broader areas of society. There will always be an element of rationing needed when it comes to health services. What is unethical is to present rationing as an alternative prior to considering and actually trying all the alternatives possible to design a more just system. The notion of distributive justice as developed in this work challenges the country not to consider rationing as a primary solution to problems that are created, not by lack of resources, but by lack of equity in the distribution of those limited resources. It is evident in American health care that there could be a more just and equitable distribution of medical resources if the medical needs of all would be the priority. With the successes of programs like Medicare, it is clear that the country could do a much better job to share the community health resources in a way that the whole population would benefit, while trying to curtail any kind of fraud regarding funds dedicated to health care and promoting a more equitable distribution.[96] This is especially true when we see that American society tends to spend what may be considered excessively on much less basic and important things.[97]

Another interesting notion that must be considered when discussing the need for rationing is the fact that by definition rationing

---

[95]ETZIONI A., *"Health Care Rationing: A Critical Evaluation,"* Health Affairs 10(2): 90, Summer 1991.

[96]In 1997 it was determined that the amount of money that was taken from Medicare by fraud was equivalent to the deficit that was needed in order to cover the expenses of the program for that year.

[97]THOMASMA D.C., *"Establishing the Moral Basis of Medicine,"* Journal of Medicine and Philosophy 15(3): 252, June 1990.

assumes that the optimal kind of distribution has been attempted. In other words, there is no point in considering the need for rationing until the effort has been made to distribute the limited resources as equitably as possible. Only then rationing makes sense. Otherwise what would happen is that rationing would only deprive more people of the need since there would already be a percentage that was not receiving any goods to begin with. It is similar to the case mentioned before in connection to employment-based insurance in which it was pointed out that if there is an unjust distribution of work, then distributing health care insurance based on the person's job would only create a domino effect in which the injustice would, not only be continued, but magnified. There is no way that someone in his or her right conscience could claim that everything has been attempted regarding health care. Obviously the financial interests of so many people involved in one way or another in health care provision are more important than taking care in an equitable way of the needs of the population. Many experts in the field of health care are convinced that reductions in other kinds of spending plus a better and more cost effective health planning are sufficient to overcome the problems faced by the health care system today.[98] Only when this has been attempted it can be said that rationing has been done with an orientation toward the common good and that it is free of wrongful discrimination. This is even more urgent to consider when it has been estimated that ten percent of health care spending is currently wasted on the administrative apparatus needed to sustain our present system while with a national health program there could be substantial savings without having to ration care any further or having to place more constraints on patients and doctors.[99] The 14% of the gross domestic product (GDP) we spend presently on health care should be sufficient to provide universal coverage while retaining a high quality of care if a strategy of structural change can keep spending under control by reversing the patterns of investment and behavior that would

---

[98]THOMASMA D.C., *"Establishing the Moral Basis of Medicine,"* Journal of Medicine and Philosophy 15(3): 252, June 1990.

[99]HIMMELSTEIN D.U., WOOLHANDLER S., *"Cost Without Benefit: Administrative Waste in U.S. Health Care,"* New England Journal of Medicine 314: 443, February 13, 1986.

threaten any kind of health care system.[100]

c. The dilemma of equity vs. utility

One of the most difficult problems facing distributive justice within the context of American health care has to do with how to solve cases in which different principles are in conflict among themselves. This acknowledges the fact that even if a more just health care system is implemented in the country, it does not mean that all the problems of health care will be solved. The scarcity of resources is a real problem as highlighted above, and even when there is no question that before trying rationing as a solution there must be a certain assurance that all the possible structures for the system have been studied and considered, there is no guarantee that the structural change will completely solve the problem of scarcity of resources. Our contention is that a restructuring of the system, as will be proposed later, will bring about a much more efficient system with less waste and better results in order to provide better health care for the whole population. There will always be issues for which there is no easy solution due to the lack of resources needed to respond to the demand. One example of this is organ transplants.

Recently there has been much attention given to the different principles in biomedical ethics while relatively little attention has been paid to the critical task of resolving conflicts among the different principles. Regarding access to health care, one of the major conflicts involving principles occurs between justice and utility. Justice can also be referred to as "equity." To phrase this problem in the form of a simple question: What are we to do when there is a conflict between being just to everyone in the population and maximizing the results of a certain medical treatment for that same population? Or saying it in another way: Should we as a society sacrifice utility for the sake of equality? How can the principle of distributive justice as defined, help us to answer these questions? In order to answer them it is important to first define more clearly the problem.

There are different kinds of principles that must be considered. Some principles have to do with the consequences of certain actions. For example, the principles of beneficence and nonmaleficence have to do with maximizing the good and minimizing the bad. Other principles have to do with the formal structure of an action. Examples of these are the

---

[100]STARR P., *The Logic of Health Care Reform: Why and How the President's Plan Will Work*, p. 28.

principle of veracity, which focuses on an act of truth-telling, or the principle of fidelity, which focuses on the act of promise-keeping. One author has named these two kinds of principles as consequence-maximizing principles and nonconsequentialist principles respectively.[101]

Among the consequence-maximizing principles there are found the principles that can be defined as utilitarian. Social utility takes into consideration the benefits and the harms for all who are affected by certain actions or rules. Individual utility would limit relevant benefits or harms to the individual patient. As mentioned before, the principles of beneficence and nonmaleficence are also major consequence-maximizing principles.

Among the nonconsequentialist principles, that do not focus primarily on maximizing consequences, are found the principles of autonomy (sometimes better expressed as respect for autonomy), respect for persons (which is closely related to autonomy and includes elements such as veracity and fidelity, as mentioned above), and justice.

Having placed justice in its proper place among principles, being a nonconsequentialist one, it is important to explain how is this important principle supposed to be implemented. If the principles of veracity and fidelity, which are grouped under respect for persons, for example, provide an alternative to the consequence-maximizing individual beneficence principle, it is also possible that there is a nonconsequence-maximizing principle at the social level that offers an ethical alternative to social beneficence. As one egalitarian author has put it: "Justice is also social in character; however, rather than focusing on the mere maximization of good consequences, it focuses on the pattern of distribution."[102]

Just as there are different versions of the principle of utility, as we saw before with the differences between social and individual utility, in the same way it could be said that there are differences in the principle of justice. Earlier in this work, for example, we discussed the ideas of John Rawls about what was called the "maximin" principle. This was the justice principle that defended a certain distribution of goods as just, as long as the inequalities improved the condition of the least well off. We

---

[101]VEATCH R., *"Resolving Conflicts Among Principles: Ranking, Balancing, and Specifying,"* Kennedy Institute of Ethics Journal 5(3):200, September 1995.

[102]Ibid., p. 205.

mentioned as well how other egalitarians saw distribution as just, only when goods are distributed more equally.[103] In essence, each different theory of justice will offer a solution to the problem of conflicting principles according to their main tenets. Obviously the simplest answer would be to hold a single-principle theory such as pure libertarianism or pure utilitarianism. Yet, there are problems with this approach since when dealing with health issues there are different goods to be pursued such as the patient's good, medical good, society's good, etc. Even when it comes to emphasizing the patient's good, there are many factors that come into play here such as medical, legal, financial, familial, and other such factors, that in a way make the patient the only one who can figure out what course of action would maximize the total good. Another problem with a single-principle theory approach is that it is very difficult to measure medical goods and the promotion of the patient's well-being. The total well-being of a patient is not always equivalent to just the medical good. In other words, following a single-principle theory would leave out too much of the moral life.

We have seen in unit two the problems with Rawls' solution. The pure egalitarian solution is more realistic but it falls short of providing an equal distribution since it only calls for a "more equal distribution." Faced with these problems, some other writers have suggested an approach of balancing the competing principles.[104] The problems with this approach is that everyone can always argue that one principle is more weighty than another without any way to reach a solution. Many counter-intuitive implications can arise from this approach. The quantification of principles creates a certain kind of repugnance and a lack of realism in the interpretation of some ethicists.[105]

---

[103]For this see VEATCH R., *The Foundations of Justice: Why the Retarded and the Rest of Us Have Claims to Equality.* New York: Oxford University Press, 1986.

[104]One example of this is given by W.D. Ross who identifies seven "*prima facie* duties" or principles which are impossible to rank, but they can be "balanced" by considering the weight of each duty in particular moments. See VEATCH R., *"Resolving Conflicts Among Principles: Ranking, Balancing, and Specifying,"* Kennedy Institute of Ethics Journal 5(3):208, September 1995.

[105]See BRODY B., *Life and Death Decision Making.* New York: Oxford University Press, 1988.

One other possibility for resolving conflicts among principles is to try to rank them according to priority. Each principle that takes precedence over another must be completely satisfied before the next principle can come into play. Earlier in the text we saw how Rawls attempted to order the principles in his theory, placing justice over utility. The problem with this approach is that, unless we are willing to work with a very reduced number of principles, it is very difficult to assign a lexical order that would apply to every situation. Robert Veatch suggests a mixing of these approaches in the following way: First the consequence-maximizing principles must be balanced by giving them equal weight. Then the same must be done for the nonconsequentialist principles, giving them equal weight as well. The third and most critical step according to Veatch is to rank the effect of the nonconsequentialist principles over the consequence maximizing ones. What this does is that it treats the principle of beneficence as an imperfect obligation. The principle of beneficence by itself could never justify breaking or taking precedence over a nonconsequentialist principle such as fidelity to promises, telling the truth, or respecting autonomy. Each of these nonconsequentialist principles must be satisfied first. Only then a nonconsequentialist principle, such as justice, could take precedence over the principle of fidelity to promises. By balancing the principle of justice against the principle of promise-keeping gives the basis for breaking the promise. This is something that the principle of beneficence or nonmaleficence will not do by themselves. Nonconsequentialist principles are perfect obligations. It is nonconsequentialist principles that can provide the exceptional case in which another nonconsequentialist principle will be overruled according to how they rank among themselves.[106] Veatch concludes by saying:

> My conclusion is that the appropriate manner for the resolution of conflict among competing principles is the specification of norms in a mixed strategy that involves both some lexical ordering and some balancing. In cases of conflict, one should balance among nonconsequentialist principles and between the consequence-maximizing ones and then lexically rank the claims of the combined package of nonconsequentialist principles over the

---

[106] VEATCH R., *"Resolving Conflicts Among Principles: Ranking, Balancing, and Specifying,"* Kennedy Institute of Ethics Journal 5(3):211-215, September 1995.

combined package of consequentialist ones.[107]

When it comes to the conflict between the principles of justice and utility in health care, it would be clear from the above discussion of Robert Veatch's ideas that justice, being a nonconsequentialist principle, would take priority over utility. No doubt that Veatch would be willing to sacrifice a utilitarian approach which would maximize the good of the majority in order to satisfy the principle of a more just distribution of health care services.[108] What is never addressed by Veatch in his work is why this is so. In other words, why are nonconsequentialist principles to be ranked always above the consequence-maximizing principles? If a reason could be given for this, then those who tend to place consequence-maximizing principles, such as beneficence, above nonconsequentialist principles, such as autonomy (a utilitarian approach), would have an explanation why their ranking of principles is wrong. At the same time, those who try to say that in essence beneficence is connected to autonomy since this last one is itself a good, even though not an absolute good (the approach of someone like Edmund Pellegrino), would realize that the reason they can say this is because there is another nonconsequentialist principle, such as justice, that prevents the absolutization of autonomy, since it ranks above autonomy. Translating these principles into the justice / utility debate related to health care we could say that there is no example that could be given in which the claim that maximizing the utility of health care is itself part of justice since being just in essence maximizes the utility of medical goods. Autonomy may be a good in itself, but this is not the reason why it takes precedence over beneficence. In the same way justice may be a good in itself but this is not the reason why it should be considered before utility. The reason why this should be considered so is because justice, like autonomy and any other nonconsequentialist principle, using Veatch's terminology, responds to an obligation that can never be superseded by a utilitarian, maximizing principle, but only by a

---

[107] VEATCH R., *"Resolving Conflicts Among Principles: Ranking, Balancing, and Specifying,"* Kennedy Institute of Ethics Journal 5(3):217, September 1995.

[108] The author had specific conversations with Dr. Veatch about this very issue in which this point was clearly made. Veatch was willing to accept a decrease in the utility of certain medical procedures for the sake of a more egalitarian distribution of medical services.

higher obligation. Within the theory presented here, in which distributive justice is seen as the only implementation possible for a theory of justice that conceives the social dimension of the human person and the existence of a common good recognizable by society, providing health care in a just way to the whole population with the resources available in society, is as close as we can get to an absolute obligation over which only the sacredness and value of life itself can have a higher rank. It can be said that in a certain way Veatch recognizes this, since in the chart in which he discusses the difference between the two kinds of principles, he distinguishes them by saying that the nonconsequentialist principles are different from the consequence-maximizing principles because they are based on obligations and not in consequence maximizing.[109] Just health care is an obligation of every society, always considering the resources available, but at the same time always striving to achieve the most equitable distribution according to a proportional equality in which the priority would be providing health care and not the utilization of health care for other purposes.

---

[109]See the chart entitled Figure 1 in VEATCH R., *"Resolving Conflicts Among Principles: Ranking, Balancing, and Specifying,"* Kennedy Institute of Ethics Journal 5(3):212, September 1995.

TEN

FOUR PROPOSALS FOR PROMOTING
JUST ACCESS TO CARE

The principles of the common good and distributive justice have been shown to provide a much needed basis for an understanding of the moral and societal obligation for the provision of health care. Especially in the United States, where it seems that today there are more people asking, "What do I have a right to do?" rather than "What is the right thing to do?," it is important to show that there are certain societal obligations that cannot be ignored if we want to build a just society. Just health care is one of the most essential elements today in helping to achieve this transformation.

There are four concrete proposals that will help in concluding this unit and in offering some simple but practical means by which the common good implemented through distributive justice in health care can take place in the United States and thus offer just access to everyone.

1. Universal Access

We saw in the first chapter how universal coverage in health care does not necessarily mean universal access. Both of these goals are far from being achieved in the United States where more than 37 million people lack coverage and many more lack timely access to health services. When early in the 1960's the country was devoting approximately 6% of the gross domestic product (GDP) to health and medical care for a population of less than 200 million Americans, policy makers believed that universal access could be achieved as social policy with a few more percentage points of GDP. In that time Sweden, where health planners advocated 10% of societal resources, was often cited as a prototype. Today, when over 14% of the GDP is being dedicated to health care with foreseen increases in the future, such an investment has not solved the problem.

Universal access to health care means the availability of the highest-quality health care possible for all. In order to achieve this it is evident that there is a kind of overall commitment needed that involves many different aspects. A structural change in the system can only happen if all the components of the system are taken into consideration. For example, we have seen how the lack of primary care in the U.S. has been one of the main obstacles in better access to care, and how in other countries there is an explicit commitment to universal access to care by having a high percentage (40 to 50 percent) of all clinical physicians as general practitioners. This percentage is very low in the U.S. (15%) as we have already seen and analyzed. If there is going to be systemic change in health care provision in the U.S., all these factors must be considered.

Universal access to health care as a goal does something very important. As the U.S. Catholic bishops have pointed out, it links the health care of the poor and the working classes with the health care of those with greater resources in a way that the development of a two-tiered system is prevented from happening, and at the same time better quality of care is provided.[110] Universal access facilitated in this way will begin to tear down the walls that at this time obstruct access even to a decent minimum of health care, not to mention other more expensive necessary procedures. This will reduce as well the socio-economic status health gradient which shows that individuals lower in the socio-economic status hierarchy have less access to medical care.

Universal access to health care also means that equal access to medical treatment will be independent of employment. Health care provision connected to employment makes it seem as if almost there is a penalty for not working. Once a person has a job today through which he or she is insured, leaving that work as well may become a problem due to the lack of willingness of other companies to provide health care coverage for individuals after certain age or when a pre-existing medical condition is present. We have seen the origins of employer-based insurance, and how there was no consideration at the time of the moral and ethical questions that should be raised when health is the concern. The whole arrangement was one of economic convenience at the time, through which now the injustices and discriminatory practices already present in the working world are spread even more. A universal health insurance protection is a moral imperative in the United States today and integral to

---

[110]U.S. BISHOPS, *Resolution on Health Care Reform,* Origins 23(7):101, July 1, 1993.

any effort to create a just health care system. Some authors have called the principle of universal access "the soul of health care system reform."[111]

To provide universal access to health care is in itself a choice-expanding policy that would help in eliminating many of the ways that liberty in seeking health care has been curtailed in today's American society. A program that provides this kind of access to care can be designed taking into consideration the circumstances in the United States, and in the process increase the real options Americans have.

2. A Single-Payer System

In order to implement a system that would provide universal access to health care according to the special circumstances which face today's societies, there is evidence that a single-payer system would offer the best way to achieve it. As has been mentioned before, if the principles of the common good and distributive justice are going to be considered, a patient-centered system must be the primary concern. The duplication of procedures and administrative waste that comes about as part of a multi-payer system is one of the first things that should become obvious to the community. A single-payer system has been shown to do away with much of this waste which would allow the significant percentage of the gross domestic product (GDP) already being invested in health care to be used more effectively and efficiently.

A single-payer system would create a monopsony which could function in different ways. In Germany, for example, insurers are organized into a single bargaining unit who work out a global budget for health care goods and services. In Canada, the government is the single purchaser of health care in the country with the global budget for health care constituting the totality of expenditures for a state or region which would be divided among those who provide health care services. The government has an extensive role to play in both of these alternatives. In the German example there is still a certain level of competition, which some people claim is beneficial for a more efficient health care system, the difference being that instead of a free market with no restraints, the government functions as a guarantor of fair competition under equal terms.

---

[111] BROCK D.W., DANIELS N., *"Ethical Foundations of the Clinton Administration's Proposed Health Care System,"* Journal of the American Medical Association 271(15): 1189, April 20, 1994.

What the free market strategies attempt in an oblique way, a single-payer system tries to accomplish in a straightforward way. This is done by the government explicitly limiting resources available to providers through the establishment of fixed budgets.[112]

A single-payer system's superiority in helping to effectively contain costs in health care is empirically demonstrable. The U.S. has relied mainly upon managed care strategies to control health care costs. While leaving many people outside a reasonable health care safety net, the United States now spends more on health care than any other country in the world. When compared to other countries it is evident that the reason for this is the multiplicity of payers who continually duplicate efforts and confuse providers by operating with a much higher level of administrative costs than countries with single payer-systems.

There is an ideological resistance in the U.S. to a single-payer system possibly from the people that would most benefit from it. During the 1980's the income of American doctors grew rapidly. By the mid nineties their median salary was over $139,000, while surgeons' median salary was $233,800. This has been in sharp contrast to very minimal increases in workers' salaries. In countries with a single-payer system, such as Germany, physicians' salaries have actually fallen from six to three and a half times the wage of an average German worker.[113] This trend has allowed for a greater sense of societal stability than the one experienced in the United States with the widening gap between the "haves" and "have-nots" in the population. The American public sees itself increasingly burdened by medical costs and deprived of insurance by the present system. This affects not only poor people but people all over the socio-economic spectrum. Small businesses in particular and self-employed entrepreneurs have been hurt directly by the dramatic increases in health care costs. The present health care system in the United States has proven to be too constraining, and physicians are beginning to realize that offering themselves as free economic agents for managed care purposes has an adverse effect on the very meaning of their profession. Many are beginning to recognize the advantages of a well-structured, globally budgeted, single-payer system in giving them an increased sense of clinical autonomy for the welfare of their patients while at the same

---

[112]JOST T.S., TANENBAUM S.J., *"Selling Cost Containment,"* American Journal of Law and Medicine 19(1-2):101, 1993.

[113]Ibid., p. 103.

time increasing their collective economic power in exchange for an entrepreneurial freedom which they have traditionally enjoyed in the past, but that today, due to the complexities inherent in the system, has been turned over to administrators whose main interests are far from the immediate well-being of their patients.

A national health service providing insurance for all Americans under a single-payer system could generate substantial savings in health care. This would eliminate the entire private health insurance industry, much of the current bureaucracy found in hospitals and nursing homes, and some of the expenses of doctor's offices. The percentage of the gross domestic product (GDP) dedicated to health care could be administered by this national health service, which would in turn work with the state governments by giving each hospital an annual payment to cover operating expenses and the doctors on a fee-for-service basis. The whole billing process would be simplified because hospitals would require virtually no billing department and minimal internal accounting. With a unified insurance system, physicians' billing would be simplified as well. The overhead costs of insurance could be reduced dramatically as well as the hospitals' administrative costs.[114] Another alternative regarding physicians' salaries would be for the national health service, working through the state governments, to pay a salary or capitation fee. Because of this there would be no insurance overhead.[115] In Canada, self-employed physicians have professional expenses that average 36% of their gross

---

[114] In the Canadian system, for example, the overhead of the universal public insurance averages 2.5% of program costs. This represents one quarter of the overhead of private insurers in the U.S. (8%). In Canada insurance overhead and hospital administration together consume only 6% of total health resources. See HIMMELSTEIN D.U., WOOLHANDLER S., *"Cost Without Benefit: Administrative Waste in U.S. Health Care,"* New England Journal of Medicine 314: 443, February 13, 1986.

[115] In Great Britain, for example, the National Health Service pays doctors a capitation fee. Administrative costs there account for 5.7% of hospital expenses while central administration of the system accounts for 2.6%. These account for 6% of total health costs. See HIMMELSTEIN D.U., WOOLHANDLER S., *"Cost Without Benefit: Administrative Waste in U.S. Health Care,"* New England Journal of Medicine 314: 443, February 13, 1986.

income, while in England they average 29% of gross income.[116]

3. Greater Involvement of the States

It has been already mentioned several times that the subsidiarity principle is a very important one in the theology of the church. This principle holds that higher organizations should not interfere or try to solve the problems that can be handled at a lower, ground-roots level. At the same time it has been shown how health care provision in the United States today is such a complicated system of varied interests and pursuits that it is impossible to provide just access to health care without some kind of governmental intervention. The current aversion present in the American society against any kind of governmental intervention, should be seen as a tendency that needs to be corrected. Even though traditionally the Catholic Church has never been statist in the solutions it has promoted, it can never be said that it has been anti-government. Government is one of the tools to foster the common good of all the citizens, and its role is an essential one in any democratic society. Therefore, when it relates to health care, the principle of subsidiarity would apply in what can be called an "inversed" way. This means that just health care would require some kind of government assistance if the principle of subsidiarity is going to be implemented requiring the higher level to provide what cannot be efficiently provided by the lower one. One way, though, that the principle of subsidiarity understood in its original form may be applied to health care matters in the U.S. is if there is an increased emphasis on the role of the individual fifty states. Collaborative partnerships with local and state governments on the part of the federal government is seen by many as the key to the future success in providing universal access to health care.[117]

It has been shown how one of the major problems with health care provision through the individual states has been created due to a multi-payer system. The states have been assigned the role of regulating

---

[116] HIMMELSTEIN D.U., WOOLHANDLER S., *"Cost Without Benefit: Administrative Waste in U.S. Health Care,"* New England Journal of Medicine 314: 443, February 13, 1986.

[117] CHAPMAN T.W., *"Challenge of Poverty: Some Advice for Advocates of Managed Competition,"* Hospitals and Health Networks 67(13): 56, July 5, 1993.

Medicaid funds, and the inequalities that have been shown from state to state have been one of the major concerns in facilitating access to the poor. This multiple financing system has forced individual states to increase the percentage above the poverty line over which they would consider providing funds to the poor. This percentage is such a high one, that in essence it ends up defeating its very purpose. With a single-payer system the states could have an expanding role in administering the health care budget, and distribute it in such a way that it would truly benefit the diverse population compositions present in the individual states of the nation. This type of assistance would be in agreement with the notion of proportional equality. With the collaboration of the states, the vast amount of money that is apportioned to health care could be more efficiently and effectively distributed to take care of the needs of all. At the local and state levels citizens could have more of a say so and control of the way these funds are distributed. One example of this kind of participation which was mentioned before is the way that the state of Oregon devised community discussions about health care policy prior to the more formal political process. Despite the shortcomings of the Oregon plan, as discussed before, this is one very positive element that would promote active participation from the state population in dealing with their health care particular needs and regional problems. In this way the demographic needs of each state would be addressed in a more direct way, and the whole system would be brought closer to the people that it will affect.

4. Preventive Over Defensive Care

When health care is treated as a market commodity, with a terminology appropriate for a commercial enterprise, and with great emphasis being placed on the rights of the different parties involved, it lends itself to a system that will be obsessed with the legal and juridical ramifications instead of a system that builds on a social obligation to facilitate health care in a timely fashion. The fact that the United States, despite having five percent of the world's population, is home to seventy percent of the world's lawyers, makes health care one of the primary sources of income for many in the legal profession.[118] Current fictional novels have picked up this theme by providing plots that place lawyers

---

[118]HOLLOWELL J.W., *"The Health Care Crisis—How We Got There,"* Virginia Medical Quarterly 120(4):224, Fall 1993.

hunting for clients in the hospitals while doctors spend much of their time in the courts. This has given rise to what has been called "defensive medicine," in which physicians have to protect themselves against frivolous law suits by ordering all kinds of unnecessary medical tests and procedures. This kind of approach to health care affects the costs in such a way that it in turn requires more money to pay for medical practice in general. As it has been shown, these high costs of medical care have been one of the decisive factors in keeping people away from timely access to the system. Guaranteed health care through a system that would offer universal access through a single-payer system with the collaboration of the individual states of the nation would provide a true incentive, or at least remove the present disincentive, to seek preventive care before illness strikes and to seek treatment earlier when it does. This type of approach may very well lower the overall costs of health care, while at the same time provide for a more healthy population whose work productivity will be greater and its general quality of life enhanced. The notion that a healthier population is truly a national asset in innumerable ways, has been one slow to come in the United States. Preventive care would create a greater sense of civic fellowship and social solidarity.

Today in the U.S. very few insurance plans emphasize and pay for routine preventive care. Preventive measures in the country are inadequate for every sector of the population and only accounts for 2.3% of health care spending, as it was discussed in chapter two.[119] Currently, the United States spends too much on high-tech acute care and not enough on preventive measures. A system that would place less emphasis on the financial aspects of health care and would be more attentive to the health care needs of the population would utilize the enormous monetary resources dedicated to health care in a more intelligent and effective way. Preventive measures to provide better health to the population will cease being measured simply in terms of statistical lives, but on the merits of the actual effects of good preventive medicine on the good health of the population. The lack of incentives to recognize the effects of good preventive medicine comes in part from the current structure of health care in the U.S. in which statistical lives of healthy people are not a source of income for health care providers.

---

[119]HIMMELSTEIN D.U., WOOLHANDLER S., *"Pitfalls of Private Medicine: Health Care in the U.S.A.,"* Lancet 2(8399): 393, August 18, 1984.

CONCLUSION

Through the chapters of this work we have ventured into the confounding world of health care in the United States of America. These chapters gave a historical sense of the development of medical care in the country from the beginning of its relatively short history. At the same time they have portrayed the astounding advances in the field to the point of making health care an irreplaceable and unique service for the population. Through the statistical data given, which continues to be the subject of deep study even to this day, it was shown how America is having colossal problems with providing adequate access to health care to all citizens. These problems are not simply coming from one factor or one front but from many different inequitable situations which affect a significant number in the population. The components that have created such an unequal access to care were studied in detail.

With this problem of limited access to health care as a documented reality, there was a search for the basic philosophies and theories that have brought the situation to where it is today. Different definitions were studied about "rights" and "health" while at the same time unearthing one of the most crucial problems in the way the problem with unequal access to health care is being confronted today. This problem is the devaluing of the notion of "right" in American society, and the need to balance this with a view of a societal obligation to provide equitable health care. Since none of the modern philosophical theories and ethical thinkers appear to give a comprehensive answer to the access problem in health care, the development of a new theory was presented. This theory would be based on a societal obligation to provide just health care instead of pressing for a possibly misunderstood notion of a right to health care. The main problem with this approach of pressing for a societal obligation was seen to be the difficulty in finding the principle or principles upon which such obligation would be based. The difficulty of finding such principles has become greater due to the pluralist society in which we live today.

The search for these principles upon which to base a social obligation to provide health care was undertaken within the Catholic Christian tradition. The author's Roman Catholic tradition has something to do with this choice, but it has been admitted even by Protestant ethicists that Catholics have produced the most systematically developed and officially formulated version of Christian ethics.[1] Within the Catholic Christian tradition two pre-modern principles were presented as offering a basis for a societal obligation to provide just health care. These principles were the ones of the common good and distributive justice. Both of these principles have seen a resurgence in the ethical literature of recent times. Two of the most significant debates in modern ethical discussions have to do with these principles. A historical survey, the teaching of the Church's magisterium, and the present day debate were presented for both principles. A theory of justice based on these two principles was then developed and offered as including three specific contributions within the tradition of the Church: A social understanding of the person, a humane understanding of society (the common good), and a just distribution according to needs.

This theory was then applied to the present health care system in the United States after highlighting the main problems that the system faces and the many solutions that have been suggested. The Catholic theory of justice offered a moral basis for health care reform in which the object was to highlight several universal principles that could be acknowledged within a pluralistic society. These universal principles based on the common good include five elements: the nature of health care, the stewardship of resources, the need for universal access, comprehensive similar benefits, and the integrity needed to be preserved in the physician-patient relationship. An application of this moral basis to the American context followed by highlighting six important steps that need to take place: the patient should be a priority, the need for a comprehensive approach to health care, the importance of a correct understanding of the role of government, the need to emphasize care over administration, the importance of promoting local responsibility, and the need for the terminology to change into a more socially-minded one. These aspects coming from an appreciation of the common good then were made concrete through an application based on the principle of distributive justice in which the three related problems of treating health care merely as a market commodity, seeking for premature rationing, and not being able to prioritize the different principles, were discussed. Finally, four proposals were presented that would reform the current system and provide just health care to the whole population. These

---

[1]GUFTANSON, J.M., *Protestant and Roman Catholic Ethics: Prospects for Rapprochement,* Chicago: University of Chicago Press, 1978.

Conclusion 313

proposals are: universal access to health care, the establishment of a single-payer system, a greater role for the individual states in the nation, and the promotion of preventive care over defensive care. Each of these proposals will encounter a tremendous challenge due to the wall of individualism that exists in the present arrangement for health care provision in the country. Nevertheless, the signs indicate that the health care situation, particularly in regards to access to medical care, is not improving but getting worse. Our hope is that the principles studied in this work may offer ethical guidance when the inescapable changes in health care provision take place.

* * * * ** * *

On Saturday, October 11, 1997, European leaders meeting in Strasbourg, France, agreed during a two day summit to create a new court of human rights. There was a final declaration in the meeting that called for a new plan of action toward the continent's downtrodden and ill-treated.[2] This was seen as an intensified effort to move toward a Europe that would be more democratic, more just, and with a constant concern for human dignity. This 40-nation Council of Europe, which was founded in 1949, reaffirmed in their final document of the summit their commitment to the principles of democracy, respect for human rights and the rule of law, and its role for setting the standards in these matters for all of Europe. The protection of the human person was placed at the heart of the resolutions achieved.

In the United States of America democracy, justice, and human dignity have always been part of the original blueprint that gave birth to a great nation. There is always a need to evaluate the national progress in securing those great ideals for everyone, and when elements that interfere with those laudable goals are identified, no time should be wasted, no words remain unspoken, no efforts saved, in correcting the situation.

Throughout this work we have ventured into the vast territory of health care reform, especially in what concerns access to medical care and services. The long and successful history of health care in the United States is beyond doubt one of the great chapters in the history of the country. The fact that in a relatively short period of time, health care has begun serving interests that defeat its own purpose and meaning, should

---

[2]See ULBRICH J., *"Europeans Call for Ban on Cloning,"* in *The Times Picayune,* Sunday, October 12, 1997, p. A-15.

be enough of a catalyst to motivate the whole society to see that it is not simply a matter of multiple rights that is at stake, but the very way we exist as a society and the obligations that such a society must fulfill. The challenge ahead is not to lose sight of that blueprint developed by the founding fathers of the nation in which democracy, justice, and human dignity were the only ways to secure the true freedom of all citizens. Providing for the health care of the population in a just way is one of the essential ways through which a society promotes human dignity, self realization, and freedom.

BIBLIOGRAPHY

General Works and Articles

Books:

ADAY, L.A.; ANDERSEN, R.; FLEMING, G.V., *Health Care in the U.S.: Equitable for Whom?* Beverly Hills, California: Sage Pub. 1980.
_____, *Access to Medical Care in the United States: Who Has It, Who Doesn't.* Chicago: Pluribus Press, University of Chicago 1984.
ARROW, Kenneth Joseph, *Social Choice and Justice.* Cambridge, Mass.: Belknap Press, 1983.
ASHLEY, Benedict M.; O'ROURKE, Kevin D., *Ethics of Health Care.* The Catholic Health Association of the United States, 1986.
BENESTAD, J. Brian; BUTLER, Francis J. (Eds.), *Quest for Justice. A Compendium of Statements of the United States Catholic Bishops on the Political and Social Order 1966-1980.* National Conference of Catholic Bishops, United States Catholic Conference, 1981.
BIGONGIARI, Dino (ed.), *The Political Ideas of St. Thomas Aquinas.* New York: Hafner Press, London: Collier Macmillan Publishers, 1974 (10th ed.).
BONIFAZI, Duilio; ALICI, Luigi, *Il Pensiero del Novecento. Filosofia, Scienza, Cristianesimo.* Brescia: Editrice Queriniana, 1982.
BROWN, Alan, *Modern Political Philosophy: Theories of the Just Society.* Harmondsworth, Middlesex, England; New York, N.Y., U.S.A.: Penguin, 1986.
BRUNNER, Emil, *Justice and the Social Order.* New York: Harper, 1945.
CABREY, Kathryn A., *An Ethical Perspective on the Allocation of Scarce Medical Resources as Exemplified in the Federal Financing of Care to Renal Patients.* Thesis (Ph.D.) Georgetown University. 1982. (420pp.).
THE CATHOLIC HEALTH ASSOCIATION, *No Room in the Marketplace: The Health Care of the Poor.* (As approved by the CHA Board of Trustees April 24, 1986), St. Louis, MO., 1986.
COLEMAN, John A., (ed.), *One Hundred Years of Catholic Social Thought: Celebration and Challenge.* Maryknoll, New York: Orbis Books, 1991.

COPELAND, Warren R., *Economic Justice: The Social Ethics of U.S. Economic Policy.* Nashville: Abingdon Press, 1988.
CURRAN, Charles E., *American Catholic Social Ethics: Twentieth-Century Approaches.* Notre Dame, London: University of Notre Dame Press, 1982.
DANIELS, Norman (ed.), *Reading Rawls: Critical Studies on Rawls' A Theory of Justice.* New York: Basic Books 1975.
DEUTSCH, Morton, *Distributive Justice: A Social-Psychological Perspective.* New Haven: Yale University Press, 1985.
DIUMENAE Y PUJOL, Luis, *Cuestiones Actuales de Moral.* Madrid: San Pio X, 1992.
DOUGHERTY, Charles J., *Back to Reform: Values, Markets, and the Health Care System.* New York: Oxford University Press 1996.
DWORKIN, Ronald, *Taking Rights Seriously.* Cambridge: Harvard University Press, 1977.
EDWARDS, Richard L., (Editor-in-Chief); HOPPS, June Gary (Associate Editor-in-Chief), *Encyclopedia of Social Work.* 19th edition. Washington D.C.: NASW Press, 1995.
FREIDSON, Eliot, *Profession of Medicine.* New York: Dood, Mead 1970.
FRY, John, and HASLER, John C., *Primary Health Care 2000.* Churchill Livingstone, Edinburgh, London, Melbourne and New York 1986.
FRY, John; LIGHT, Donald; RODNICK, Jonathan and ORTON, Peter, *Reviving Primary Care A US-UK Comparison.* Radcliffe Oxford and New York: Medical Press, 1995.
FUCHS, Victor R., *Who Shall Live? Health, Economics, and Social Choice.* New York: Basic Books, Inc., 1974.
FURFEY, Paul Hanly, *Fire on the Earth.* New York: Macmillan, 1936.
_____, *Three Theories of Society.* New York: Macmillan, 1937.
_____, *A History of Social Thought.* New York: Macmillan, 1942.
GALSTON, William A., *Justice and the Human Good.* Chicago: University of Chicago Press, 1980.
GARDNER, E. Clinton, *Justice and Christian Ethics.* Cambridge, New York: Cambridge University Press, 1995.
GLEASON, Philip, *The Conservative Reformers: German-American Catholics and the Social Order.* Notre Dame, Indiana: University of Notre Dame Press, 1968.

GLOVER, Jacqueline J., *The Role of Physicians in Cost Containment: An Ethical Analysis.* (Thesis Ph. D.) Georgetown University, Washington D.C., 1988, (184 pp.).
GOODIN, Robert E., *Protecting the Vulnerable: A Reanalysis of Our Social Responsibilities.* Chicago: University of Chicago Press, 1985.
GORDON, Scott, *Welfare, Justice, and Freedom.* New York: Columbia University Press, 1980.
GOROVITZ, Samuel et al, (eds.), *Moral Problems in Medicine.* New Jersey: Prentice-Hall Inc., 1976.
GREMILLION, Joseph (presentor), *The Gospel of Peace and Justice: Catholic Social Teaching Since Pope John.* Maryknoll, N.Y.: Orbis Books 1976.
GUERRY, Emile Most Reverend, *The Social Doctrine of the Catholic Church.* New York, London, Boston: Alba House, 1961.
GUFTANSON, James M., *Protestant and Roman Catholic Ethics: Prospects for Rapprochement,* Chicago: University of Chicago Press, 1978.
HART, Stephen, *What Does the Lord Require?: How American Christians View Economic Justice.* New York: Oxford University Press, 1992.
HELD, Virginia, *Rights and Goods: Justifying Social Action.* New York: Free Press; London: Collier Macmillan, 1984.
HOCHSCHILD, Jennifer L., *What's Fair?: American Beliefs About Distributive Justice.* Cambridge, Mass.: Harvard University Press, 1981.
HOLLAND, Joe, *Social Analysis: Linking Faith and Justice.* Maryknoll, N.Y.: Orbis Books, 1983.
JONAS, Steven, *Health Care Delivery in the United States.* New York: Springer Publishing Co., 1986 [3rd edition].
KAPLAN, Morton A., *Justice, Human Nature, and Political Obligation.* New York: Free Press, 1976.
KUENNE, Robert E., *Economic Justice in American Society.* Princeton, N.J.: Princeton University Press, 1993.
LAND, Philip S., *Catholic Social Teaching: As I Have Lived, Loathed, and Loved It.* Chicago: Loyola University Press, 1994.
LAW, Sylvia A., *Blue Cross: What Went Wrong?* New Haven: Yale University Press:, 1976 (2nd ed.).
LEBACQZ, Karen, *Six Theories of Justice: Perspectives from Philosophical and Theological Ethics.* Minneapolis: Augsburg Pub. House, 1986.

LIO, Ermenegildo, *Morale e Beni Terreni. La Destinazione Universale dei Beni Terreni nella "Gaudium et Spes" e in Alcune Fonti.* Roma: Città Nuova Editrice, 1976.
LUCAS, J.R. *On Justice.* Oxford: Clarendon Press, 1980.
LUCASH, Frank S. (ed.), *Justice and Equality Here and Now.* Ithaca: Cornell University Press, 1986.
MAGILL, Gerard; HOFF, Marie D., (eds.), *Values and Public Life.* Lanham, New York, London: University Press of America, 1995.
MAINELLI, Vincent P. (ed.), *Social Justice!: The Catholic Position.* Washington D.C.: Consortium Press, 1975.
MARTIN, Rex, *Rawls and Rights.* Lawrence, Kan.: University Press of Kansas, 1985.
MCCUEN, Gary E. (ed.), *American Justice: Is America a Just Society?* Anoka, Minn.: Greenhaven Press, 1975.
MESSNER, Johannes, *Social Ethics: Natural Law in the Western World.* St. Louis: B. Herder, 1965 (3rd. Ed.).
MICHELMAN, Irving S., *The Moral Limitations of Capitalism.* Aldershot; Brookfield, USA: Avebury, 1994.
MILLER, William D., *A Harsh and Dreadful Love: Dorothy Day and the Catholic Worker Movement.* New York: Liveright, 1973, paperback ed. Garden City, New York: Doubleday Image Books, 1974.
NATHAN, N.M.L., *The Concept of Justice.* London: Macmillan Press, 1971.
NOVAK, Michael,*The Catholic Ethic and the Spirit of Capitalism.* New York: Free Press; Toronto: Maxwell Macmillan Canada; New York: Maxwell Macmillan International, 1993.
PIZZORNI, Reginaldo M., *Giustizia e Carita.* Roma: Città Nuova: Pontificia Universita Lateranense, 1995 (3rd ed.).
POLAINO-LORENTE, Aquilino (ed). *Manual de Bioética General,* Madrid: Ediciones RIALP, 1994.
THE POPE JOHN CENTER, *Scarce Medical Resources and Justice.* Braintree, Mass., 1987.
ROEMER, John E., *Egalitarian Perspectives: Essays in Philosophical Economics.* Cambridge; New York: Cambridge University Press, 1994.
ROEMER, Milton I., *An Introduction to the U.S. Health Care System.* New York: Springer Publishing Co., 1986 [2nd edition].
ROSSER, James M.; MOSSBERG, Howard E., *An Analysis of Health Care Delivery.* New York: John Wiley & Sons, 1977.

RYAN, John A., *A Living Wage: Its Ethical and Economic Aspects.* New York: Macmillan, 1906; rev. ed. 1920.
_____ , *Distributive Justice: The Right and Wrong of Our Present Distribution of Wealth.* New York: Macmillan, 1916; rev. ed. 1927; 3rd. Ed., 1942.
_____ , *The Church and Socialism and Other Essays.* Washington: The University Press, 1919.
RYAN, John A.; MOORHOUSE, F.X. Millar (eds.), *The State and the Church.* New York: Macmillan, 1920.
_____ , *Seven Troubled Years, 1930-36: A Collection of Papers on the Depression and on the Problems of Recovery and Reform.* Ann Arbor, Michigan: Edwards Brothers, 1937.
RYAN, John A.; BOLAND, Francis J., *The Norm of Morality Defined and Applied to Particular Actions.* Washington, D.C.: National Catholic Welfare Conference, 1952.
SHACTMAN, David; ALTMAN, Stuart H., *Market Consolidation, Antitrust, and Public Policy in the Health Care Industry: Agenda for Future Research.* Princeton, New Jersey: Robert Wood Johnson Foundation 1995.
SHELP, Earl (ed.), *Justice and Health Care.* Dordrecht, Holland / Boston, U.S.A. / London, England: D. Reidel Publishing Company, 1981, Vol 8.
SMURL, James F., *The Burdens of Justice: Social Issues in Crisis.* Chicago: Loyola University Press, 1994.
SOLOMON, Robert C.; MURPHY, Mark C., (eds.), *What is Justice? Classic and Contemporary Readings.* New York: Oxford University Press, 1990.
STARFIELD, Barbara M.D., *Primary Care. Concept, Evaluation, and Policy.* New York - Oxford: Oxford University Press, 1992.
STEFANINI, Luigi, *Personalismo Sociale.* Roma: Edizioni Studium, 1979 (2a ed).
STEIDL-MEIER, Paul, *Social Justice Ministry: Foundations and Concerns.* New York: Le Jacq Publishing Inc., 1984.
STEWART, Jane Emmert, *Home Health Care.* St. Louis, Toronto, London: The C.V. Mosby Company, 1979.
THOMAS AQUINAS, *Summa Theologiae.* Blackfriars edition, New York: McGraw-Hill Book Co., 1964.
VIANO, Carlo Augusto (a cura de), *Teorie Etiche Contemporanee.* Torino: Bollati Boringhieri editore, 1990.

WEIGEL, George; ROYAL, Robert, (eds.), *A Century of Catholic Social Thought: Essays on "Rerum Novarum" and Nine Other Key Documents.* Ethics and Public Policy Center, Washington D.C., 1991.
WELLMAN, Carl, *Welfare Rights.* Totowa, N.J.: Rowman and Littlefield, 1982.
WILLIAMS, Oliver F.; HOUCK, John W., *Catholic Social Thought and the New World Order.* University of Notre Dame Press, Notre Dame, London, 1993.
WOGAMAN, J. Philip, *Economics and Ethics: A Christian Inquiry.* Philadelphia: Fortress Press, 1986.
WOLFF, Robert P., *Understanding Rawls: A Reconstruction and Critique of A Theory of Justice.* Princeton, N.J.: Princeton University Press, 1977.
WOLFF, Jonathan, *Robert Nozick: Property, Justice, and the Minimal State.* Stanford, California: Stanford University Press, 1991.
ZWEIG, Michael, (ed.), *Religion and Economic Justice.* Philadelphia: Temple University Press, 1991.

Articles:

AARON, Henry J., *"Issues Every Plan to Reform Health Care Financing Must Confront."* Journal of Economic Perspectives 8(3): 31-43, 1994 Summer.
———————, *"Thinking Straight about Medical Costs."* Health Affairs: 7-13, 1994 Winter.
ABRAMS, F.R., *"Patient Advocate or Secret Agent?"* Journal of the American Medical Association 256 (13): 1784-5, Oct. 3, 1986.
AGICH, George J. (ed.), *Responsibility in Health Care,* in Philosophy and Medicine, H.Tristram Engelherdt Jr., Stuart F. Spicker (eds.), Dordrecht, Holland / Boston, U.S.A. / London, England: D. Reidel Publishing Company, 1982, Vol 12.
ANDERSEN, Ronald M., *"Revisiting the Behavioral Model and Access to Medical Care: Does It Matter?"* Journal of Health and Social Behavior, Vol. 36 (March): 1-10, 1995.
ANDERSON, R.J., *"How to Preserve Ethical Values, Equal Access While Seeking New Efficiency."* Health Management Quarterly:16-20, 1986 3rd. Quarter.
ANNAS, G.J., *"All the President's Bioethicists."* Hastings Center Report 9(1): 14-5, Feb., 1979.

APOLEBY, J.; YATES, J., *"Data Briefing. Waiting for Fairness."* Health Service Journal 105 (5439): 34-5, February 9, 1995.

AROSKAR, Mila Ann, *"Ethics in Nursing and Health Care Reform: Back to the Future?"* Hastings Center Report 24(3): 11-12, May, 1994.

BATTISTELLA, R.M.; KUDER, J.M., *"Universal Access to Health Care: A Practical Perspective."* Journal of Health and Human Resources Administration 16 (1): 6-34, 1993 Summer.

BECK, L.C.; KALOGREDIS, V.J., *"Successful Group Must Agree on Basic Philosophy."* Pennsylvania Medicine 80(10): 28-9, Oct., 1977.

BECKER, Marshall H., *"A Medical Sociologist Looks at Health Promotion."* Journal of Health and Social Behavior, Vol 34: 1-46, 1993.

BELL, Nora K., *"The Scarcity of Medical Resources: Are There Rights to Health Care?"* Journal of Medicine and Philosophy 4(2): 158-169, June, 1979.

BERGEN, Stanley S. Jr., *"President Clinton's Health Care Reform Proposal: The American Health Security Act of 1993."* Trends in Health Care, Law and Ethics 8(4): 47-9, 1993 Fall.

BESHAROV, D.J.; SILVER, J.D., *"Rationing Access to Advanced Medical Techniques."* Journal of Legal Medicine 8(4): 507-32, Dec., 1987.

BESS, D.R., *"Philosophy, Prescriptions, and Politics."* Journal of the American Medical Association 243(6): 525-7, Feb. 8, 1980.

BEVAN, G.; CHARLTON, J., *"Making Access to Health Care More Equal: The Role of General Medical Services."* [published erratum appears in Br Med J (Clin Res Ed) 1987 Nov. 21: 295 (6609): 1349]. British Medical Journal Clinical Research Ed. 295 (6601):764-7, Sept., 26, 1987.

BIRCH, S.; ABELSON, J., *"Is Reasonable Access What We Want? Implications Of, and Challenges to, Current Canadian Policy on Equity in Health Care."* International Journal of Health Services 23 (4): 629-53, 1993.

BLANKENAU, R., *"Universal Access? Undocumented Residents and Reform: How Will We Pay for Their Care?"* Hospitals and Health Networks 67 (19):36, 38, 40-1, Oct. 5, 1993.

BLENDON, Robert, et al., *"Satisfaction With Health Systems in Ten Nations."* Health Affairs:185-90, 1990 Summer.

BLOCK, Lester E., *"Rx for Health-Care Woes."* Barron's: 61, June 27, 1994.

BOLENSKI, J.D., *"Paradigm Shift in American Health Care: Are We Ready for the Comprehensive System?"* Health Matrix 1(2): 259-65; discussion 267-73, 1991 Summer.

BOYLE, Joseph M., *"A Catholic Perspective on Morality and the Law."* Journal of Law and Religion 1(1):227-240, Summer 1983.

BREITBART, V.; CHAVKIN, W.; WISE, P.H., *"The Accessibility of Drug Treatment for Pregnant Women: a Survey of Programs in Five Cities."* American Journal of Public Health 84 (10): 1658-61, Oct., 1994.

BRISTOW, L., *"Choosing the Right Medicine—AMA's Lonnie Bristow, MD, Talks Reform."* (Interview by Dennis L. Breo, published erratum appears in Journal of the American Medical Association 27:271(16): 1240, April, 1994). Journal of the American Medical Association 271 (7): 562-7, Feb. 16, 1994.

BRODY, Howard, *"Framing the Health Reform Debate."* Hastings Center Report 24(3): 7-8, May, 1994.

BROMBERG, M.D., *"Economics, Ethics, and Access: the Perspective of Investor-Owned Hospitals."* National Forum On Hospital and Health Affairs :83-93, 1983.

BROOKS, A.P., *"Establishing a Statewide Primary Care Network: The PrimaryOne Experience."* Medical Interface 8(3): 60-3, March, 1995.

BRUDER, P.T., *"Ethical Dilemmas and the Hospital Pharmacist."* Topics in Hospital Pharmacy Management 10(3): 39-46, Nov., 1990.

BUCHANAN, Joan L.; LEIBOWITZ, Arleen; KEESEY, Joan, *"Medicaid Health Maintenance Organizations: Can They Reduce Program Spending?"* Medical Care 34(3):249-263.

BULMER, M., *"A Contrast to the American Model: The British Tradition of Social Administration Moral Concerns at the Expense of Scientific Rigor."* Hastings Center Report 11(2): 35-42, April, 1981.

BUNKER, J.P., *"Distributive Justice and the Risks and Benefits of Ophthalmology."* International Ophthalmology Clinics 20(4): 159-67, 1980 Winter.

BURKE, E.C., *"Clinton's Health Care Reform Proposals. First Lady Brings Encouraging News to AMA Annual Meeting."* Minnesota Medicine 76 (7): 5, July, 1993.

BURKLE, W.S., *"Cimetidine's Low Price: Can We Afford It?"* American Journal of Hospital Pharmacy 47(11): 2534-5, Nov., 1990.

BURNUM, J.F., *"Primary Care Within the Academic Tradition."* Journal of the American Medical Association 233(9): 974-5, Sept. 1, 1975.

BYRD, W.M.; CLAYTON, L.A., *"The 'Slave Health Deficit'. Racism and Health Outcomes."* Health Pac Bulletin 21(2): 25-8, 1991 Summer.

CAHILL, Lisa Sowle, *The Catholic Tradition: Religion, Morality, and the Common Good.* Journal of Law and Religion. 5(1): 75-94, 1987.

CALLAHAN, Daniel, *"Our Fear of Dying."* Newsweek 122(14): 67, Oct. 4, 1993.

CARLISLE, D.M.; LEAKE B.D.; SHAPIRO, M.F., *"Racial and Ethnic Differences in the Use of Invasive Cardiac Procedures Among Cardiac Patients in Los Angeles County, 1986 Through1988."* American Journal of Public Health 85 (3): 352-6, March, 1995.

CARTER, Jimmy; FRAME, Randy, *"The Church's Preventive Medicine."* Christianity Today 38(7): 30-33, June 20, 1994.

CASHMAN, Suzanne B.; FULMER, Hugh S.; STAPLES, Lee, *"Community Health: Beyond Care for Individuals."* Social Policy 24(4): 52-62, 1994 Summer.

CAWS, P., *"What Does Anyone Owe Anyone?"* Mount Sinai Journal of Medicine 62(2): 89-93; discussion 116-23, March, 1995.

CHAPMAN, C.B.; TALMADGE, J.M., *"The Evolution of the Right to Health Concept in the United States."* Pharos of Alpha Omega Alpha 34(1): 30-51, January, 1971.

CHERNOMAS, R., *"Comments on Birsh and Abelson's 'Is Reasonable Access What We Want?'"* International Journal of Health Services 24 (2): 371-2, 1994.

CHILDRESS, James F., *"Priorities in the Allocation of Helath Care Resources."* Soundings 62(3): 257, Fall 1979.

CHRISTENSEN, C.N., *"Federal Regulation: Philosophy and Practice."* Annals of Internal Medicine 89(5 Pt 2 Suppl): 835-7, Nov., 1978.

COMER, J.; MUELLER, K., *"Access to Health Care: Urban-Rural Comparisons From a Midwestern Agricultural State."* Journal of Rural Health 11 (2): 128-36, 1995 Spring.

CONNORS, E.J., *"Catholic Health Care: Future Blueprint."* Health Progress 67(9): 31-3, 61, Nov., 1986.

CONRAD, Ann P., *"The Health Care Policy Pendulum: An Ethical Perspective."* Social Thought 8: 25-38, 1982 Winter.

CORNELIUS, L.J., *"Ethnic Minorities and Access to Medical Care: Where Do They Stand?"* [published erratum appears in Journal of the

Association for Academic Minority Physicians 1993: 4(2): 66] Journal of the Association for Academic Minority Physicians 4(1): 16-25, 1993.

COTTON, P., *"Growing Access Crisis Threatens Health System."* Medical World News 28 (14): 30-2, 34-6, 39-40, July 27, 1987.

_____, *"Preexisting Conditions 'Hold Americans Hostage' to Employers and Insurance."* Journal of the American Medical Association 265(19): 2451-2453, May 15, 1991.

COX, William J., *"National Health Care: Catholic Hospitals Rethink Their Stand."* Liguorian 71: 24-8, 1983 Fall.

CULVER, A.J.; WAGSTAFF, A., *"Equity and Equality in Health and Health Care."* Journal of Health Economics 12 (4): 431-57, Dec., 1993.

CUNNINGHAM P.J.; CORNELIUS L.J., *"Access to Ambulatory Care for American Indians and Alaska Natives: the Relative Importance of Personal and Community Resources."* Social Science and Medicine. 40 (3): 393-407, Feb., 1995.

CUTLER, David M., *"A Guide to Health Care Reform."* Journal of Economic Perspectives 8(3): 13-29, 1994 Summer.

DALEN, J.E.; SANTIAGO, J., *"Insuring the Uninsured is Not Enough."* Archives of Internal Medicine 151(5): 860-2, May, 1991.

DANIEL, S.L.; DERIZIER, N., *"The Woman no One Would Take."* Urban Health 14(1): 22-3, Jan., 1985.

DANIELS, Norman, *"Health Care Needs and Distributive Justice."* Philosophy and Public Affairs: 146-179, Spring 1981.

_____, *"Principles for National Health Care Reform."* Hastings Center Report 24(3): 8-9, May, 1994.

DARLING, H., *"The Role of the Federal Government in Assuring Access to Health Care."* Inquiry 23 (3): 286-95, 1986 Fall.

DAVIS, C.K., *"Who Will Pay? The Economic Realities of Health Care Reform."* Scholarly Inquiry for Nursing Practice 6(3): 217-9, 1992 Fall-Winter.

DAVITT, Joan K.; KAYE, Lenard W., *"Supporting Patient Autonomy: Decision Making in Home Health Care."* Social Work 41(1): 41-50, Jan., 1996.

DELUCA, D.M., *"The Ethics of Health Service Delivery: A Challenge to Public Health Leadership."* Asia-Pacific Journal of Public Health 3(3): 195-9, 1989.

DENTZER, S., *"Untangling Universal Coverage."* US News and World Report 117 (2): 47, July 11, 1994.

DETWILLER, Lloyd F., *"Balancing Need, Demand Resources: Key to Canada's NHI Survival."* Hospital Progress 61: 11-12, Nov., 1980.

DE VILLE, Kenneth, *"Parties to the Social Contract? Justice, Proposition 187 and Health Care For Undocumented Immigrants."* Trends in Health Care, Law and Ethics 10(1-2): 113-118, 1995 Winter.

DICKENSON, Donna, *"Is Efficiency Ethical? Resource Issues in Health Care"* in *Introducing Applied Ethics,* Almond, Brenda (ed.), Cambridge: Blackwell, 1995.

DOHERTY, R.B., *"Scoring Clinton: Can He Expand Access and Cut the Deficit?"* Internist 34 (3): 22-4, March, 1993.

DOUGHERTY, Charles J., *"Setting Health Care Priorities: Oregon's Next Steps."* Hastings Center Report., May-June, 1991, at special supp. 1-16.

EDDY, D.M., *"Clinical Decision Making: From Theory to Practice. Cost-Effectiveness Analysis. A Conversation With My Father."* Journal of the American Medical Association 267(12): 1669-75, March 25, 1992.

_____, *"Clinical Decision Making: From Theory to Practice. Rationing Resources While Improving Quality. How to Get More For Less."* [Comment in: Journal of the American Medical Association April 5, 1995; 273(13):995; discussion 996-7. Comment in: JAMA. April 5, 1995 :273(13): 995-6; discussion 996-7, Comment in JAMA. April 5, 1995: 273(13): 996; discussion 996-7] JAMA. 272(10): 817-24, Sept. 14, 1994.

ELLIS, P.A., *"Role of Ethics in Modern Healthcare: 1."* British Journal of Nursing 2(2): 144-6, Jan 28- Feb 10, 1993.

ENGELHARDT, H.T. Jr., *"The Birth of the Medical Humanities and the Rebirth of the Philosophy of Medicine: The Vision of Edmund D. Pellegrino."* Journal of Medicine and Philosophy 15(3): 237-41, June, 1990.

ENGOREN, M., *"Health System Reform: Will Controlling Cost Require Rationing Services?"* [Comment on: Journal of the American Medical Association July 27, 1994: 272(4): 324-8] Journal of the American Medical Association 273(4): 285; discussion 286, Jan. 25, 1995.

EVANS, C.A. Jr., *"Immigrants and Health Care: Mounting Problems."* Annals of Internal Medicine 122 (4): 309-10, Feb. 15, 1995.

EVANS, M. Stanton, *"Why There Is a Health Care Crisis."* Consumers' Research Magazine 77(6): 10-15+, June, 1994.

FARMER, Paul, *"Medicine and Social Justice."* America 173(2): 13-17, July 15, 1995.
FEATHER, N.T., *"Human Values and Their Relation to Justice."* Journal of Social Issues 50(4):129-151, 1994 Winter.
FEIN, Rashi, *"The Politics of Health Reform."* Dissent 41(1): 43-51, 1994 Winter.
FEINGOLD, Eugene, *"Health Care Reform—More Than Cost Containment and Universal Access."* American Journal of Public Health 84(5): 727-8, May, 1994.
FERRERA, M., *"The Rise and Fall of Democratic Universalism: Health Care Reform in Italy, 1978-1994."* Journal of Health Politics, Policy and Law 20 (2): 275-302, 1995 Summer.
FINNS, J.J.; BACCHETTA, M.D., *"Framing the Physician-Assisted Suicide and Voluntary Active Euthanasia Debate: The Role of Deontology, Consequentialism, and Clinical Pragmatism."* Journal of American Geriatrics Society 43(5): 563-8, May, 1995.
FLAHERTY, K.M., *"Insurance for People With AIDS Remains Problematic Despite ADA."* Journal of Law, Medicine and Ethics 21 (3-4):397-9, 1993 Fall-Winter.
FLEISCHMAN, Alan R., *"Physicians and Ethics in the Health Care Reform Debate."* Hastings Center Report 24(3): 10-11, May, 1994.
FLEMING, S.T.; WILLIAMSON, H.A. Jr.; HICKS, L.L.; RIFE, I., *"Rural Hospital Closures and Access to Services."* Hospital and Health Services Administration 40 (2): 247-62, 1995 Summer.
FREEMAN, H.E.; COREY, C.R., *"Insurance Status and Access to Health Services Among Poor Persons."* Health Services Research 28 (5): 531-41, Dec., 1993.
FREEMAN, H.P., *"The Impact of Clinical Trial Protocols on Patient Care Systems in a Large City Hospital. Access For the Socially Disadvantaged."* Cancer 72 (9 Suppl): 2834-2838, Nov. 1, 1993.
FRENZEN, P.D., *"Health Insurance Coverage in U.S. Urban and Rural Areas."* Journal of Rural Health 9 (3): 204-14, 1993 Summer.
FRIEDERS, Michaeleen, *"Multiplicity health care system: accountability at three levels."* Hospital Progress 63: 44-5+, Sept., 1982.
FRIEDMAN, Emily. *"Fact, Fallacy and Fairness: The Ethics of Health Care Reform."* California Hospitals. 6(6):19-20, Nov.-Dec., 1992.
FUCHS, V.R., *"The 'Competition Revolution' in Health Care."* Health Affairs 7 (3): 5-24, 1988 Summer.

FUNKHOUSER, S.W.; MOSER, D.K., *"Is Health Care Racist."* Advances in Nursing Science. 12 (2): 47-55, Jan., 1990.
GAERTNER, Wulf, *"Distributive Justice: Theoretical Foundations and Empirical Findings."* European Economic Review 38(3-4): 711-20, Apr., 1994.
GAMBLE, Vanessa Northington, *"Conversations With History."* Women's Review of Books 10(5): 30, Feb., 1993.
GEELHOED, G.W., *"Access to Care in a Changing PracticeEnvironment."* Bulletin of the American College of Surgeons 70(6): 11-15, June, 1985.
GIFFORD, J.F. Jr.; ANLYAN, W.G., *"Sounding Board. The Role of the Private Sector in an Economy of Limited Health Care Resources."* New England Journal of Medicine 300 (14): 790-3, April 5, 1979.
GILBERT, F.I. Jr.; NORDYKE, R.A., *"The Case for Restructuring Health Care in the United States: The Hawaii Paradigm."* Journal of Medical Systems 17 (3-4): 283-8, Aug., 1993.
GILBERTSON E.E., *"A Call for Advocacy and Rededication to 'Health Care For All'."* Urban Health 12 (3): 43-4, March, 1983.
GILL, D.G.; INGMAN, S.R.; CAMPBELL, J., *"Health Care Provision and Distributive Justice: End Stage Renal Disease and the Elderly in Britain and America."* Social Science and Medicine 32(5): 565-77, 1991.
GINZBERG, Eli, *"Improving Health Care For the Poor. Lessons From the 1980s."* Journal of the American Medical Association 271 (6): 464-7, Feb. 9, 1994.
GOLD, M.; CHU, K.; FELT, S.; HARRINGTON, M.; LAKE, T., *"Effects of Selected Cost-Containment Efforts: 1971-1993."* Health Care Financing Review 14 (3): 183-225, 1993 Spring.
GOLDING, Martin P., *"Justice and Rights: A Study in Relationship."* In Shelp, Earl [editor], Justice and Health Care. Dordrecht, Holland / Boston, U.S.A. / London, England: D. Reidel Publishing Company, 1981, Vol 8. pp. 23-35.
GOLDSTICK, D., *"Distributive Justice and Utility."* The Journal of Value Inquiry 25(1): 65-71, Jan., 1991.
GORDON, David, *"Philosophy - Theories of Distributive Justice by John E. Roemer."* Library Journal 121(6): 83, Apr 1, 1996.
GOTTLIEB, S.R., *"Ensuring Access to Health Care: What Communities Can Do to Make a Difference Through Private Sector Coalitions."* Inquiry 23 (3): 322-9, 1986 Fall.

GROSSMAN, E.G., *"Comparing the Options For Universal Coverage."* Health Affairs 13 (2): 84-100, 1994 Spring (II).
GUTTMACHER, S., *"Poor People, Poor Care."* Health Pac Bulletin 15 (4): 15-17, Jul-Aug, 1984.
HAAS, J.S.; UDVARHELYI, I.S.; MORRIS, C.N.; EPSTEIN, A.M., *"The Effect of Providing Health Coverage to Poor Uninsured Pregnant Women in Massachusetts."* Journal of the American Medical Association 269 (1): 87-91, Jan. 6, 1993.
HAFNER-EATON, C., *"Patterns of Hospital and Physician Utilization Among the Uninsured."* Journal of Health Care for the Poor and Underserved 5 (4): 297-315, 1994.
HAGGERTY, R.J., *"The Limits of Medical Care."* New England Journal of Medicine 313 (6): 383-4, Aug. 8, 1985.
HAMPTON, G.M., *"Have Health Care Professionals Adopted the Marketing Concept?"* Health Marketing Quarterly 10(1-2): 5-32, 1992.
HART, H. L. A., *"Rawls On Liberty and Priority."* In Reading Rawls, pp. 230-252. Edited by Norman Daniels. New York: Basic Books, Inc., 1975.
HARTLEY, D.; QUAM, L.; LURIE N., *"Urban and Rural Differences in Health Insurance and Access to Care."* Journal of Rural Health 10 (2): 98-108, 1994 Spring.
HARTWELL, S.W. Jr., *"Bioethics, Medicine, and the Moral Ground."* Physician Executive 16(3): 23-4, May-Jun., 1990.
HARVEY, Birt, *"Toward a National Child Health Policy."* Journal of the American Medical Association 264 (2): 252-3, July 11, 1990.
_____, *"A Proposal to Provide Health Insurance to All Children and All Pregnant Women."* New England Journal of Medicine 323 (17): 1216-20, Oct. 25, 1990.
HEHIR, J.Bryan, *"Health Care for All: A Catholic Perspective."* Commonweal 120(9): 7-9, May 7, 1993.
HENRIOT, P.J., *"Catholic Health Care. Competing and Complementary Models."* Health Progress 66(7): 36-40, Sept., 1985.
HERZLINGER, R.E., *"The Failed Revolution in Health Care—The Role of Management."* Harvard Business Review 67(2): 95-103, Mar-Apr., 1989.
HEUSSNER, Ralph C. Jr., *"Peddling Drugs to Docs."* Minnesota Medicine 77(6): 24-31, June, 1994.
HIMES, M.J., "The Catholic Health Care Facility: Its Role as Church." Hospital Progress 63(2): 31-5, 52, Feb., 1982.

HIMMELSTEIN, David U.; WOOLHANDLER, Steffie, *"Care Denied: US Residents Who Are Unable to Obtain Needed Medical Services."* American Journal of Public Health 85 (3): 341-4, March, 1995.

HOEFLER, J.M.; THAI, K.V., *"The Politics and Economics of Health Care Finance: Tough Questions and No Easy Answers."* Journal of Health and Human Resources Administration 16 (2): 121-43, 1993 Fall.

_____, *"Politics and Economics of Health Care Finance: A Symposium."* Journal of Health and Human Resources Adm. 16 (2): 115-20, 1993 Fall.

HOLAHAN, J.; MOON, M.; WELCH, W.P.; ZUCKERMAN, S., *"An American Approach to Health System Reform."* Journal of the American Medical Association 265(19): 2537-40, May 15, 1991.

HOWELL, Leon, *"Our Clinton Watch."* Christianity and Crisis 53(1): 4, Feb.1, 1993.

HUGHES, J., *"Ultimate Justification: Wittgenstein and Medical Ethics."* Journal of Medical Ethics 21(1): 25-30, Feb., 1995.

HUGHES, T.F.; ECKEL, F.M., *"Ethical Issues Associated With Managed Care Pharmacy Services."* Topics in Hospital Pharmacy Management 10(3): 30-8, Nov., 1990.

HULL, Robert, *"Distributive Justice and the Minnesota Health Access Initiative."* The Journal of Medical Humanities 16(2): 93-103, 1995 Summer.

HURLEY, R.E., *"The Purchaser-Driven Reformation in Health Care: Alternative Approaches to Leveling Our Cathedrals."* Frontiers of Health Service Management 9(4): 5-35; discussion 45, 1993 Summer.

HUTCHINSON, R.A.; SCHUMOCK, G.T., *"Need to Develop a Legal and Ethical Base for Pharmaceutical Care."* Annals of Pharmacotherapy 28(7-8): 954-6, Jul-Aug., 1994.

IRWIN, Sarah, *"Age Related Distributive Justice and Claims on Resources."* British Journal of Sociology 47(1):68-92, March, 1996.

JACOBS, Michael S., *"Recent Developments in Antitrust Law and Their Implications for the Clinton Health Care Plan."* Journal of Law, Medicine and Ethics 21(2): 163-72, 1993 Summer.

JENNINGS, Bruce; CALLAHAN, David; WOLF, Susan M., *"The Professions: Public Interest and Common Good."* Hastings Center Report 17:6, February, 1987.

JOHNSON, R.L.; GILL, S.L., *"U.S. Needs a New Vision of National Health Policy."* Health Progress 70(6): 24-8, Jul-Aug., 1989.
JOHNSSON, Julie; MCILRATH, Sharon, *"Reform Deals Threaten Universal Coverage Bid."* American Medical News 37(24): 1,29, June 27, 1994.
JOHNSSON, Julie, *"Kennedy Bill Marks Senate's First Step Toward Reform."* American Medical News 37(24): 28, June 27, 1994.
JONES, E.I., *"Effects of Competition of Access to Care: Will New Trends in Competition Limit Access to Health Care For Blacks."* Journal of the National Medical Association 77(12): 967-8, December, 1985.
JONSSON, B., *"Improving Patient Care: Consequences For Resource Allocation."* Cardiology 84(6): 420-6, 1994.
JUSTICE, Diane E., *"The Aging Network: A Balancing Act Between Universal Coverage and Defined Eligibility."* Generations 19(3): 58-62, 1995 Fall.
KASSIRER, J.P., *"Managed Care and the Morality of the Marketplace."* New England Journal of Medicine 333(1): 50-2, July 6, 1995.
KEE, F.; GAFFNEY, B.; CANAVAN, C.; LITTLE, J.; MCCONNELL, W.; TELFORD, A.M.; WATSON, J.D., *"Is Choice of General Practitioner Important for Patients Having Coronary Artery Investigations?"* Quality in Health Care 3(1): 17-22, March, 1994.
KELLEY, M.A.; PERLOFF, J.D.; MORRIS, N.M.; LIU, W., *"Access to Primary Care Among Young African-American Children in Chicago."* Journal of Health and Social Policy 5 (2): 35-48, 1993.
KELLY, J., *"Evolution of a 'Right to Health Care'."* Medical World News. Spec No: 60-2, 65-70, January, 1985.
KELLY, Margaret J., *"Health Care Facility; Platform for Social Justice."* Hospital Progress63: 50-3, May, 1982.
KELLY, W.N.; KRAUSE, E.C.; KROWINSKI, W.J.; SMALL, T.R., *"National Survey of Ethical Issues Presented to Drug Information Centers."* American Journal of Hospital Pharmacy47(10): 2245-50, October, 1990.
KENNEY, Jay, *"Market Oriented Health Policy: An Analysis of the Pro-Competition Strategy."* Social Thought 9: 15-29, 1983 Summer.
KENT, C., *"Perspectives. Health Reform and the Poor: Empty Promises or a Promising Blueprint?"* Faulkner and Grays Medicine and Health 47(47): suppl 4 p., December 6, 1993.

KERTESZ, L., *"Enrollment, Access Woes Cited at Some Medicare Risk HMOs."* Modern Healthcare 25(12): 6, March 20, 1995.

KESSEL, R.A., *"Ethical and Economic Aspects of Governmental Intervention in the Medical Care Market."* Washington: American Enterprise Institute for Public Policy Research, May 12, 1977.

KIDSON, C., *"Equity, Poverty and the Economics of Health Care Consumption."* Southeast Asian Journal of Tropical Medicine and Public Health 25(4): 615-7, December, 1994.

KING, Gary, *"A New Frontier But the Same Old Problem."* Journal of Law, Medicine and Ethics 22(2): 138-40, 1994 Summer.

KINZER, D.M., *"Care of the Poor Revisited."* Inquiry 21(1): 5-16, 1984 Spring.

KINZER, D., *"Criteria and Guidelines for Reforming the United States Health Care System."* New England Journal of Medicine 322:467, 1990.

KLINGHOFFER, M.; ORIENT, J.M., *"Civil Defense in the United States: Evolution and Regression."* Southern Medical Journal 79(2): 135-40, February, 1986.

KOHN, D., *"The Role of Business Process Reengineering in Health Care."* Topics in Health Information Management 14(3): 1-6, February, 1994.

KOLLER, Christopher F., *"Health, Justice, Community - Health Care Reform: A Catholic View by Philip S. Keane."* Commonweal 121(12): 26-7, June 17, 1994.

LAMONT, Julian, *"The Concept of Desert in Distributive Justice."* Philosophical Quarterly44(174):45-64, January, 1994.

LEE D.W.; GILLIS, K.D., *"Physician Responses to Medicare Payment Reform: an Update on Access to Care."* Inquiry 31(3): 346-53, 1994 Fall.

LEE, P.R.; MOSS, N.; KRIEGER, N., *"Measuring Social Inequalities in Health. Report on the Conference of the National Institutes of Health."* Public Health Reports 110(3): 302-5, May-June, 1995.

LEVIN, Lowell S., *"If Medicine Doesn't Affect Health Much, What Does?"* Social Policy 24(4): 46-48, 1994 Summer.

LEVIT, Katharine R.; LAZENBY, Helen C., *"Health Care Spending in 1994: Slowest in Decades."* Health Affairs 15(2): 130-44, 1996 Summer.

LEWIN, J.C.; SYBINSKY, P.A., *"Hawaii's Employer Mandate and Its Contribution to Universal Access."* Journal of the American

Medical Association 269(19): 2538-43, May 19, 1993.
LEWIS, I.J., *"Control of Health Care Costs: Freedom, Justice, and the Political Order."* Man and Medicine 5(4): 273-90, 1980.
LONG, S.H.; MARQUIS, M.S., *"The Uninsured 'Access Gap' and the Cost of Universal Coverage."* Health Affairs 13(2):211-20, 1994 Spring (II).
LOUGHLIN, M., *"Dworkin, Rawls and Reality."* Health Care Analysis 3(1): 37-43, February, 1995.
LOWE, Michael; KERRIDGE, Ian H.; MITCHELL, Keneth R., *"'These Sorts of People Don't Do Very Well': Race and Allocation of Health Care Resources."* Journal of Medical Ethics 21(6): 356-60, December, 1995.
LUCK, M.F., *"A Philanthropic Philosophy for the 21st Century."* Journal / Association for Healthcare Philanthropy:27-9, 1994 Spring.
MAC SHEOIN, T., *"Unethical Behavior in an Ethical Industry? Critical Coverage of the Pharmaceutical Industry, 1983-1984."* International Journal of Health Services 16(1): 41-62, 1986.
MARINER, W.K., *"Rationing Health Care and the Need for Credible Scarcity: Why Americans Can't Say No."* American Journal of Public Health 85(10): 1439-45, Oct., 1995.
MARQUIS, M.S.; LONG, S.H., *"Uninsured Children and National Health Reform."* Journal of the American Medical Association 268(24): 3473-7, Dec. 23-30, 1992.
MARQUIS, M.S.; BUCHANAN, J.L., *"How Will Changes in Health Insurance Tax Policy and Employer Health Plan Contributions Affect Access to Health Care and Health Care Costs?"* Journal of the American Medical Association 271(12): 939-44, Mar. 23-30, 1994.
MATTAI, Giuseppe. *"Un percorso etico sempre attuale: La Giustizia."* Asprenas 43 (1): 43-54, 1996.
MATZ, R., *"Health System Reform: Will Controlling Cost Require Rationing Services?"* [Comment on: Journal of the American Medical Association Jul. 27, 1994: 272(4): 324-8] JAMA 273(4): 285-6, Jan. 25, 1995.
MAY, William F.; FOEGE, William, *"The Ethical Foundations of Health Care Reform."* Christian Century 111(18): 572-576, Jun. 1, 1994.
MAYER, J.D., *"International Perspectives on the Health Care Crisis in the United States."* Social Science and Medicine 23 (10): 1059-65, 1986.

MCCLURE, L.W., *"Who Needs History?"* Academic Medicine 70(6): 461-2, June, 1995.
MCCORMICK, Brian, *"New Managed Care Mantra: Doctor Control."* American Medical News 37(24): 3, 27, June 27, 1994.
MCCORMICK, Richard A., *"Bioethical Issues and the Moral Matrix of U.S. Health Care."* Hospital Progress 60(5): 42-5, May, 1979.
_____., *"Value Variables in the Health-Care Reform Debate."* America 168(19: 7-13, May 29, 1993.
MCCULLOUGH, Lawrence B., *"The Right to Health Care."* Ethics in Science and Medicine 6(1): 1-9, 1979.
MCMILLION, Charles W., *"Health Care for All? Paying for Health Care Reform."* Harvard Business Review 72(2): 12-13, March, 1994.
MCNAMEE, Mike, *"The New Math of Health-Care Reform."* Business Week 3345: 47, Nov. 8, 1993.
MCNEIL B.J., *"Socioeconomic Forces Affecting Medicine: Times of Increased Retrenchment and Accountability."* Seminars in Nuclear Medicine 23 (1): 3-8, Jan., 1993.
MENZEL, Paul T., *"Healthy Realism - Health Care Politics, Policy and Distributive Justice: The Ironic Triumph by Robert P. Rhodes."* Hastings Center Report 23(2): 44-45, March, 1993.
MEYER, Harris, *"House Backs Flexible System Reform Tactics."* American Medical News 37(24): 1,22, June 27, 1994.
MEYER, J.A.; SILOW-CARROLL, S.; SARDEGNA, C.J., *"Universal Access to Health Care. A Comprehensive Tax-Based Approach."* Archives of Internal Medicine 151(5): 917-22, May, 1991.
MIKOCHIK, S.L., *"When Life Becomes Optional: A Comment on Kevin O'Rourke's Approach to Forgoing Life Support."* Issues in Law and Medicine 10(3): 343-51, 1994 Winter.
MILLER, Bruce L., *"Responsibility and Public Policy in Health Care: Commentary on Essays by Williams and Rich."* In AGICH, George J. (ed), Responsibility in Health Care. [Philosophy and Medicine, H.Tristram Engelherdt Jr., Stuart F. Spicker (eds.)] Dordrecht, Holland / Boston, U.S.A. / London, England: D. Reidel Publishing Company, 1982, Vol 12.
MILLER, G.J., *"The Nation's Health Deficit and Its Political Economy."* Lancet 344(8934): 1419-20, Nov. 19, 1994.
MOKUAU, N., Fong, R., *"Assessing the Responsiveness of Health Services to Ethnic Minorities of Color."* Social Work in Health Care 20(2): 23-34, 1994.

MOONEY, A., *"The Great Society and Health: Policies for Narrowing the Gaps in Health Status Between the Poor and the Nonpoor."* Medical Care 15(8): 611-9, August, 1977.

MOORE, R.M. Jr.; KACZMAREK, R.G.; HAMBURGER, S., *"Prenatal Ultrasound: Are Socially Disadvantaged Groups Afforded Equal Access?"* Journal of Health Care for the Poor and Underserved 1(2): 229-36, 1990 Fall.

MORISON, R.S., *"Rights and Responsibilities: Redressing the Uneasy Balance."* Hastings Center Report 4(2): 1-4, April, 1974.

MORREIM, E.Haavi, *"Access Without Excess."* Journal of Medicine and Philosophy 17(1): 1-6, February, 1992.

_____, *"Moral Justice and Legal Justice in Managed Care: The Ascent of Contributive Justice."* Journal of Law, Medicine and Ethics 23(3): 247-265, 1995 Fall.

MORRIS, J.N., *"Social Inequalities Undiminished."* Health Visitor 53(9): 361-5, Sept., 1980.

MOSKOP, J.C., *"Rawlsian Justice and a Human Right to Health Care."* Journal of Medicine and Philosophy 8(4): 329-38, Nov., 1983.

MUNDIGER, M.O., *"Health Service Funding Cuts and the Declining Health of the Poor."* New England Journal of Medicine 313 (1): 44-7, July 4, 1985.

MURDOCK, Deroy, *"But Medisave Would Benefit Patients and the Economy."* Insight on the News 10(25): 37-38, June 20, 1994.

MURPHY, E.A., *"Some Epistemological Aspects of the Model in Medicine."* Journal of Medicine and Philosophy 3(4): 273-92, Dec., 1978.

NATIONAL CONFERENCE OF CATHOLIC BISHOPS, *"A Pastoral Letter on Health and Health Care."* Origins 11: 396-402, December 3, 1981.

NICHOLSON, R.H., *"Truth Lies Somewhere, If We Knew But Where."* Hastings Center Report 23(5): 5, Sept.-Oct., 1993.

NICKEL, J.W., *"Should Undocumented Aliens Be Entitled to Health Care?"* Hastings Center Report 16(6): 19-23, Dec., 1986.

NOLAN. B., *"Economic Incentives, Health Status and Health Services Utilisation."* Journal of Health Economics 12 (2): 151-69, July, 1993.

NORTON E.C.; STAIGER D.O., *"How Hospital Ownership Affects Access to Care for the Uninsured."* Rand Journal of Economics 25(1): 171-85, 1994 Spring.

NUTTER, Donald O. et al, *"Restructuring Health Care in the United States: A Proposal for the 1990s."* Journal of the American Medical Association 265(19):2516-2520, May 15, 1991.

NUTTER, D.W., *"Access to Care and the Evolution of Corporate, For-Profit Medicine."* New England Journal of Medicine 311(14): 917-9, Oct. 4, 1984.

OBERMAN, Linda, *"Reform Efforts Continue, Despite Red Ink."* American Medical News 37(24): 4, June 27, 1994.

_____, *"Reform's Cost-Benefit Balancing Act."* American Medical News 37(18): 3, 35, May 9, 1994.

O'CONNELL, L.J., *"Ethicists and Health Care Reform: An Indecent Proposal?"* Journal of Medicine and Philosophy 19(5): 419-24, Oct., 1994.

O'CONNOR, J.J. Card., *"The Right to Health Care."* Origins 15: 186-8, Sept. 5, 1985.

O'CONNOR, J.J. Card., *"The Sanctity of Life and the Right to Adequate Health Care."* New Oxford Review 53: 15-17, March, 1986.

O'KEEFFE, J.E., *"Health Care Financing: How Much Reform is Needed?"* Issues in Science and Technology 8(3): 42-9, 1992 Spring.

OSWALD, N., *"Survival of the Safety Net. A Look at Clinton's Health Care Plan."* Health Pac Bulletin 23(3): 25-7, 1993 Fall.

OZAR, D.T., *"Social Ethics, the Philosophy of Medicine, and Professional Responsibility."* Theoretical Medicine 6(3): 281-94, Oct., 1985.

PACI, P.; Wagstaff, A., *"Equity and Efficiency in Italian Health Care."* Health Economics 2 (1): 15-29, April, 1993.

PARKER, B.R., *"A Measure of the Effects of Competition in the U.S. Health Care Sector During the 1980s."* International Journal of Health Planning and Management 4(2): 125-37, April-June, 1989.

PARKIN, D.; HENDERSON, J., *"How Important is Equality of Access to Hospital? A Case Study of Patients' and Visitors' Travel Costs."* Hospital and Health Services Review 83 (1): 23-7, Jan., 1987.

PASSWATER, D., *"For-Profit Health Care: An Ethical Dilemma."* Health Values 13(3): 15-21, May-June, 1989.

PAULY, Mark V., *"Universal Health Insurance in the Clinton Plan: Coverage as a Tax-Financed Public Good."* Journal of Economic Perspectives 8(3): 45-53, 1994 Summer.

PELLEGRINO, E.D., *"Rationing Medical Care: The Need for Distributive Justice."* Internist 19(8): 5, Oct., 1978.

PEREIRA, J., *"The Economics of Inequality in Health: A Bibliography."* Social Science and Medicine 31(3): 413-20, 1990.

PETRONIS, K.R.; CARROLL, C.E.; HELD, P.J.; PORT, F.K., *"Effect of Race on Access to Recombinant Human Erythropoietin in Long-Term Hemodialysis Patients."* Journal of the American Medical Association 271 (22): 1760-3, June 8, 1994.

PHILLIPS, Peter, *"Justice Enfleshed in Every Community."* Priest and People 3: 55-8, 1989 Fall.

PILARCZYK, D.E., *"The Catholic Health Facility: Would You Know One If You Saw One?"* Hospital Progress 63(8): 30-3, August, 1982.

POPP, R., *"Health Care for the Poor: Where Has All the Money Gone?"* Journal of Nursing Administration 18(1): 8-12, Jan., 1988.

POWELL, M.L. 3rd., *"Access to Health Care: Cost is the Primary Barrier."* Rhode Island Medicine 77 (9): 316-7, Sept., 1994.

PURTILO, Ruth B., *"Interdisciplinary Health Care Teams and Health Care Reform."* Journal of Law, Medicine and Ethics 22(2): 121-26, 1994 Summer.

REINHARDT, U. E., "The Importance of Quality in the Debate on National Health Policy." In J.B. Couch (ed) *Health Care Quality Management for the 21st Century Tampa: The American College of Physician Executives,* 1991.

_____, *"Health Care of the Poor: Symposium on CHA's Task Force Report. An American Paradox."* Health Progress 67(9): 42, Nov., 1986.

_____, *"Reorganizing the Financial Flows in American Health Care."* Health Affairs. [Supplement], 1993.

_____, *"Managed Competition in Health Care Reform: Just Another American Dream, or the Perfect Solution?"* Journal of Law, Medicine and Ethics 22(2): 106-20, 1994 Summer.

_____, *"Coverage and Access in Health Care Reform."* New England Journal of Medicine 330(20): 1452-53, May 19, 1994.

RICE, D.P., *"Ethics and Equity in U.S. Health Care: The Data."* International Journal of Health Services 21(4): 637-51, 1991.

RINES, J.T., *"Prospective Payment: Unanswered Ethical Questions."* Journal - American Medical Record Association 56(3): 20-4, March, 1985.

RIVO, M.L.; SATCHER, D., *"Improving Access to Health Care Through Physician Workforce Reform. Directions for the 21st. Century."* Journal of the American Medical Association 270 (9): 1074-8,

Sept. 1, 1993.
ROACH, John Robert, Cardinal, *"Social Justice: Reviving the Common Good."* Origins 20:585-93, Feb 14, 1991.
ROBERTS, S.V.; GLASTRIS, P.; IMPOCO, J.; HETTER, K., *"Shutting the golden door."* US News and World Report 117(13): 36-40, Oct. 3, 1994.
ROEMER, M.I., *"Optimism on Attaining Health Care Equity."* Medical Care 18 (7): 775-81, July, 1980.
ROSEN, S., *"Beyond Doctors: Workers in Health-Care Reform."* Social Policy 24 (4): 40-5. 1994 Summer.
ROSSER, W.W., *"Why Academic Primary Care Physicians Should Fight for a Universally Accessible Health Care System."* Family Medicine 24(3): 176-7, 185, March-April, 1992.
ROTHMAN, D.J., *"The Rising Cost of Pharmaceuticals: An Ethicist's Perspective."* American Journal of Hospital Pharmacy 50(8 Suppl 4): 810-2, Aug., 1993.
ROWLAND, D.; SALGANICOFF, A., *"Commentary: Lessons from Medicaid—Improving Access to Office-Based Physician Care for the Low-Income Population."* American Journal of Public Health 84 (4): 550-2, April, 1994.
RUBINSTEIN, David, *"Capitalism, Social Mobility, and Distributive Justice."* Social Theory and Practice 19(2): 183-204, 1993 Summer.
RUBLEE, D.A., *"Medical Technology in Canada, Germany, and the United States."* Health Affairs 8 (3): 178-81, 1989 Fall.
RUIZ, P., *"Access to Health Care for Uninsured Hispanics: Policy Recommendations."* Hospital and Community Psychiatry 44 (10): 958-62, Oct., 1993.
RUSSELL, Louise, *"Opportunity Costs in Modern Medicine."* Health Affairs 11(2):162-69, 1992 Summer.
SASS, H.M., *"Justice, Beneficence, or Common Sense?: The President's Commission's Report on Access to Health Care."* Journal of Medicine and Philosophy 8(4): 381-8, Nov., 1983.
SAUNDERS, William P., *"Health Care Delivery in Light of the Gospel Challenge."* Linacre 51:34-8, 1984 Fall.
SAYER, A., *"Prices of Equitable Access: The New Massachusetts Health Insurance Law."* Hastings Center Report 18 (3): 21-5, June-July, 1988.
SCHAFER, A., *"Comments on Birch and Abelson's 'Is Reasonable Access What We Want?'"* International Journal of Health Services 24(2):

373-5, 1994.
SCHALL, J.V., *"The Costs of Mercy."* Linacre 51: 105-11, May, 1984.
SCHIEBER, G.J.; POULLIER, J-J.; GREENWALD, L.M., *"Health Care Systems in Twenty-Four Countries."* Health Affairs: 22-38, 1991 Fall.
SCHLESIGNER, M.; BENTKOVER, J.; BLUMENTHAL, D.; CUSTER, W.; MUSACCHIO, R.; WILLER, J., *"Multihospital Systems and Access to Health Care."* Advances in Health Economics and Health Services Research 7:121-40, 1987.
SCHORR, A.L., *"What is Reform in Health Care?"* Social Work 37(3): 263-5, May, 1992.
SCHRAMM, C.J., *"Health Care Financing for All Americans."* Journal of the American Medical Association 265(24): 3296-9, June 26, 1991.
SCHROEDER, Steven A., *"Time to Confront Health Care Rationing."* Minnesota Medicine 77(11): 8-9, Nov., 1994.
SCHWARTZ, Michael C., *"Economics 101 for Bishops."* Crisis 8: 26-31, Mar., 1990.
SCHWARTZ, R.L., *"Life Style, Health Status, and Distributive Justice."* Health Matrix 3(1): 195-217, 1993 Spring.
SCHWARTZ, L.R.; HAMMER, L.M.; VEATCH, R.M., *"Dispensing Medication Without Receiving Payment."* American Journal of Hospital Pharmacy 51(13): 1680; discussion 1680-3, July 1, 1994.
SCITOVSKY, A.A.; CAPRON, A.M., *"Medical Care at the End of Life: The Interaction of Economics and Ethics."* Annual Review of Public Health 7:59-75, 1986.
SECUNDY, M.G., *"Strategic Compromise: Real World Ethics."* Journal of Medicine and Philosophy 19(5): 407-17, Oct., 1994.
SEMKOW, B.W., *"Limited Information, Medical Entitlements and Distributive Justice."* Social Science and Medicine 21(10): 1187-92, 1985.
SEMPLE, J., *"Bentham's Utilitarianism and the Provision of Medical Care."* Clio Medica 23: 30-45, 1993.
SHAPIRO, S.H., *"Privatization and Commercialization of Health Care Financing and Delivery: Ethical Issues."* Journal of Health Administration Education 6(2): 273-85, 1988 Spring.
SHELP, Earl E., *"Justice: A moral test for health care and health policy."* In Shelp, Earl (ed), Justice and Health Care. Dordrecht, Holland / Boston, U.S.A. / London: England: D. Reidel Publishing Company, 1981, Vol 8. pp. 213-229.

SHELTON, R.L., *"Human Rights and Distributive Justice in Health Care Delivery."* Journal of Medical Ethics 4(4): 165-71, Dec., 1978.
SIEVERTS, S., *"What About the Uninsured?"* Health Management Quarterly:5-8, 1985 Summer.
SILVERS, A., *"Damaged Goods: Does Disability DisQALYfy People From Just Health Care?"* Mount Sinai Journal of Medicine 62(2): 102-11; discussion 116-23, March, 1995.
SI NAHR, J.; SMITH, L.; GOTTLIEB, S.R., *"How Can We Equitably Share Health Care's Obligation to the Poor?"* Health Management Quarterly:16-9, 1985 Summer.
SISK, Jane E.; GLIED, Sherry A., *"Innovation Under Federal Health Care Reform."* Health Affairs 13(3): 82-97, 1994 Summer.
SMITH, J.E., *"Ethical Issues Raised by the Human Genome Project."* American Journal of Hospital Pharmacy 50(9): 1945-50, Sept., 1993.
SPIEGLER, M.H., *"Health Care Rationing in the United States: Are We There Yet?"* Journal of the American Optometric Association 63(9): 638-42, Sept., 1992.
SPILLMAN, B.C., *"The Impact of Being Uninsured on Utilization of Basic Health Care Services."* Inquiry 29 (4): 457-66, 1992 Winter.
SPINELLO, Richard A., *"Ethics, Pricing and the Pharmaceutical Industry."* Journal of Business Ethics 11(8): 617-626, Aug., 1992.
STERN, Paul, *"Citizenship, Community and Pluralism: The Current Dispute on Distributive Justice."* Praxis International 11(3): 261-297, Oct., 1991.
STERNFELD, Leon, *"HMOs and People With MS."* Inside MS 12(1): 19, 1994 Winter.
STONE, Deborah A., *"The Struggle for the Soul of Health Insurance."* Journal of Health Politics, Policy and Law 18(2): 287-317, 1993 Summer.
St. Peter, R.F.; Newacheck, P.W.; Halfon, N., *"Access to care for poor children. Separate and unequal?"* Journal of the American Medical Association 267 (20): 2760-4, May 27, 1992.
SUMMERFIELD, M.R., *"Dangers of Compromising Drug Distribution."* American Journal of Health-System Pharmacy 52(7): 752-3, April 1, 1995.
SUMMERS, J., *"Healthcare Reform: Beginning the Ethical Debate."* Journal of Healthcare Materiel Management 12(3): 52, 55-6, March, 1994.

TENERY, Robert M. Jr., *"Don't Confuse Universal Access with Universal Coverage."* American Medical News 37(18): 21, May 9, 1994.
THUROW, L.C., *"Learning to Say 'No'."* New England Journal of Medicine 311 (24): 1569-72, Dec. 13, 1984.
THOMASMA, David C., *"An Apology for the Value of Human Lives."* Hospital Progress 63 (4): 49-52, 68, April, 1982.
TODD, James S., *"Challenge to Medicine: Meshing Science and Social Reality."* American Medical News 22(4): suppl 13, Jan. 26, 1979.
TORRENS, James S., *"Health Care: Your Money or Your Life."* America 169(18): 6-9, Dec. 4, 1993.
TRAD, Paul V., *"Health Care Reform: The Entitlement to Psychotherapeutic Services."* American Journal of Psychotherapy 48(1): 1-4, 1994 Winter.
TRESOLINI, C.P.; SHUGARS, D.A.; LEE, L.S., *"Teaching an Integrated Approach to Health Care: Lessons From Five Schools."* Academic Medicine 70(8): 665-70, Aug., 1995.
UNDERWOOD, S.M.; HOSKINS, D.; CUMMINS, T.; MORRIS, K.; WILLIAMS, A., *"Obstacles to Cancer Care: Focus on the Economically Disadvantaged."* Oncology Nursing Forum 21 (1): 47-52, Jan.-Feb., 1994.
UPCHURCH, G.; EARP J.A.; BLALOCK S.J., *"Access to Medications for the Low-Income North Carolina Citizens. Without Funds, How Can They Follow Doctor's Orders?"* North Carolina Medical Journal 55 (5): 173-7, May, 1994.
VAN DOORSLAER, E.; WAGSTAFF, A.; CALONGE, S.; CHRISTIANSEN, T.; GERFIN, M.; GOTTSCHALK, P.; JANSSEN, R.; LACHAUD, C.; LEU, R.E.; NOLAN, B. et al., *"Equity in the Delivery of Health Care: Some International Comparisons."* Journal of Health Economics 11(4): 389-411, Dec., 1992.
VEATCH, Robert M., *"Justice in Health Care: The Contribution of Edmund Pellegrino."* Journal of Medicine and Philosophy 15(3): 269-87, June, 1990.

_____, *"Rationing: Why Justice Requires Multiple Insurance Plans."* National Forum: Phi Kappa Phi Journal 73(3): 22-24+, 1993 Summer.

_____, *"What Counts as Basic Health Care? Private Values and Public Policy."* Hastings Center Report 24(3): 20-21, May, 1994.

VEATCH, Robert M., *"Healthcare Rationing Through Global Budgeting: The Ethical Choices."* Journal of Clinical Ethics 5(4): 291-6, 1994 Winter.
VLADECK, B.C., *"Equity, Access, and the Costs of Health Services."* Medical Care 19 (12 Suppl): 69-80, Dec., 1981.
WAGNER, L., *"Government Should Ensure Health Access."* Modern Health Care 20 (28):4, July 16, 1990.
WALLACE, P.E., *"Access to Healthcare and the Long-Stay Patient. A Case Study."* Hospital Topics 73 (1): 28-34, 1995 Winter.
WALLEY, Robert L., *"A New Health Care Initiative Within the Church."* Linacre 51: 71-9, 1984 Fall.
WATSON, Sidney Dean, *"Minority Access and Health Reform: A Civil Right to Health Care."* Journal of Law, Medicine and Ethics 22(2): 127-37, 1994 Summer.
WEBER, Leonard J., *"Ethics Commission Access Report Urges Adequate Care for All; A Commentary on Secondary Access to Health Care."* Hospital Progress 65: 62-5, July-August, 1984.
_____, *"Infant Treatment Decisions: Ethics and Cost."* Health Progress 65 (11): 28-31, Dec., 1984.
WEIL, T.P., *"A Universal Access Plan: A Step Toward National Health Insurance?"* Hospital and Health Services Administration 37(1): 37-51, 1992 Spring.
WEISSMAN, J.S.; EPSTEIN, A.M., *"The Insurance Gap: Does it Make a Difference?"* Annual Review of Public Health 14: 243-70, 1993.
WHITNEY, H.A. Jr., *"Pharmacy Morality, II: The Darkside of Alternative Medicine."* Journal of Pharmacy Technology 10(2): 49-50, March-April, 1994.
WHITTLE, J.; CONIGLIARO, J.; GOOD, C.B.; LOFGREN, R.P., *" Racial Differences in the Use of Invasive Cardiovascular Procedures in the Department of Veterans Affairs Medical System."* New England Journal of Medicine 329 (9): 621-7, Aug. 26, 1993.
WIATROWSKI, W.J., *"Who Really Has Access to Employer-Provided Health Benefits?"* Monthly Labor Review 118 (6): 36-44, June, 1995.
WIENER, Joshua M., *"Getting it Right on Health Care Reform."* Brookings Review 12(1): 5, 1994 Winter.
WIKLER, D., *"Forming and Ethical Response to For-Profit Health Care."* Business and Health 2(3): 25-9, Jan.-Feb., 1985.
WILENSKY, G., *"Access to Care: Where Are the Holes in the Net? The Plight of the Uninsured."* Health Matrix 3 (3): 8-10, 1985 Fall.

WILLIAMS, Bernard, "*Persons, Character and Morality,*" in *The Identities of Persons,* ed. Amelie O. Rorty, Los Angeles: University of California Press, 1976.
WILLIAMS, A.P.; SCHWARTZ, W.B.; NEWHOUSE, J.P.; BENNETT, B.W., "*How Many Miles to the doctor?*" New England Journal of Medicine 309 (16): 958-63, Oct. 20, 1983.
WILSON, George, "*Health Care Reform and 'Market Forces'.*" America 170(13): 6-7, April 16, 1994.
WILSON, John; HARGROVE, Barbara. "*Habits of the Heart.*" Book Review. Religious Studies Review. 14: 304-316, 1988.
WOLFE, S., "*Ethics and Equity in Canadian Health Care: Policy Alternatives.*" International Journal of Health Services 21(4):673-80, 1991.
WOLFF, Adam, "*Practice Parameters in Health Reform: New State Approaches Precede Clinton Plan.*" Journal of Law, Medicine and Ethics 21(3-4): 394-7, 1993 Fall.
WOOLHANDLER, S.; HIMMELSTEIN, D.U., "*Resolving the Cost / Access Conflict: The Case for a National Health Program.*" Journal of General Internal Medicine 4 (1): 54-60, 1989 Jan-Feb.
YANKELOVICH, Daniel, "*The Debate That Wasn't: The Public and the Clinton Plan.*" Health Affairs [Spring 1995]: 7-23.
YOUNG, Jeffrey T; GORDON, Barry, "*Distributive Justice as a Normative Criterion in Adam Smith's Political Economy.*" History of Political Economy 28(1): 1-25, 1996 Spring.
ZOLOTH, A.M., "*The Need for Ethical Guidelines for Relationships Between Pharmacists and the Pharmaceutical Industry.*" American Journal of Hospital Pharmacy 48(3): 551-552, March, 1991.

Selected Works and Articles for Chapter One: Health Care in the U.S.A.

Books:
ANDERSEN, Ronald M.; RICE, Thomas H.; KOMINSKI, Gerald F., *Changing the U.S. Health Care System.* San Francisco:Jossey-Bass Publishers 1996.
BEAUCHAMP, Tom L.; CHILDRESS, James F., *Principles of Biomedical Ethics.* New York, Oxford: Oxford University Press, 1994 (4th ed).

Bibliography 343

BORDLEY, James III; MCGEHEE, Harvey A., *Two Centuries of American Medicine*. Philadelphia: W.B. Saunders Co., 1976.
CHURCHILL, Larry R., *Rationing Health Care in America*. Notre Dame, Indiana: University of Notre Dame Press, 1987.
DOUGHERTY, Charles J., *American Health Care. Realities, Rights, and Reform*. New York, Oxford: Oxford University Press, 1988.
DUFFY, John, *The Healers: A History of American Medicine*. Urbana, Chicago, London: University of Illinois Press, 1976.
ENCYCLOPEDIA OF SOCIAL WORK, 19th edition. NASW Press, Washington D.C., 1995.
FREEMAN, H.E.; LEVINE, S.; REEDER, L.G.(eds.), *Handbook of Medical Sociology* (3rd. Ed.). Englewood Cliffs, N.J.: Prentice Hall, 1979.
HOLLINGSWORTH, J. Rogers, *A Political Economy of Medicine: Great Britain and the United States*. Baltimore, London: The John Hopkins University Press, 1986.
JONAS, Steven, *An Introduction to the U.S. Health Care System*. New York: Springer Publishing Co., 1992 [3rd edition].
KISSICK W.L., *Medicine's Dilemmas. Infinite Needs Versus Finite Resources*. New Haven, London: University Press, 1994.
KOVNER, Anthony R (Ph.D.), *Health Care Delivery in the United States*. New York: Springer Publishing Co., 1990 (4th ed.).
MARKS, Geoffrey; BEATTY, William K., *The Story of Medicine in America*. New York: Charles Scribner's Sons, 1973.
MENZEL, Paul T., *Strong Medicine: The Ethical Rationing of Health Care*. Oxford: Oxford University Press, 1990.
NATIONAL CENTER FOR HEALTH STATISTICS, Health United States, 1996-97, Hyattsville, Md.: Public Health Service, 1996-97.
PACKARD, Francis R., *History of Medicine in the United States (2 volumes)*. New York: Paul B. Hoeber Inc., 1931.
PELLEGRINO, Edmund D.; THOMASMA, David C., *A Philosophical Basis of Medical Practice. Toward a Philosophy and Ethic of the Healing Professions*. Oxford, New York: Oxford University Press:, 1981.
RAFFEL, Marshall W.; RAFFEL, Norma K., *The U.S. Health System: Origins and Functions*. New York: John Wiley & Sons, 1989 [3rd edition].
RHODES, Robert P., *Health Care: Politics, Policy, and Distributive Justice. The Ironic Triumph*. Albany: State University of New York Press, 1992.

RYDER, C.F., *Changing Patterns in Home Care.* Washington D.C.: PHS Pub. No. 1657, June 1967.
SOCIAL SECURITY AMENDMENTS OF 1965, U.S. Congress, Public Law 89-97, July 30, 1965.
SPIEGEL, Allen D., *Home Healthcare: Home Birthing to Hospice Care.* Owings Mills, MD: National Health Publishing, 1983.
STARR, Paul, *The Social Transformation of American Medicine.* New York: Basic Books, Inc. Publishers, 1982.
_____, *The Logic of Health Care Reform: Why and How the President's Plan Will Work.* New York: Whittle Books, 1992.
TRATTNER, W.I., *From Poor Law to Welfare State: A History of Social Welfare in America.* New York: Free Press, 1989 (4th ed.).
U.S. HOUSE OF REPRESENTATIVES, Committee on Ways and Means. *Overview of Entitlement Programs. (Background material and data on programs within the jurisdiction of the Committee on Ways and Means).* Washington D.C.: U.S. Government Printing Office. Green Books for 1992 (May 15), 1993 (July 7), and 1994 (July 15).
VETERANS ADMINISTRATION, *Annual report, 1984.* Washington D.C.: U.S. Government Printing Office. 1984.
VETERANS HEALTH SERVICES AND RESEARCH ADMINISTRATION. *Integrated Psychiatric Care Planning Guidelines, Criteria and Standards.* Washington, D.C.: Department of Veterans Affairs, 1991.
WARHOLA, C.F.; RYDER, C.F., *Planning for Home Health Services: A Resource Handbook.* Washington D.C.: DHHS. Pub. No. HRA 80-14017, August, 1980.
WEISS, Lawrence D., *No Benefit: Crisis in America's Health Insurance Industry.* Boulder:Westview Press, 1992.
WILLIAMS, Stephen J. and TORRENS, Paul (Eds.), *Introduction to Health Services.* New York: Delmar Publishers Inc. 1993 (4th ed.).
YOSHIKAWA, T. T., *United States Department of Veterans Affairs: Health Care for the Aging Veteran.* L'Annee Gerontolique (Paris), 1992.

Articles:

ADLER, N.E., BOYCE, W.T., CHESNEY, M.A., FOLKMAN, S., SYME, S.L., *"Socioeconomic Inequalities in Health. No Easy Solution."* Journal of the American Medical Association 269 (24): 3140-5,

Jun 23-30, 1993.

ANGELL, Marcia, *"The Beginning of Health Care Reform: The Clinton Plan."* New England Journal of Medicine 329(21): 1569-1570, Nov. 18,1993.

AYANIAN, John Z., *"Heart Disease in Black and White."* New England Journal of Medicine 329 (9): 656-8, Aug. 26, 1993.

BAKER, D.W.; STEVENS, C.D.; BROOK, R.H., *"Patients Who Leave a Public Hospital Emergency Department Without Being Seen by a Physician. Causes and Consequences."* Journal of the American Medical Associatio 266(8):1085-90, Aug 28, 1991.

BASHSHUR, R.L.; HOMAN, R.K.; SMITH, D.G., *"Beyond the Uninsured: Problems in Access to Care."* Medical Care 32 (5): 409-19, May, 1994.

BAYER, R.; CALLAHAN, D.; CAPLAN, A.L.; JENNINGS, B., *"Toward justice in health care."* American Journal of Public Health 78(5): 583-8, May, 1988.

BEAUCHAMP, D.E., *"Public Health as Social Justice."* Inquiry 13(1): 3-14, March, 1976.

BEAUCHAMP, T.L.; FADEN, R.R., *"The Right to Health and the Right to Health Care."* Journal of Medicine and Philosophy 4(2): 118-31, 1979 June.

BERNSTEIN, Aaron (In New York with Bureau Reports), *"'Now We Have No Insurance'—As Health Costs Spiral, Small Businesses Stop Covering Workers,"* Business Week, November 26, 1990, p. 187.

BINDMAN, A.B.; KEANE, D.; LURIE, N., *"A Public Hospital Closes. Impact on Patients' Access to Care and Health Status."* Journal of the American Medical Association 264 (22): 2899-2904, Dec. 12, 1990.

BLUSTEIN, J.; WEITZMAN, B.C., *"Access to Hospitals with High-Technology Cardiac Services: How is Race Important?"* American Journal of Public Health 85 (3): 345-51, March, 1995.

BROOKS, D.D.; SMITH, D.R.; ANDERSON, R.J., *"Medical Apartheid. An American Perspective."* Journal of the American Medical Association 266(19): 2746-9, Nov. 20, 1991.

BRUNGS, Robert A., *"Toward a Theology of Health Care."* Review for Religious 45: 24-44, Jan-Feb, 1986.

BUTLER, J.A.; ROSENBAUM, S.; PALFREY, J.S., *"Ensuring Access to Health Care for Children with Disabilities."* New England Journal of Medicine 317 (3): 162-5, Jul 16, 1987.

CHERKASKY, Martin., *"The Montefiore Hospital Home Care Program,"* American Journal of Public Health 39(2): 163-166, February, 1949.

CHURCHILL, L.; HAUERWAS, S.; SMITH, H., *"Medical Care for the Poor: Finite Resources, Infinite Need."* Health Progress 66(10): 32-5, Dec., 1985.

COHEN, Wilbur J., *"The Long, Difficult Road to Enactment."* Health Progress 66: 22-3, Jul-Aug, 1985.

CURTIS, R., *"The Role of State Governments in Assuring Access to Care."* Inquiry 23 (3): 277-85, 1986 Fall.

DANIELS, Norman, *"Equity of Access to Health Care: Some Conceptual and Ethical Issues."* Milbank Memorial Fund Quarterly - Health and Society 60(1): 51-81, 1982 Winter.

DAVIS, K., *"Inequality and Access to Health Care."* Milbank Memorial Fund Quarterly 69(2):253-73, 1991.

DAVIS, K.; ROWLAND, D., *"Uninsured and Underserved: Inequities in Health Care in the United States,"* Milbank Quarterly 61 (1983): 149-176.

DOWELL, M.A., *"Hill-Burton: the Unfulfilled Promise."* Journal of Health Politics, Policy and Law 12 (1): 153-75, 1987 Spring.

EDDY, D.M., *"Health System Reform. Will Controlling Costs Require Rationing Services?"* Journal of the American Medical Association 272(4): 324-8, July 27, 1994.

EDITORIAL, *"Black-White Disparities in Health Care."* Journal of the American Medical Association 263 (17): 2344-6, May 2, 1990.

ENTHOVEN, Alain C., *"Managed Competition: an Agenda for Action."* Health Affairs 7 (3): 25-47, 1988 Summer.

ESCARCE, J.J.; EPSTEIN, K.R.; COLBY, D.C.; SCHWARTZ, J.S., *"Racial Differences in the Elderly's Use of Medical Procedures and Diagnostic Tests."* American Journal of Public Health 83 (7): 948-54, July, 1993.

FALCONE, D.; BROYLES, R., *"Access to Long-Term Care: Race as a Barrier."* Journal of Health Politics, Policy and Law 19 (3): 583-95, 1994 Fall.

FLEMING, Steven T., *"Primary Care, Avoidable Hospitalization and Outcomes of Care: A Literature Review and Methodological Approach."* Medical Care Research and Review, Vol. 52, No. 1: 88-108, 1995.

FRIEDMAN, Emily, *"The Uninsured. From Dilemma to Crisis."* Journal of the American Medical Association 265(19): 2491-5, May 15,

1991.

FRIEDMAN, Emily, *"Making Room in the Marketplace."* Health Progress 71(10): 16-20, 23, Dec., 1990.

_____, *"The Weird New Healthcare Boat. Titanic or Good Ship Lollipop?"* Health Progress 70(1): 32-8, Jan-Feb, 1989.

GINZBERG, Eli., *"Access to Health Care for Hispanics."* Journal of the American Medical Association 265(2): 238-41, January 9, 1991.

GINZBERG, E.; OSTOW, M., *"Beyond Universal Health Insurance to Effective Health Care."* Journal of the American Medical Association 265(19): 2559-62, May 15, 1991.

HAYWARD R.A.; SHAPIRO, M.F.; FREEMAN, H.E.; COREY, C.R., *"Inequities in Health Services Among Insured Americans. Do Working-Age Adults Have Less Access to Medical Care Than the Elderly?"* New England Journal of Medicine 318 (23): 1507-12. June 9, 1988.

HIMMELSTEIN, David U.; WOOLHANDLER, Steffie, *"Pitfalls of Private Medicine: Health Care in the USA."* Lancet 2 (8399): 391-4, August 18, 1984.

JECKER, Nancy S., *"Can an Employer-Based Health Insurance System be Just?"* Journal of Health Politics, Policy and Law 18(3): 657-673, 1993 Fall.

JOHNSON J.L.; PRIMAS, P.J.; COE, M.K., *"Factors that Prevent Women of Low Socioeconomic Status From Seeking Prenatal Care."* Journal of the American Academy of Nurse Practitioners 6 (3): 105-11, March, 1994.

MANNING, W.G.; LIEBOWITZ, A.; GOLDBERG, G.A., *"A Controlled Trial of the Effect of a Prepaid Group Practice on Use of Services,"* New England Journal of Medicine 310 (1984):1505-1510.

ROWLAND, D.; LYONS, B.; EDWARDS, J., *"Medicaid: Health Care of the Poor in the Reagan Era,"* Annual Review of Public Health 9 (1988): 427-450.

SAFRAN, D.G.; TARLOV, A.R.; ROGERS, W.H., *"Primary Care Performance in Fee-For-Service and Prepaid Health Care Systems: Results from the Medical Outcomes Study,"* Journal of the American Medical Association 271(1994):1579-1586.

SCHROEDER, Steven A., *"The Medically Uninsured - Will They Always be with Us?"* New England Journal of Medicine 334(17): 1130-33, 1996.

SHAPIRO, M.F.; WARE, J.E.; SHERBOURNE, C.D., *"Effects of Cost Sharing on Seeking Care for Serious and Minor Symptoms: Results of a*

Randomized Controlled Trial," Annals of Internal Medicine 104 (1986):246-251.

STEVENS, Patricia E., *"Who Gets Care? Access to Health Care as an Arena for Nursing Action."* Scholarly Inquiry for Nursing Practice 6(3): 185-200, 1992 Fall-Winter.

WORTHEN, D.M., *"The Partnership Between the VA and U.S. Medical Schools,"* VA Practitioner, June 1984: 53-58.

**Selected Works and Articles for Chapter Two:
Theories and Principles Influencing Health Care Delivery in the United States**

Books:

BLUM, Henrik., *Planning for Health Development and Application of Social Change.* New York: Behavioral Publishers, 1974.

CARLEN, Claudia, *The Papal Encyclicals.* (Several Volumes by Years) Raleigh: McGrath Publishing Co., 1981.

COHEN, Morris R, *American Thought.* Glencoe, Illinois: The Free Press, 1954.

DREITZEL, H.P., *The Social Organization of Health.* New York: Macmillan Press 1971, pp. v-xvii.

ENTHOVEN, Alain C., *Health Plan. The Only Practical Solution to the Soaring Cost of Medical Care.* Mass.: Addison-Wesley Publishing Co., 1980.

FLETCHER, Joseph, *Humanhood: Essays in Biomedical Ethics.* Buffalo: Prometheus Books, Inc., 1979.

GLENDON, Mary Ann, *Rights Talk: The Impoverishment of Political Discourse.* New York: The Free Press, 1991.

GROB, Gerald N; BILLIAS, George Athan, *Interpretations of American History: Patterns and Perspectives,* Vol. I., New York: The Free Press, 1982 (4th ed).

HAKSAR, Vinit, *Equality, Liberty and Perfectionism.* Oxford: Oxford University Press, 1979.

MACKINNON, Barbara, (ed.) *American Philosophy: A Historical Anthology.* Albany: State University of New York Press, 1985.

MILL, John S., *Utilitarianism.* In John Stuart Mill, John M. Robson (ed.), New York: St. Martin's Press, 1966.

MUELDER, Walter G.; SEARS, Laurence, *The Development of American Philosophy.* Boston: Houghton Mifflin Company, 1940.

NOZICK, Robert, *Anarchy, State and Utopia.* New York: Basic Books, Inc., 1974.
PARSONS, T. *Patients, Physicians, and Illness.* Gartly Jaco (Ed.), New York: Free Press, 1972, pp. 107-127, (2nd ed).
PELLEGRINO, Edmund D.; THOMASMA, David C., *For the Patient's Good. The Restoration of Beneficence in Health Care.* New York, Oxford: Oxford University Press, 1988.
PRESIDENT'S COMMISSION FOR THE STUDY OF ETHICAL PROBLEMS IN MEDICINE AND BIOMEDICAL AND BEHAVIORAL RESEARCH, *Securing Access to Health Care.* Washington D.C.: U.S. Government Printing Office, 1983.
RAWLS, John, *A Theory of Justice,* Cambridge, MA: Harvard University Press, 1971.
TAYLOR, Charles, *Philosophy and the Human Sciences,* Cambridge, N.Y.: Cambridge University Press, 1985.
VEATCH, Robert M., *A Theory of Medical Ethics.* New York: Basic Books, Inc., 1981.

Articles:

BERNARDIN, J.L. Card., *"The Consistent Ethic of Life and Health Care Systems."* Linacre 52:335-42, Nov., 1985.
BLANK, R.H., *"Rationing Medicine: Hard Choices in the 1990s."* American Journal of Gastroenterology 87(9): 1076-84, Sept., 1992.
BOUCHARD, Charles E., *"Healthcare Reform's Moral, Spiritual Issues. The Problems Are Not Just Political."* Health Progress:54-60, May - June, 1996.
BROCK, D.W.; DANIELS, N., *"Ethical Foundations of the Clinton Administration's Proposed Health Care System."* Journal of the American Medical Association 271(15): 1189-96, April 20, 1994.
BUCHANAN, Allen, *"Justice: A philosophical Review."* Shelp, Earl [editor], Justice and Health Care. Dordrecht: Holland / Boston, U.S.A. / London, England: D. Reidel Publishing Company, 1981, Vol 8. pp. 3-21.
CALLAHAN, D., *"Symbols, Rationality, and Justice: Rationing Health Care."* American Journal of Law and Medicine 18(1-2): 1-13, 1992.

CARNEY, Kim, *"Cost Containment and Justice."* In Shelp, Earl [editor], Justice and Health Care. Dordrecht, Holland / Boston, U.S.A. / London, England: D. Reidel Publishing Company, 1981, Vol 8. pp. 161-178.
CHILDRESS, James F., *"A right to Health Care?"* Journal of Medicine and Philosophy 4(2):132-147, June, 1979.
DANIELS, Norman, *"Rights to Health Care and Distributive Justice: Programmatic Worries."* Journal of Medicine and Philosophy 4(2): 174-91, June, 1979.
DICKERSON, John F., *"Dr. Clinton Scrubs Up."* Time, December 8, 1997.
DUFFY, T.P., *"Rationing Health Care: Its Impact and Implications for Hematology-Oncology."* Yale Journal of Biology and Medicine 65(2): 75-82, Mar.-Apr., 1992.
ENGELHARDT, H. Tristram, *"Health Care Allocations: Responses to the Unjust, the Unfortunate, and the Undesirable."* In Shelp, Earl [editor], Justice and Health Care. Dordrecht, Holland / Boston, U.S.A. / London, England: D. Reidel Publishing Company, 1981, Vol 8. pp. 121-137.
ETZIONI, Amitai, *"Health Care Rationing: A Critical Evaluation."* Health Affairs 10(2):88-95, 1991 Summer.
GOLDFIELD, N., *"Why We Cannot Agree on the Direction of Health Reform: An Exploration of American Values."* Physician Executive 18(4): 16-22, Jul. - Aug., 1992.
HAMMONDS, Keith H., *"Hit Where It Hurts: Why HMO Profits Are Shrinking Fast."* Business Week, October 27, 1997, pp. 42-43.
HEHIR, J.Bryan, *"Policy Arguments in a Public Church: Catholic Social Ethics and Bioethics."* Journal of Medicine and Philosophy 17(3): 347-64, June, 1992.
KELMAN, S., *"The Social Nature of the Definition Problem in Health."* International Journal of Health Services 5(4): 625-642, 1975.
KILNER, Jonh F., *"Health-care Resources, Allocation of."* Encyclopedia of Bioethics, Vol. 2, (Revised Edition), Warren Thomas Reich [Editor in Chief], New York: Simon & Schuster, 1995, pp. 1067-1084.
LARSON, Erik, *"The Soul of an HMO."* Time. :45-52, Jan. 22, 1996.
MCCULLOUGH, Lawrence B., *"Justice and Health Care: Historical Perspectives and Precedents."* In Shelp, Earl [editor], Justice and Health Care. Dordrecht, Holland / Boston, U.S.A. / London, England: D. Reidel Publishing Company, 1981, Vol 8. pp.51-71.

MECKLER L., *Panel Endorses "Bill of Rights" for Health Care*, The Times Picayune, November 20, 1997, p. A-20.

NATIONAL CONFERENCE OF CATHOLIC BISHOPS, *"Resolution on Health Care Reform."* Origins 23(7): 97-102, 1993.

OUTKA, Gene, *"Social Justice and Equal Access to Health Care,"* in *Contemporary Issues in Bioethics,* Tom Beauchamp and Le Roy Walters (eds.), Encino, California: Dickenson Publishing Co., Inc., 1978.

_____, *"Social Justice and Equal Access to Health Care."* Perspectives in Biology and Medicine 18(2): 185-202, 1975 Winter.

PAULY, Mark et al., *"A Plan for 'Responsible National Health Insurance'."* Health Affairs: 5-25, 1991 Spring.

RAWLS, John, *"A Kantian Conception of Equality."* Cambridge Review 96:2225, pp. 94-99, Feb., 1975.

SADE, Robert M., *"Medical Care as a Right: A Refutation."* In Ethics in Medicine, pp. 573-576. Edited by Stanley-J. Reiser, Arthur J. Dyck and William J. Curran. Cambridge: The M.I.T. Press, 1977.

SIEGLER, Mark, *"A Right to Health Care: Ambiguity, Professional Responsibility, and Patient Liberty."* Journal of Medicine and Philosophy 4(2): 148-157, June, 1979.

VAN DER WILT, G.J., *"Cost-Effectiveness Analysis of Health Care Services, and Concepts of Distributive Justice."* Health Care Analysis 2(4): 296-305, Nov., 1994.

WILDAVSKY, Aaron, *"Resolved, that Individualism and Egalitarianism be Made Compatible in America: Political-Cultural Roots of Exceptionalism,"* in *Is America Different,* Byron E. Shafer (ed.), Oxford:Clarendon Press, 1991.

WILLIAMS, Bernard, *"Conflict of Values,"* in *The Idea of Freedom,* Alan Ryan (ed.), Oxford: Oxford University Press, 1979.

_____, *"The Idea of Equality,"* in *Justice and Equality,* Hugo A. Bedau (ed.), Englewood Cliffs, New Jersey: Prentice Hall, Inc., 1971.

Selected Works and Articles for Chapter Three:
A Catholic Theory of Justice

Books:

BELLAH, Robert N. et al., *Habits of the Heart: Individualism and Commitment in American Life.* Berkeley, Los Angeles, London: University of California Press, 1985.

BENTHAM, Jeremy, *An Introduction to The Principles of Morals and Legislation.* With an introduction by Laurence J. Lafleur, New York: Hafner Press, 1948.

BERNA, A. et al, *Curso de Doctrina Social Católica.* Madrid: BAC 1967.

BLOOM, Allan (translation with notes and interpretive essay), *The Republic of Plato.* New York, London: Basic Books Inc., 1968.

CALVEZ, Jean-Yves; PERRIN, Jacques, *The Church and Social Justice.* Chicago: Henry Regnery Company, 1961.

CARLEN, Claudia, *The Papal Encyclicals.* (Several Volumes by Years) Raleigh: McGrath Publishing Co., 1981.

CICERO, Marcus Tullius, *On the Commonwealth.* Translated with notes and Introduction by G.H. Sabine and S.B. Smith, Columbus: The Ohio State University Press, 1929.

COLEMAN, John; BAUM, Gregory, *Rerum Novarum: A Hundred Years of Catholic Social Teaching.* London: SCM Press, *Concilium* 1991/5.

COPLESTON, Frederick, *A History of Philosophy.* Vol.1, Part 1, New York: Image Books, 1962.

DEANE, Herbert A., *The Political and Social Ideas of St. Augustine.* New York and London: Columbia University Press, 1963.

DOUGLAS, R. Bruce; HOLLENBACH, David (Editors), *Catholicism and Liberalism: Contributions to American Public Philosophy.* Cambridge University Press, 1994.

DWORKIN, Ronald, *A Matter of Principle.* Cambridge, MA and London, England: Harvard University Press, 1985.

FAIDHERBE, A.J., *La Justice Distributive.* Paris: Librairie du Recueil Sirey, 1933.

FLANNERY, Austin, *Vatican Council II: The Conciliar and Post-Conciliar Documents,* Minnesota: The Liturgical Press, 1975.

GAYDOS, Francis A., *Distributive Justice and Public Education in the United States.* (Dissertation) St. Thomas Seminary, Denver, CO, 1957.

HEBBLETHWAITE, Peter, *Paul VI: The First Modern Pope.* New York: Paulist Press, 1993.

HOBBES, Thomas, *Leviathan.* Edited by Michael Oakeshott. New York: Collier Books, 1962.

HOLLENBACH, David, Justice, *Peace, and Human Rights: American Catholic Social Ethics in a Pluralistic Context.* New York: Crossroad Publishing Co., 1988.

JOHN OF ST. THOMAS, *Cursus Theologicus,* Vol. III. Paris: Edition by Ludovicus Vives, 1883.

LOCKE, John, *An Essay Concerning the True Original Extent and End of Civil Government.* In Robert Maynard Hutchins (Editor in Chief), *Great Books of the Western World,* Vol. 35, pp. 25-81.

MACINTYRE, Alasdair, *After Virtue: A Study in Moral Theory.* Notre Dame: University of Notre Dame Press, 1984 (2nd ed.).

MADISON, James; HAMILTON, Alexander; JAY, John, *The Federalist Papers.* Edited by Isaac Kramnick. New York: Penguin Books, 1987.

MARITAIN, Jacques, *The Person and the Common Good.* New York: Charles Scribner's Sons, 1947.

MARITAIN, Jacques, *Scholasticism and Politics.* New York: The MacMillan Company, 1941.

MCKEON, Richard, (ed.) *The Basic Works of Aristotle.* New York: Random House, 1941.

MERKELBACH, Benedict H, *Summa Theologica Moralis* (Volume II), Paris: Desclee de Brouwer & Cie., 1954.

THE NEW CATHOLIC ENCYCLOPEDIA, Vol. IV, New York: McGraw-Hill Book Company, 1967.

NOVAK, Michael, *Free Persons and the Common Good.* Lanham/New York/London: Madison Books, 1989.

O'BRIEN, David J.; SHANNON, Thomas A. [editors], *Catholic Social Thought: The Documentary Heritage.* Maryknoll, New York: Orbis Books, 1992.

PINKARD, Terry, *Democratic Liberalism and Social Union,* Philadelphia: Temple University Press, 1987.

RAMSEY P., *The Patient as Person,* New Haven: Yale University Press, 1970.

RESCHER, Nicholas, *Distributive Justice,* New York: Bobbs-Merril, 1966.

REYNOLDS, Charles H.; NORMAN, Ralph V. (Editors), *Community in America: The Challenge of "Habits of the Heart."* Berkeley, Los Angeles, London: University of California Press, 1988.

SANDEL, Michael J., *Democracy's Discontent: America in Search of a Public Philosophy.* Cambridge, Mass; London, England: The Belknap Press of Harvard University Press, 1996.

──────────────, *Liberalism and the Limits of Justice.* Cambridge, London, New York, New Rochelle, Melbourne, Sydney: Cambridge University Press, 1984 (3rd edition).

SMITH, Adam, *An Inquiry Into The Nature and Causes of The Wealth of Nations.* Edited by Edwin Cannan, New York:The Modern Library, 1937.

THE STAFF OF THE POPE SPEAKS MAGAZINE (eds), *The Encyclicals and Other Messages of John XXIII.* [Commentaries by J.F. Cronin, F.X. Murphy, F. Smith], Washington D.C.: TPS Press, 1964.

WALZER, Michael (ed.), *Toward a Global Civil Society.* Providence, Oxford: Berghahn Books, 1995.

──────────────, *Spheres of Justice. A Defense of Pluralism and Equality.* New York: Basic Books, Inc. Publishers, 1983.

Articles:

BRYANT, J.H., *"Principles of Justice as a Basis for Conceptualizing a Health Care System,"* International Journal of Health Services 7(4):707-739, 1977.

FLETCHER, Joseph, *Ethics and Health Care Delivery: Computers and Distributive Justice* in VEATCH R.M. and BRANSON R (eds), *Ethics and Health Policy,* Cambridge: Ballinger Publishing Co., 1976, pp. 99-109.

HOLLENBACH, David, *"The Common Good Revisited."* Theological Studies 50:70-94, 1989.

KIRWIN, J. R, *Christianizing the New Society: A New Translation of Mater et Magistra,"* in Catholic Social Guild, *The Social Thought of John XXIII,* England: Samuel Walker Press, 1964.

LUSTIG, Andrew B, *"The Common Good in a Secular Society: The Relevance of a Roman Catholic Notion to the Healthcare Allocation Debate."* Journal of Medicine and Philosophy 18(6): 569-587, December, 1993.

WEBER, Wilhelm, *Society and State as a Problem for the Church.* In *The Church in the Modern Age,* edited by Gabriel Adrianyi et al., trans. Anselm Biggs, New York: Crossroads, 1981, pp. 229-259.

Selected Works and Articles for Chapter Four: Reforming Access to Health Care

Books:

BRODY B., *Life and Death Decision Making.* New York: Oxford University Press, 1988.

THE CATHOLIC HEALTH ASSOCIATION, *Setting Relationships Right: A Working Proposal for Systemic Healthcare Reform.* [Adopted by the Board of Trustees of the CHA of the U.S.,Feb. 20, 1992] St. Louis, MO., 1992.

KEANE, Philip, *Health Care Reform: A Catholic View,* Mahwah, New Jersey: Paulist Press 1992.

KENNEDY, Terence, *Doers of the Word,* Liguori, MO.: Triumph Books, 1996.

NATIONAL LEADERSHIP COMMISSION ON HEALTH CARE, *For the Health of a Nation,* Health Administration Press Perspectives: Ann Arbor, Michigan, 1989.

VEATCH, Robert M., *The Foundations of Justice: Why the Retarded and the Rest of Us Have Claims to Equality.* New York: Oxford University Press, 1986.

THE WHITE HOUSE DOMESTIC POLICY COUNCIL [Intro by Erik Eckholm], *The President's Health Security Plan.* New York, Toronto:Times Books, Random House, 1993.

Articles:

BERMAN, H.J.; KLEIN, D., *"Pieces of the Puzzle: Steps Toward Affordable Health Care."* Hospital and Health Services Administration 37 (1): 3-11, 1992 Spring.

BLENDON, Robert et al, *"The Beliefs and Values Shaping Today's Health Reform Debate."* Health Affairs, [Spring] (1): 274-284, 1994.

BUTLER, Stuart M., *"A Tax Reform Strategy to Deal with the Uninsured."* Journal of the American Medical Association 265(19): 2541-2544, May 15, 1991.

CHAPMAN, T.W., *"Challenge of Poverty: Some Advice for Advocates of Managed Competition."* Hospitals and Health Networks 67 (13): 56, July 5, 1993.

DE LAS HERAS, J., *"La Relación Médico-Paciente,"* in Manual de Bioética General, Polaino-Lorente, Aquilino (ed.), Madrid:Ediciones

RIALP, 1994.

ENTHOVEN, Alain C.; KRONICK, Richard, *"A Consumer-Choice Health Plan for the 1990s,"* (Two-Part Article), New England Journal of Medicine 320(1,2): 29-37; 94-101, (1989).

FEIN, Rashi, *"The Health Security Partnership: A Federal-State Universal Insurance and Cost-Containment Program,"* Journal of the American Medical Association 265: 2555-2558, May 15, 1991.

GOSTIN, Lawrence O., *"Health Care Reform in the United States."* Journal of Law, Medicine and Ethics 21(1): 6-9, 1993 Spring.

GRUMBACH, Kevin; BODENHEIMER, Thomas; HIMMELSTEIN, David; WOOLHANDLER, Steffie. *"Liberal Benefits, Conservative Spending: The Physicians for a National Health Program Proposal,"* Journal of the American Medical Association 265: 2549-2554, May 15, 1991.

HIMMELSTEIN, David U.; WOOLHANDLER, Steffie, *"A National Health Program for the United States,"* New England Journal of Medicine 320(2): 102-108, January 12, 1989.

_____, *"Cost Without Benefit: Administrative Waste in U.S. Health Care."* New England Journal of Medicine 314:441-445, February 13, 1986.

HOLLOWELL, J.W., *"The Health Care Crisis—How We Got There."* Virginia Medical Quarterly 120 (4): 222-4, 1993 Fall.

JECKER, N.S.; PEARLMAN, R.A., *"An Ethical Framework for Rationing Health Care."* Journal of Medicine and Philosophy 17(1): 79-96, February, 1992.

JOST, T.S.; TANENBAUM, S.J., *"Selling Cost Containment."* American Journal of Law and Medicine 19 (1-2): 95-119, 1993.

KILBORN P.T., *"Health Care Premiums to Surge,"* in *The Times Picayune,* Monday, October 20, 1997, p. A-7.

LAW LIBRARY OF LOUISIANA DEPOSITORY, Supreme Court Building, 301 Loyola Ave., New Orleans. Senate and House Bills (in Microfiche).

THE NEW YORK TIMES, January 29, 1992.

ROCKEFELLER, John D, *"A Call for Action: The Pepper Commission's Blueprint for Health Care Reform,"* Journal of the American Medical Association 265: 2507-2510, May 15, 1991.

_____, *"The Pepper Commission Report on Comprehensive Health Care,"* New England Journal of Medicine 323: 1005-1007, Oct. 4, 1990.

THOMASMA, David C., *"Establishing the Moral Basis of Medicine."*

Journal of Medicine and Philosophy 15(3): 245-67, June, 1990.
TODD, James S.; SEEKINS, Steven V.; KRICHBAUM, John A.; HARVEY, Lynn K., *"Health Access America—Strengthening the US Health Care System,"* Journal of the American Medical Association 265: 2503-2506, (1991).
ULBRICH J., *"Europeans Call for Ban on Cloning,"* in *The Times Picayune,* Sunday, October 12, 1997, p. A-15.
VEATCH, Robert M., *"Resolving Conflicts Among Principles: Ranking, Balancing, and Specifying."* Kennedy Institute of Ethics Journal 5(3): 199-218, September, 1995.
VEATCH, Robert M., *"Just Social Institutions and the Right to Health Care."* Journal of Medicine and Philosophy 4(2): 170-173, June, 1979.